T0259453

Cognitive-Behavioral Therapy in Youth

Guest Editors

TODD E. PETERS, MD
JENNIFER B. FREEMAN, PhD

CHILD AND ADOLESCENT PSYCHIATRIC CLINICS OF NORTH AMERICA

www.childpsych.theclinics.com

Consulting Editor
HARSH K. TRIVEDI, MD

April 2011 • Volume 20 • Number 2

SAUNDERS an imprint of ELSEVIER, Inc.

W.B. SAUNDERS COMPANY
A Division of Elsevier Inc.

Elsevier Inc. ● 1600 John F. Kennedy Boulevard ● Suite 1800 ● Philadelphia, Pennsylvania 19103-2899

http://www.childpsych.theclinics.com

**CHILD AND ADOLESCENT PSYCHIATRIC CLINICS OF NORTH AMERICA Volume 20, Number 2
April 2011 ISSN 1056–4993, ISBN-13: 978-1-4557-0428-6**

Editor: Sarah E. Barth
Developmental Editor: Jessica Demetriou

Child and Adolescent Psychiatric Clinics of North America (ISSN 1056-4993) is published quarterly by Elsevier Inc., 360 Park Avenue South, New York, NY 10010-1710. Months of issue are January, April, July, and October. Business and Editorial Offices: 1600 John F. Kennedy Boulevard, Suite 1800, Philadelphia, PA 19103-2899. Periodicals postage paid at New York, NY and additional mailing offices. Subscription prices are $275.00 per year (US individuals), $425.00 per year (US institutions), $139.00 per year (US students), $318.00 per year (Canadian individuals), $513.00 per year (Canadian institutions), $176.00 per year (Canadian students), $378.00 per year (international individuals), $513.00 per year (international institutions), and $176.00 per year (international students). International air speed delivery is included in all Clinics subscription prices. All prices are subject to change without notice. **POSTMASTER:** Send address changes to Child and Adolescent Psychiatric Clinics of North America, Elsevier Health Sciences Division, Subscription Customer Service, 3251 Riverport Lane, Maryland Heights, MO 63043. **Customer Service: 1-800-654-2452 (U.S. and Canada); 314-447-8871 (outside U.S. and Canada). Fax: 314-447-8029. E-mail: JournalsCustomerService-usa@ elsevier.com (for print support) or journalsonlinesupport-usa@elsevier.com (for online support).**

Reprints. For copies of 100 or more of articles in this publication, please contact the Commercial Reprints Department, Elsevier Inc., 360 Park Avenue South, New York, New York 10010-1710 Tel.: (212) 633-3812; Fax: (212) 462-1935, e-mail: reprints@elsevier.com.

Child and Adolescent Psychiatric Clinics of North America is covered in *MEDLINE/PubMed (Index Medicus), ISI, SSCI, Research Alert, Social Search, Current Contents,* and *EMBASE/Excerpta Medica.*

Printed and bound by CPI Group (UK) Ltd, Croydon, CR0 4YY
Transferred to Digital Print 2011

Contributors

CONSULTING EDITOR

HARSH K. TRIVEDI, MD
Associate Professor of Psychiatry, Vanderbilt University School of Medicine; and Executive Medical Director, and Chief of Staff, Vanderbilt Psychiatric Hospital, Nashville, Tennessee

CONSULTING EDITOR EMERITUS

ANDRÉS MARTIN, MD, MPH

FOUNDING CONSULTING EDITOR

MELVIN LEWIS, MBBS, FRCPSYCH, DCH

GUEST EDITORS

TODD E. PETERS, MD
Chief/Fellow in Child and Adolescent Psychiatry, The Warren Alpert Medical School of Brown University, Bradley Hospital, East Providence, Rhode Island

JENNIFER B. FREEMAN, PhD
Director of Child & Adolescent Outpatient Services, Hasbro Children's Hospital; Assistant Professor (Research), Department of Psychiatry and Human Behavior, The Warren Alpert Medical School of Brown University, Providence, Rhode Island

AUTHORS

COURTNEY L. BENJAMIN, MA
Doctoral Candidate, Department of Psychology, Temple University, Philadelphia, Pennsylvania

CAROLINE L. BOXMEYER, PhD
Research Scientist, Department of Psychology, Center for the Prevention of Youth Behavior Problems, The University of Alabama, Tuscaloosa, Alabama

GINA M. BRELSFORD, PhD
Assistant Professor, School of Behavioral Sciences and Education, Penn State University-Harrisburg, Middletown, Pennsylvania

ERNESTINE C. BRIGGS, PhD
Assistant Professor, Department of Psychiatry and the Behavioral Sciences, Duke University School of Medicine, Durham, North Carolina

DOUGLAS M. BRODMAN, BA
Graduate Student, Department of Psychology, Temple University, Philadelphia, Pennsylvania

LINDSEY BRUETT, BA
Research Assistant, Clinical and Research Program in Pediatric Psychopharmacology, MGH, Cambridge, Massachusetts

LISA W. COYNE, PhD
Assistant Professor, Psychology Department; Director, Early Childhood Research Clinic, Suffolk University, Boston, Massachusetts

COLLEEN M. CUMMINGS, PhD
Postdoctoral Fellow, Department of Psychology, Temple University, Philadelphia, Pennsylvania

PATTY DELANEY, LCSW
Research Project Clinician, Western Psychiatric Institute and Clinic; Children's Hospital of UPMC, Pittsburgh, Pennsylvania

SHANNON DORSEY, PhD
Assistant Professor, Division of Public Behavioral Health and Justice Policy, University of Washington School of Medicine, Seattle, Washington

JULIE M. EDMUNDS, MA
Graduate Student, Department of Psychology, Temple University, Philadelphia, Pennsylvania

CHRISTIANNE ESPOSITO-SMYTHERS, PhD
Department of Psychology, George Mason University, Fairfax, Virginia

CHRISTOPHER A. FLESSNER, PhD
Psychology Fellow, Division of Child and Family Psychiatry, Rhode Island Hospital, Warren Alpert School of Medicine at Brown University; Bradley Hasbro Children's Research Center, Providence, Rhode Island

INTI FLORES, BA
Children's Hospital of UPMC; Medical Student, University of Pittsburgh Medical School, Pittsburgh, Pennsylvania

ROBERT D. FRIEDBERG, PhD, ABPP
Associate Professor, Division of Child Psychiatry, Penn State Milton Hershey Medical Center/College of Medicine, Hershey, Pennsylvania

AUDE HENIN, PhD
Co-Director, Child Cognitive-Behavioral Therapy Program, Department of Psychiatry, Massachusetts General Hospital (MGH), Boston; Director of Cognitive Behavioral Therapy Research, Clinical and Research Program in Pediatric Psychopharmacology, MGH, Cambridge; Assistant Professor of Psychiatry, Harvard Medical School, Boston, Massachusetts

DINA R. HIRSHFELD-BECKER, PhD
Co-Director, Child Cognitive-Behavioral Therapy Program, Department of Psychiatry, Massachusetts General Hospital (MGH), Boston; Director of High Risk Studies and Anxiety Research, Clinical and Research Program in Pediatric Psychopharmacology, MGH, Cambridge; Associate Professor of Psychiatry, Harvard Medical School, Boston, Massachusetts

LUIS JIMENEZ-CAMARGO, MA
Doctoral Student, Department of Psychology, Center for the Prevention of Youth Behavior Problems, The University of Alabama, Tuscaloosa, Alabama

ANDREA E. KASS, BA
Department of Psychology, Washington University in St Louis, St Louis, Missouri

PHILIP C. KENDALL, PhD
Distinguished University Professor, Laura H. Carnell Professor of Psychology, Department of Psychology, Temple University, Philadelphia, Pennsylvania

KATHARINA KIRCANSKI, MA, CPhil
Division of Child and Adolescent Psychiatry, UCLA-Semel Institute for Neuroscience and Human Behavior, University of California Los Angeles, Los Angeles, California

DENA A. KLEIN, PhD
Assistant Professor of Clinical Psychiatry and Behavioral Sciences, Child Outpatient Psychiatry Department, Montefiore Medical Center, Bronx, New York

RACHEL P. KOLKO, BA
Department of Psychology, Washington University in St Louis, St Louis, Missouri

JOHN E. LOCHMAN, PhD, ABPP
Professor and Doddridge Saxon Chairholder in Clinical Psychology, Director, Department of Psychology, Center for the Prevention of Youth Behavior Problems, The University of Alabama, Tuscaloosa, Alabama

EVAN R. MARTINEZ, BA
Clinic Coordinator/Research Assistant, Psychology Department, Suffolk University, Boston, Massachusetts

HEATHER MAZURSKY, MA
Research Coordinator, Clinical and Research Program in Pediatric Psychopharmacology, MGH, Cambridge, Massachusetts

LOUISE McHUGH, PhD
Assistant Professor, Psychology, School of Human and Health Sciences, Swansea University, Swansea, United Kingdom

JAMIE A. MICCO, PhD
Psychologist, Clinical and Research Program in Pediatric Psychopharmacology, MGH, Cambridge; Child Cognitive-Behavioral Therapy Program, MGH, Boston; Instructor in Psychiatry, Harvard Medical School, Boston, Massachusetts

ALEC L. MILLER, PsyD
Professor of Clinical Psychiatry and Behavioral Sciences and Chief, Child Outpatient Psychiatry Department, Montefiore Medical Center, Bronx, New York

THOMAS H. OLLENDICK, PhD
University Distinguished Professor, Department of Psychology; Director, Child Study Center, Virginia Polytechnic Institute and State University, Blacksburg, Virginia

TARA S. PERIS, PhD
Division of Child and Adolescent Psychiatry, UCLA-Semel Institute for Neuroscience and Human Behavior, University of California-Los Angeles, Los Angeles, California

KATHARINE A. PHILLIPS, MD
Professor of Psychiatry and Human Behavior, Warren Alpert Medical School of Brown University; Director, Body Dysmorphic Disorder Program; Director of Research for Adult Psychiatry, Rhode Island Hospital, Providence, Rhode Island

JOHN C. PIACENTINI, PhD, ABPP
Division of Child and Adolescent Psychiatry, UCLA-Semel Institute for Neuroscience and Human Behavior, University of California-Los Angeles, Los Angeles, California

NICOLE P. POWELL, PhD, MPH
Research Scientist, Department of Psychology, Center for the Prevention of Youth Behavior Problems, The University of Alabama, Tuscaloosa, Alabama

CONNOR M. PULEO, MA
Graduate Student, Department of Psychology, Temple University, Philadelphia, Pennsylvania

JAMISON ROGERS, MD
Clinical Assistant Professor of Psychiatry and Human Behavior, Warren Alpert Medical School of Brown University, Providence; Attending Psychiatrist, Adolescent Inpatient Unit, Bradley Hospital, East Providence, Rhode Island

LAURA D. SELIGMAN, PhD
Associate Professor, Department of Psychology, University of Toledo, Toledo, Ohio

CARA A. SETTIPANI, MA
Graduate Student, Department of Psychology, Temple University, Philadelphia, Pennsylvania

ANTHONY SPIRITO, PhD, ABPP
Division of Clinical Psychology, Department of Psychiatry and Human Behavior, Warren Alpert Medical School of Brown University, Providence, Rhode Island

EVA SZIGETHY, MD, PhD
Children's Hospital of UPMC; Associate Professor, Department of Psychiatry; Associate Professor, Department of Pediatrics, University of Pittsburgh; Director, Medical Coping Clinic, Division of Gastroenterology, Children's Hospital of Pittsburgh, Pittsburgh, Pennsylvania

RACHEL D. THOMPSON, MA
Clinical Psychology Doctoral Candidate, Psychology Department, University of Cincinnati, Cincinnati, Ohio; Research Project Assistant, Western Psychiatric Institute and Clinic, Children's Hospital of UPMC, Pittsburgh, Pennsylvania

BRIANA A. WOODS, PhD
Health Behavior Health Education, Gillings School of Global Public Health, University of North Carolina, Chapel Hill, North Carolina

KRISTEN UHL, BS
Department of Psychiatry, Rhode Island Hospital, Providence, Rhode Island

DENISE E. WILFLEY, PhD
Professor of Psychiatry, Medicine, Pediatrics, and Psychology, Department of Psychiatry, Washington University School of Medicine, St Louis, Missouri

JENNIFER WOLFF, PhD
Department of Psychiatry and Human Behavior, Rhode Island Hospital/Warren Alpert Medical School of Brown University, Providence, Rhode Island

Contents

> Cognitive-behavioral therapies (CBTs) have been shown to be efficacious for the treatment of anxiety disorders in children and adolescents. Randomized clinical trials indicate that approximately two-thirds of children treated with CBT will be free of their primary diagnosis at posttreatment. Although several CBT treatment packages have been investigated in youth with diverse anxiety disorders, common core components have been identified. A comprehensive assessment, development of a good therapeutic relationship and working alliance, cognitive restructuring, repeated exposure with reduction of avoidance behavior, and skills training comprise the core procedures for the treatment of anxiety disorders in youth.

> Obsessive-compulsive disorder (OCD) is a common, chronic, and impairing condition in youth. Cognitive-behavioral therapy (CBT), now widely recognized as the gold standard intervention for childhood OCD, relies on exposure and response prevention, and also includes psychoeducation, creation of a symptom hierarchy, imaginal exposures, cognitive interventions, and a contingency management system. This article reviews the theoretical underpinnings of current CBT approaches, key components of treatment, developmental considerations specific to childhood OCD, and evidence supporting the use of this psychosocial intervention. The current state of knowledge will be aided by further study of predictors and mechanisms of CBT treatment response.

> Several cognitive-behavioral therapy (CBT) approaches are available for treating child and adolescent posttraumatic stress disorder (PTSD). These treatments include common elements (eg, psychoeducation, gradual exposure, relaxation). This review (1) delineates common elements in CBT approaches for treating child and adolescent PTSD; (2) provides a detailed review of three CBT approaches with substantial evidence of effectiveness; and (3) describes promising practices in the area of CBT approaches to treating child and adolescent PTSD. Cultural and implementation considerations are also included.

> Eating disorders and obesity in children and adolescents involve harmful behavior and attitude patterns that infiltrate daily functioning. Cognitive-behavioral therapy (CBT) is well suited to treating these conditions, given

the emphasis on breaking negative behavior cycles. This article reviews the current empirically supported treatments and the considerations for youth with weight control issues. New therapeutic modalities (ie, enhanced CBT and the socioecologic model) are discussed. Rationale is provided for extending therapy beyond the individual treatment milieu to include the family, peer network, and community domains to promote behavior change, minimize relapse, and support healthy long-term behavior maintenance.

Body dysmorphic disorder (BDD) usually begins during early adolescence and appears to be common in youth. BDD is characterized by substantial impairment in psychosocial functioning and high rates of suicidality. Cognitive-behavioral therapy (CBT) tailored to BDD is the best tested and most promising psychosocial treatment for adults. CBT has been used for youth with BDD, but has not been systematically developed for or tested in youth. This article focuses on CBT for BDD in adults and youth; possible adaptations and the need for treatment research in youth; and prevalence, clinical features, diagnosis, recommended pharmacotherapy, and treatments that are not recommended.

This article focuses on the use of cognitive-behavioral therapy (CBT) strategies for children and adolescents with externalizing disorders. Following a description of risk factors for youth antisocial behavior, several components common to CBT interventions for youth with externalizing behaviors will be described. Using the Coping Power Program as a model, child treatment components including Emotion Awareness, Perspective Taking, Anger Management, Social Problem Solving, and Goal Setting will be reviewed. CBT strategies for parents of youth with disruptive behaviors will also be described. Finally, the article summarizes the evidence for the effectiveness of CBT strategies for externalizing disorders and presents specific outcome research on several programs that include CBT techniques.

This article provides an overview of cognitive-behavioral therapy (CBT) for repetitive behavior disorders. Because tic disorders and trichotillomania are the most often studied and most debilitating of these conditions, this article focuses on the efficacy of CBT for these 2 conditions. An overview of CBT for children presenting with these concerns is provided. This review focuses particularly on habit reversal training, which is at the core of most CBT-based interventions. Two recent empirical studies on the immense

across a broad range of psychiatric disorders and behavioral health issues, yet the literature looking at the adaptation of ACT for youth populations is still nascent. This article provides an outline of key components of ACT, a brief overview of the history and development of ACT, adaptations for children, the theoretical underpinnings of ACT, assessment and therapy, and a review of the evidence-based literature to date.

FORTHCOMING ISSUES

RECENT ISSUES

RELATED INTEREST

THE CLINICS ARE NOW AVAILABLE ONLINE!

Access your subscription at:
www.theclinics.com

Foreword

The ABC's of Psychotherapy

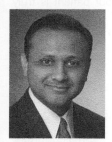

Harsh K. Trivedi, MD
Consulting Editor

As each issue of *Child and Adolescent Psychiatric Clinics of North America* is being considered, one question that weighs heavily on my mind is which topics we need to cover. Having a strong public health component in my decision-making process, I have attempted to focus on topics that can truly have a major impact on our patients and our practices. Examples of this include the recent issues on Adolescent Substance Use Disorders as well as Leadership and Management Core Competencies. These are topics that interface with our clinical practices on a routine basis. The public health component is that they are also topics for which there is a great unmet need. Likewise, if our skillset is honed, we may be in a better position to beneficially impact the lives of our patients. While I believe in the power of psychotherapy as well as the importance of multiple different modes of psychotherapy (such as psychoanalysis, psychodynamic psychotherapy, interpersonal psychotherapy, dialectical behavioral therapy, group therapy, and family therapy to name a few), there is one specific modality that requires specific attention at this time.

Cognitive-behavioral therapy (CBT), for me, is that modality. Despite the prevalence of research studies that show the efficacy of CBT for a number of conditions affecting youth, most of us (even in academic centers) have experienced the difficulty of finding true "research-quality" CBT therapists. And this is an important point. Just as a scalpel in the hands of an inexperienced surgeon will not produce the same results as someone who has done 40,000 bladder resections, there is very much an art and science to the skillful and expert practice of CBT.

It is for this reason that I am quite excited about this current issue of *Child and Adolescent Psychiatric Clinics of North America*. For those who are familiar with the field, you will quickly recognize how impressive the lineup of contributing authors truly is. Many of these folks are the ones who have written the manuals, have conducted the research studies, have proven the efficacy, and/or are the expert practitioners of CBT for that specific application. I am grateful to Todd Peters and Jennifer Freeman for their wonderful leadership and vision in assembling such a rich offering of topics and articles

Child Adolesc Psychiatric Clin N Am 20 (2011) xiii–xiv
doi:10.1016/j.chc.2011.01.016
1056-4993/11/$ – see front matter © 2011 Elsevier Inc. All rights reserved.

childpsych.theclinics.com

for this issue. I am also most appreciative of each of our authors for sharing their expertise on this topic.

While each of us will not become the expert provider in CBT, it is important to understand the many beneficial applications of CBT in youth. Likewise, it is important to understand what makes for good CBT and how to know if your patient is truly receiving high-quality CBT. Last, as we learn the ABC's of CBT, there is also the hope that this knowledge will allow for better care of our patients and the ability to hone our clinical skills as well.

Harsh K. Trivedi, MD
Vanderbilt Psychiatric Hospital
1601 23rd Avenue South, Suite 1157
Nashville, TN 37212, USA

E-mail address:
harsh.k.trivedi@vanderbilt.edu

Preface

Cognitive-Behavioral Therapy in Youth

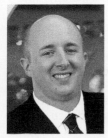 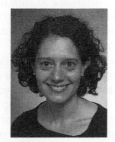

Todd E. Peters, MD   Jennifer B. Freeman, PhD
Guest Editors

"I'm going to do CBT to that child."
"CBT is easy—all you have to do is read a manual with the family."
"You don't have to care about all that other stuff when you are doing CBT."

These phrases, or others like them, are uttered by clinicians in outpatient clinics, inpatient units, and psychiatry/psychology training programs around the country, demonstrating the common misperception that cognitive-behavioral therapy, or CBT, is "done" by a therapist "to" a patient. These beliefs often eliminate the notion of a therapeutic working relationship between a therapist and his or her patients and their families, which is essential to developing an understanding of the family system and structure in which the child's symptoms are thriving. Some mental health professionals feel that CBT is a robotic, "choose-your-own-adventure" style of therapy that is based solely on handouts and manuals.

The true practice of CBT is a far departure from a strictly manualized treatment. Dating back to the origins of CBT, practitioners and researchers have understood the importance of the therapeutic bond between clinicians and their patients. This bond fosters a therapeutic environment to tackle maladaptive cognitions and engage in exposure exercises in an effort to modify beliefs or behaviors causing intrapersonal and interpersonal conflicts.

This issue of the *Child and Adolescent Psychiatric Clinics of North America* was established to provide a comprehensive look at the history and practice of CBT in youth and its evidence base across multiple childhood disorders. An additional goal of this issue is to dispel the misunderstandings of the practice of CBT that abound in the community. We hope to demonstrate that CBT is a fluid process, not a rigid or inflexible style of therapy, focused on linking cognitions to thoughts and behaviors that may have become problematic over time. The authors who contributed to this issue are true leaders in the field of CBT in children and adolescents (albeit, not an exclusive list by any means).

Child Adolesc Psychiatric Clin N Am 20 (2011) xv–xvi
doi:10.1016/j.chc.2011.01.015   **childpsych.theclinics.com**

As you will see, some clinical disorders in youth, such as depression and anxiety, have a rich history of evidenced-based data backing CBT as a first-order treatment, whereas others, such as body dysmorphic disorder, have limited empirical data. Also included are areas that may be more problematic for some practitioners, including working with very young children and those with comorbid medical issues.

We end this issue by reviewing other areas of research, including more cognitive-based (less behavioral) therapy as well as acceptance and commitment therapy. Interwoven throughout the articles are summaries of general session structure, which may provide a helpful review for those reading this work. The articles also examine future avenues for CBT development in their respective areas.

We intend for this issue to be a stand-alone summary of the current data and practice of CBT in youth, which we hope will serve as an invaluable resource for the new trainee or experienced clinician alike. As stated in Harsh Trivedi's Foreword to this issue, you will not become an expert CBT clinician by reading this issue; however, we expect that you will leave with a thorough understanding of the evidence-based practice of CBT in youth across multiple spectrums. We are very grateful for all of the time and effort that went into this issue, from the incredible group of authors to the staff at *Child and Adolescent Psychiatric Clinics of North America* who made this all possible. We also send a warm thank you to Dr Harsh Trivedi, for allowing us to contribute to this journal.

Todd E. Peters, MD
The Warren Alpert Medical School of Brown University
Bradley Hospital
1011 Veterans Memorial Parkway
East Providence, RI 02915, USA

Jennifer B. Freeman, PhD
Hasbro Children's Hospital
Department of Psychiatry and Human Behavior
The Warren Alpert Medical School of Brown University
CORO Building, One Hoppin Street
Providence, RI 02903, USA

E-mail addresses:
Todd_Peters@brown.edu (T.E. Peters)
JFreeman@lifespan.org (J.B. Freeman)

History of Cognitive-Behavioral Therapy in Youth

Courtney L. Benjamin, MA, Connor M. Puleo, MA,
Cara A. Settipani, MA, Douglas M. Brodman, BA,
Julie M. Edmunds, MA, Colleen M. Cummings, PhD,
Philip C. Kendall, PhD*

KEYWORDS

- Cognitive-behavioral therapy • Cognitive therapy
- Behavior therapy • Children • Adolescents • History

HISTORY OF COGNITIVE-BEHAVIORAL THERAPY IN YOUTH

True to its name, cognitive-behavioral therapy (CBT) emerged as a rational amalgam of behavioral and cognitive theories of human behavior, causal and maintaining forces in psychopathology, and targets for intervention.[1] The numerous strategies that comprise CBT reflect its complex and integrative history. Following from early respondent conditioning theories,[2] CBT incorporates concepts such as extinction and habituation. CBT went on to integrate modeling and cognitive restructuring strategies from social learning[3] and cognitive theories.[4,5] In addition, Meichenbaum and Goodman's[6] focus on self-talk and D'Zurilla and Goldfried's[7] problem solving are each evident in CBT's general focus on fostering the development of personal coping strategies and mastery of emotional and cognitive processes. Consistent with a tripartite view (cognition, behavior, emotion) of psychopathology,[8] CBT targets these multiple areas of vulnerability and employs multiple avenues of intervention.

This article provides a history of CBT as applied to youth psychopathology. This history can be traced to the 1960s when the value and effectiveness of the prevailing psychodynamic perspective was questioned[9,10] and found to be lacking. Behavior therapy consequently gained prominence, but in the 1960s these therapies were initially controversial and primarily relegated to the treatment of behavior dysfunction in severely disordered children. It was not until the mid to late 1970s that the gradual

C.L.B. is supported by National Institute of Mental Health (NIMH) grant F31MH086954. Preparation of the manuscript was facilitated by NIMH grants to P.C.K. (MH80788; UO1MH63747).
Department of Psychology, Temple University, 1701 North 13th Street, Philadelphia, PA 19122, USA
* Corresponding author.
E-mail address: pkendall@temple.edu

Child Adolesc Psychiatric Clin N Am 20 (2011) 179–189
doi:10.1016/j.chc.2011.01.011
1056-4993/11/$ – see front matter © 2011 Elsevier Inc. All rights reserved.

childpsych.theclinics.com

expansion of behavioral therapies reached higher functioning clients, integrated the role of cognitive processing, and incorporated a focus on emotions. The transition did not happen at once, and it was spurred by multiple sources. In the end, social cognitive processing, the psychology of self-control, and emotion regulation were melded into behavioral interventions and, eventually, emerged as the multifaceted, widely applicable, extensively practiced, and well-researched CBT of the present day. This article offers a review of (a) the emergence of CBT from child behavioral therapies, (b) the influence of cognitive theories on these early treatments, and (c) the role of multiple perspectives and research evaluations in shaping modern CBT. The current status of CBT for various childhood disorders is described and future directions for cognitive-behavioral therapy research and dissemination offered.

It may be of interest, especially to those with intolerance for grammatical infelicities, to know the history of the hyphen in cognitive-behavioral therapy. With behavior therapy predating cognitive therapy, the label had to be combined. Would it be cognitive behavioral therapy, where "cognitive" is the descriptive adjective for therapies that are "behavioral"? Or would it be cognitive "behavior therapy" or "cognitive behavioral therapies"? With the hyphen (ie, cognitive-behavioral therapy), therapy was the noun, and "cognitive-behavioral" was the integrated descriptive adjective. In 1979, and 1981, two of the earliest books on CBT had hyphenated titles.[1,11] It may also be of interest to note that "social," "developmental," and "emotional" are other terms that are aptly part of an extended hyphenated label. Cognitive-behavioral-social-developmental-emotional therapy would be more accurate, but it struggles rather than rolls off the tongue, is rejected by publishing houses that want to capitalize on "hot" labels (eg, stick with CBT), and some might even see it as stitched together in a Frankensteinian fashion. Use of the umbrella term "CBT" prevented the wrestling match that would have no doubt been necessitated by those who would have ordered the adjectives differently.

Theoretical Influences

Behavior therapy

Before there was CBT, there was behavioral therapy—an initially controversial and underestimated approach that ultimately paved the way for empirically supported treatments for mental health disorders of youth. For example, the Mowrers'[12] "bell-and-pad" procedure for the treatment of enuresis is an often-cited example of an early behavioral intervention (and it remains a first-line treatment for enuresis). Although clinical applications of behavioral strategies did not begin in earnest until the 1960s, the initial work set the stage—by targeting and addressing observable behavior and by measuring outcomes—for later child cognitive-behavioral interventions.

Respondent conditioning explanations of behavior influenced early behavior therapy, particularly for the treatment of anxiety. In respondent conditioning, a conditioned stimulus (CS) closely precedes an unconditioned stimulus (UCS) that elicits an unconditioned response (UCR) of fear. After repeated pairings, the CS alone will elicit the conditioned response (CR) of fear. Internal sensations or cues (eg, physiologic arousal) have also come to be recognized as conditioned stimuli.[13] Although the theory is powerful, it remains a somewhat incomplete explanation of human distress.[14] However, respondent conditioning was historically important in birthing notions of exposure tasks for the treatment of anxiety, now a well-established example, if not hallmark, of modern CBT for child anxiety.[15]

Respondent conditioning theories brought the concepts of extinction, habituation, and counterconditioning to the attention of developers of treatments for youth. Initial treatments for child anxiety, for example, followed from these early behavioral perspectives. Extinction of a conditioned fear occurs by way of repeated experience with the CS (eg, bees) in the absence of the UCS (eg, bee sting). Habituation naturally occurs, and after long periods in the presence of the feared stimulus without the anticipated negative outcome, the stimulus no longer elicits the same heightened levels of arousal. Wolpe and Lazarus'[2] systematic desensitization, based on counterconditioning, advocated for reciprocal inhibition (engaging in an anxiety-antagonistic response, such as relaxation, during exposure trials). Research found that anxiety decreased across exposure trials even in the absence of anxiety inhibitory responses[16] and that gradual exposure (often more palatable to clients) may not be necessary for anxiety reduction to occur.

Operant learning theory[17] played a major role in behavioral therapy as well as child CBT. In operant theory, behaviors are facilitated by environmental contingencies that follow their occurrence. Children's behavior may be positively reinforced, even unintentionally or unknowingly, by attention from caregivers in the child's environment. Negative reinforcement may also occur by the removal of demands placed on the child. Children's independent, developmentally appropriate behavior may even be punished by caregivers. These contingencies play a major role in the shaping of behavior over time. Environments low in predictable and preferred contingencies may lead to decreased self-efficacy and maladjustment.

Early applications of operant theory (eg, applied behavioral analysis) were geared toward more severe or challenging child clients[18] for whom traditional talk and play therapies were considered inappropriate. Much early behavioral therapy focused on the application of operant contingencies for increasing desired behaviors (eg, shaping, reinforcement) and reducing undesired behaviors (eg, reinforcing incompatible behaviors, time-out). These principles have influenced treatments for childhood behavior problems. As discussed by Kazdin,[19] early operant conditioning procedures were applied to child-parent interactions. As a result of extensive research, often involving direct observations of parent-child interactions, Patterson[20] determined that inconsistent parenting strategies found in families of disruptive children actually reinforce aggressive and antisocial behavior. Specifically, Patterson observed patterns of coercion between parents and behaviorally dysregulated children. In his model, a parent responds to a child's disruptive behaviors with ineffective discipline practices, such as scolding, threatening, and/or physical discipline. The child then "counterattacks," or increases disruptive, aggressive behavior, and the parent often backs down, thereby reinforcing the child's disruptive behavior.[20–22] Forgatch and Patterson[23] influenced the field by directing practitioners to help parents be consistent in their contingencies, and to use fewer ineffective punishment strategies. At present, the Parent Management Training Oregon Model[24] (PMTO) is considered a "well-established" treatment for children with disruptive behavior.[25]

Many behavioral procedures continue to be used within CBT, even if initially conceptualized within a behavioral perspective. Over time, behavioral therapy began to address the thought processes and cognitive skills that were seen as involved in the implementation and receipt of contingency management and came to be implemented among less severe populations. This shift to higher-functioning youth and to an increased awareness of the role of cognition was an important part of the transition to CBT. It is also worth noting that many behavioral interventions, and cognitive-behavioral interventions, were initiated and researched with children in mind. These therapies were not borrowed adult treatments, or downward extensions of adult treatments applied with children. To their credit, cognitive-behavioral therapies with youth were intentionally developmentally sensitive and research-informed interventions.

Shift toward cognitive-behavioral therapy

CBT has been defined as a purposeful combination of the demonstrated efficiencies and methodological rigor of behavioral procedures with the cognitive-mediational processes that influence adjustment.[1] In the 1970s, internal thought processes (eg, self-talk[6]) began to be viewed as both targets and mechanisms of change,[18] with an emphasis on improving cognitive skills rather than modifying behavior. Two early reports of CBT with children[26,27] were combinations of self-instructional training, with coping modeling and a response cost contingency. As promise was seen in efforts to incorporate children's developing cognitive abilities into behavior modification to produce therapeutic change,[28] cognitive processes became integrated with behavioral interventions. By incorporating cognition, the behavioral model fostered more broad and effective behavior change strategies.

Meyers and Craighead[18] identified several forces that led the shift toward interventions that were cognitive-behavioral in nature. One force, cognitive psychology, was a factor that affected behavior therapy with children through (a) modeling, (b) self-instruction training, and (c) problem solving. The cognitive information processing explanation of modeling, or observational learning, holds that even in the absence of respondent or operant contingencies, an individual can learn by viewing another person's behavior. Although modeling was historically identified with behavior therapy, Bandura's[29] explanation of modeling effects highlighted attention and retention, which are cognitive processes drawn from an information-processing model of cognitive psychology, as among the major factors that influenced observational learning. Bandura's account of modeling, which ushered in a cognitive explanation for a portion of behavior therapy, and his discussion of the role of symbolic cognitive processes in behavior change, were springboards for the theoretical advance of CBT.[18] Indeed, various behavior therapy interventions began to be understood from both an information-processing and a more general cognitive viewpoint.[30]

Self-instruction training[6] was another avenue through which cognitive psychology had some impact on behavior therapy. Self-instruction emerged to teach impulsive children how to control their behavior. The program drew from the language-development sector of cognitive developmental psychology, particularly the work of Luria[31] and Vygotsky,[32] who suggested that children learn to control their own behavior by overt and eventually covert speech. Researchers and clinicians continue to draw from the cognitive developmental literature to incorporate cognitive strategies and enhance behavior therapy procedures. For example, the literature on social cognition has contributed to notions of self-talk[33] and social skills training, and to our understanding of mechanisms of behavior change.

Problem solving,[7] though once linked with behavioral learning, has a cognitive information-processing flavor. Problem solving within CBT for youth[34] focuses on internal thought processes as one mechanism of change. Several early programs for youth employed problem solving.[35–37] As evidence of its lasting impact, many current empirically supported programs for youth have a problem-solving focus.[38–41] The emphasis on modifying thought processes as a means for producing both behavioral and cognitive change illustrates the integration of CBT and cognitive developmental psychology.

Interventions that targeted self-control were described as a third force behind CBT for youth.[18] Explanations of self-control procedures were increasingly cognitive in nature,[42,43] with influential articles supporting the role of internal factors in self-control. Principles of self-control were being applied to work with children in the mid-1970s, as theoretical advances (eg, Bandura's[3] self-efficacy) buttressed the relationship between overt and covert events. Studies of self-control and self-efficacy advanced the testing of private cognitive experiences in ways that could be integrated within behavioral paradigms.[1]

The emerging successes of cognitive therapy for adult disorders influenced the psychological treatment of children. A core assumption of cognitive therapy is that maladaptive cognitive processes produce psychological disorders, which can be alleviated by modifying these cognitive processes. Ellis'[5] irrational thinking and Beck's[44] cognitive distortions are examples of the key notions, and the key people, who influenced CBT. Specifically, Ellis and Harper[45] proposed that people engage in maladaptive behavior and/or experience negative mood states because they engage in irrational thought processes. Thus, they argued that the focus in therapy is changing maladaptive ways of thinking (given that a person's thoughts lead one to experience negative emotions). Beck[44] similarly maintained that maladaptive cognitions (assumptions and beliefs about oneself and the world) are associated with psychological disturbance. Many research evaluations have supported cognitive therapy with adults,[46,47] and clinical work with children has been influenced by, and frequently refers to, the work of Beck and Ellis.

The theories of Beck and Ellis, and the emerging empirical support for their clinical procedures, contributed to growing acceptance that cognitive attitudes, beliefs, expectancies, and attributions are critical for producing, understanding, and modifying the behavior of individuals with psychopathology.[1] Given the increasing number of studies supporting therapeutic benefit for cognitive therapy, an increasing focus was placed on assessing and understanding cognition[11] despite traditional difficulties with isolating and measuring such phenomena. The position that cognition is subject to the laws of learning[48,49] led to attempts to apply functional analytical assessment and contingency-based interventions to the modification of cognition. Although controversy existed regarding this approach, such efforts nonetheless provided an avenue for behaviorists to enter the cognitive arena. Some of the early cognitive therapy with adults relied on persuasion and reason, though later efforts underscored the benefit of prospective hypothesis testing and behavioral tasks (ie, homework, behavioral activation). The results of rigorous methodological research evaluations spurred further interest.[50,51]

The integration of the strategies of cognitive and behavioral therapy thrived due to the desirability and viability of this combination to produce clinically meaningful outcomes. Indeed, without the favorable research evaluations, the approach would not have gained interest from practitioners nor maintained itself among researchers. Simply put, the use of contingencies to facilitate a child's engagement in exercises that produce cognitive change was both data-supported and clinically appealing.

Expanding CBT

Although its initial impetus was the wedding and integrating of cognitive (eg, thoughts influence behavior and emotion) and behavioral (eg, research evaluation, contingencies) traditions, CBT rapidly evolved and emerged as a treatment informed by a wider set of models. CBT grew and materialized to address salient disorders in youth, as well as developmental vulnerabilities toward psychopathology. Just as the role of cognition has, in its pioneering fashion, come to be incorporated into behavioral therapy, so too have forces related to social environments, genetic vulnerabilities, therapeutic processes, and familial and peer relationships.

As an illustration of expanding models, consider Clark and Watson's[52] tripartite model as an explanation for the extensive overlap of the otherwise seen as separate disorders, anxiety and depression. The tripartite model describes how anxiety and depression share a common component, negative affect, which accounts for symptom overlap. Negative affect is the sense of high objective distress and includes a variety of affective states such as being angry, afraid, sad, worried, and guilty. The model suggests that negative affect is a shared dispositional vulnerability for emotional psychopathology, specifically anxiety and depression. By contrast, low positive affect is a factor specific to depression and autonomic arousal is a factor specific to anxiety.[52] CBT for addressing emotional disorders, in sync with the tripartite model,[53] also targets overlapping features. However, Barlow suggested that anxiety is different from autonomic arousal.[54] He proposed that negative affect is a pure manifestation of the emotion of anxiety, while autonomic arousal is a manifestation of the emotion of fear. Despite small differences, autonomic arousal, high levels of general distress and negative affect, and low positive affect are seen as important predisposing traits of emotional psychopathology.[54] Targeting and treating these salient factors across disorders is a strategic approach that has been accepted within CBT.

Barlow[8] described a triple-vulnerability model of emotional disorders: (1) a general genetic vulnerability, (2) a general psychological vulnerability characterized by a diminished sense of control, and (3) a specific psychological vulnerability resulting from early learned experiences. This diathesis-stress model is consistent with how children may develop a sense of diminished control through experiences both with their own highly reactive arousal system or high negative affectivity and with uncontrollable life events.[13] Once a diminished sense of control is developed, a child is more likely to perceive other events as uncontrollable, even those for which the child could potentially manage. For example, overcontrolling, unresponsive, and unpredictable family environments can foster a sense of uncontrollability and an external locus of control, a major psychological vulnerability.[13,55,56] A specific psychological vulnerability can arise from early socialization experiences with the family or peers, and can contribute to experiencing psychopathology in particular areas. In accordance with this vulnerability model, CBT approaches for youth incorporate parent training with an increased focus on contextual issues and the development of children's mastery over their own environment.

CURRENT STATUS AND FUTURE DIRECTIONS

Disorder-specific applications of CBT for children and adolescents have enjoyed widespread application. A search of key terms "cognitive behavioral therapy" and "children" on PsycInfo, an online database of psychological literature, revealed 1192 articles, 1156 of which were published since 1990. Increased interest in and research on CBT has firmly established its presence in clinical child and adolescent psychology and psychiatry. The initial book on CBT with children and adolescents[57] is now in its fourth edition,[58] with numerous chapters describing CBT procedures for specific disorders.

True to its ties with the empirical methods of behavior therapy, CBT with children and adolescents continues to be guided by empirical research. Studies of the nature of specific disorders inform treatment procedures, and evaluations of treatments applied to real cases inform dissemination and practice. To date, an impressive series of empirical research reports support the use of CBT for the treatment and prevention of various psychological disorders in youth. The American Psychological Association Task Force on Promotion and Dissemination of Psychological Procedures[59] established criteria for use in determining whether treatments can be considered empirically supported (see also the criteria of Chambless and Hollon[60]). Based on the criteria, treatments can be categorized as "well established," "probably efficacious," "possibly efficacious," or "experimental." CBT has emerged as the treatment with the most empirical support for numerous internalizing disorders in youth.[61–64] Specific modalities of CBT have been categorized as "well established," such as child-only groups and child groups plus a parent component for youth with depressive disorders.[62] A specific CBT protocol for youth exposed to traumatic events, Trauma-Focused CBT,[65] is also considered "well established."[64] Many other CBT protocols have been categorized as "probably efficacious"[64] for the treatment of internalizing disorders, including the Coping Cat Program[66] for anxiety and phobic disorders, school-based group CBT[67] for exposure to traumatic events,[63] and individual exposure-based CBT[68,69] for obsessive-compulsive disorder.[61] Although less support has been found for the use of CBT for externalizing disorders in youth, group CBT is considered a "well established" treatment for adolescent substance abuse[70] and some CBT protocols, such as Anger Control Training[71] and Rational-Emotive Mental Health Program,[72] are considered "probably efficacious" for the treatment of disruptive behaviors in youth.[25] Overall, CBT is often considered the "first line of defense" in the treatment of psychological disorders in youth.

Although additional work is necessary to strengthen the efficacy of CBT for youth, researchers have called for a shift toward examining the mediators, moderators, and predictors of treatment outcome.[73–75] This call implores researchers to go beyond evaluating the degree to which treatment works and to move toward examining why and for whom it works.[76] Future research has many worthy candidates of investigations. Potential mediating variables worthy of exploration include the individual components of treatment protocols, therapeutic process variables such as therapeutic alliance and child involvement, and within-client change processes.[77] Future work is also necessary to delineate whether certain pretreatment characteristics, comorbid conditions, and treatment formats moderate or predict outcome. Given the ever-increasing use of technology in society, a particular area ripe for research includes the use of computer technology in CBT protocols.[78,79]

A pressing concern and an area requiring empirical support is how best to disseminate CBT to community practice.[80] The growing empirical support of the efficacy of CBT does not guarantee its use. "Bridging the gap" between research evidence and clinical practice is an endeavor requiring effort from all parties involved, including researchers, practitioners, policymakers, and mental health consumers.[81] It can be argued that the pursuit of dissemination constitutes the next article in the history of CBT. Engagement in this endeavor will likely lead to global improvements in the mental health care of youth.

SUMMARY

CBT represents an integration of behavioral, cognitive, and other (eg, developmental, social) theories of human behavior and psychopathology. The numerous strategies that comprise CBT reflect its complex and integrative history and include conditioning, modeling, cognitive restructuring, problem solving, and the development of personal coping strategies, mastery, and a sense of self-control. CBT targets multiple areas of potential vulnerability (eg, cognitive, behavioral, or affective) and provides avenues of intervention. CBT is often considered the treatment of choice for mental health disorders in youth. Additional work is needed to understand the mediators, moderators, and predictors of treatment outcome, and to pursue the dissemination of efficacious CBT approaches.

REFERENCES

1. Kendall PC, Hollon SD. Cognitive-behavioral interventions: overview and current status. In: Kendall PC, Hollon SD, editors. Cognitive-behavioral interventions: theory, research, and procedures. New York: Academic Press; 1979. p. 1–9.
2. Wolpe J, Lazarus AA. Behavior therapy techniques. New York: Pergamon; 1966.
3. Bandura A. Social learning theory. Englewood Cliffs (NJ): Prentice Hall; 1977.
4. Beck AT. Theoretical perspectives on clinical anxiety. In: Tuma AH, Maser JD, editors. Anxiety and the anxiety disorders. Hillsdale (NJ): Lawrence Erlbaum Associates, Inc; 1985. p. 183–96.
5. Ellis A. Reason and emotion in psychotherapy. New York: Stuart; 1962.
6. Meichenbaum DH, Goodman J. Training impulsive children to talk to themselves: a means of developing self-control. J Abnorm Psychol 1971;77:115–26.
7. D'Zurilla TJ, Goldfried MR. Problem solving and behavior modification. J Abnorm Psychol 1971;78:107–26.
8. Barlow DH. Unraveling the mysteries of anxiety and its disorders from the perspective of emotion theory. Am Psychol 2000;55:1247–63.
9. Levitt E. The results of psychotherapy with children: an evaluation. J Consult Psychol 1957;21:189–96.
10. Levitt E. Psychotherapy with children: a further evaluation. Behav Res Ther 1963; 1:45–51.
11. Kendall PC, Hollon SD, editors. Assessment strategies for cognitive-behavioral interventions. New York: Academic Press; 1981.
12. Mowrer OH, Mowrer WM. Enuresis—a method for its study and treatment. Am J Orthopsychiatry 1938;8:436–59.
13. Gosch EA, Flannery-Schroeder E, Mauro CF, et al. Principles of cognitive-behavioral therapy for anxiety disorders in children. J Cognit Psychother 2006; 20:247–62.
14. Menzies RG, Clarke JC. The etiology of phobias: a nonassociative account. Clin Psychol Rev 1995;15:23–48.
15. Barrios BA, O'Dell SL. Fears and anxieties. In: Mash EJ, Barkley RA, editors. Treatment of childhood disorders. 2nd edition. New York: Guilford; 1998. p. 249–337.
16. Gillian P, Rachman S. An experimental investigation of desensitization in phobic patients. Br J Psychiatry 1974;112:392–401.
17. Skinner BF. Contingencies of reinforcement: a theoretical analysis. New York: Appleton; 1969.
18. Meyers AW, Craighead WE. Cognitive behavior therapy with children: a historical, conceptual, and organizational overview. In: Meyers AW, Craighead WE, editors. Cognitive behavior therapy with children. New York: Plenum Press; 1984. p. 1–17.
19. Kazdin AE. Parent management training. New York: Oxford University Press; 2005.
20. Patterson GR. Coercive family process. Eugene (OR): Castalia Publishing Company; 1982.
21. Patterson GR, Reid JB, Dishion T. Antisocial boys. Eugene (OR): Castalia Publishing Company; 1992.
22. Reid JB, Patterson GR, Synder J. Antisocial behavior in children and adolescents: a developmental analysis and model for intervention. Washington, DC: American Psychological Association; 2002.
23. Forgatch MS, Patterson GR. Parents and adolescents living together: part 2: family problem solving. Eugene (OR): Castalia Publishing Company; 1989.

24. Patterson GR, Reid JB, Jones RR, et al. A social learning approach to family intervention: families with aggressive children, vol. 1. Eugene (OR): Castalia Publishing Company; 1975.

25. Eyberg SM, Nelson MM, Boggs SR. Evidence-based psychosocial treatments for children and adolescents with disruptive behavior. J Clin Child Adolesc Psychol 2008;37:215–37.

26. Kendall PC, Finch AJ. A cognitive-behavioral treatment for impulsive control: a case study. J Consult Clin Psychol 1976;44:852–7.

27. Kendall PC, Finch AJ. A cognitive-behavioral treatment for impulsivity: a group comparison study. J Consult Clin Psychol 1978;46:110–8.

28. Kendall PC, Wilcox LE. A cognitive-behavioral treatment for impulsivity: concrete versus conceptual training with non-self-controlled problem children. J Consult Clin Psychol 1980;48:80–91.

29. Bandura A. Principles of behavior modification. Oxford (England): Holt, Rinehart, Winston; 1969.

30. Mahoney MJ. Cognition and behavior modification. Cambridge (MA): Ballinger; 1974.

31. Luria AR. An objective approach to the study of the abnormal child. Am J Orthopsychiatry 1961;31:1–16.

32. Vygotsky LS. Thought and language. Oxford (England): Wiley; 1962.

33. Kendall PC. On the efficacious use of verbal self-instructions with children. Cognit Ther Res 1977;1:331–41.

34. Urbain ES, Kendall PC. A review of social-cognitive problem-solving interventions with children. Psychol Bull 1980;88:109–43.

35. Allen GJ, Chinsky JM, Larcen SW, et al. Community psychology and the schools: a behaviorally oriented multilevel preventive approach. Hillsdale (NJ): Erlbaum; 1976.

36. Gesten EL, Flores de Apodaca R, Rains MH, et al. Promoting peer related social competence in young children. In: Kent MW, Rolf JE, editors. Primary prevention of psychopathology, vol. 3. Hanover (NH): University Press of New England; 1979. p. 220–47.

37. Spivak G, Shure MB. Social adjustment of young children. A cognitive approach to solving real-life problems. London: Jossey-Bass; 1974.

38. Deblinger E, Behl L, Glickman A, et al. Trauma-focused cognitive- behavioral therapy for children who have experienced sexual abuse. In: Kendall PC, editor. Child and adolescent therapy: cognitive-behavioral procedures, 4th edition. New York: Guilford Press; 2011.

39. Kendall PC. Treating anxiety disorders in youth. In: Kendall PC, editor. Child and adolescent therapy: cognitive-behavioral procedures. 4th edition. New York: Guilford Press; 2011.

40. Lochman J, Powell N, Whidby J, et al. Aggressive children: cognitive-behavioral assessment and treatment. In: Kendall PC, editor. Child and adolescent therapy: cognitive-behavioral procedures. 4th edition. New York: Guilford Press; 2011.

41. Stark K, Streusand W, Arora K. Treatment of childhood depression: the ACTION treatment program. In: Kendall PC, editor. Child and adolescent therapy: cognitive-behavioral procedures. 4th edition. New York: Guilford Press; 2011.

42. Kanfer FH. Self-monitoring: methodological limitations and clinical applications. J Consult Clin Psychol 1970;35:148–52.

43. Kanfer FH, Karoly P. Self-control: a behavioristic excursion into the lion's den. Behav Ther 1972;3:398–416.

44. Beck AT. Cognitive therapy and the emotional disorders. New York: International Universities Press; 1976.

45. Ellis A, Harper RA. A new guide to rational living. North Hollywood (CA): Wilshire Book Company; 1975.
46. Hollon SD, Beck AT. Cognitive and cognitive behavioral therapies. In: Lambert MJ, editor. Bergin and Garfield's handbook of psychotherapy and behavior change. 5th edition. New York: Wiley; 2004. p. 447–92.
47. Leahy R, editor. Contemporary cognitive therapy: theory, research, and practice. New York: Guilford Press; 2004.
48. Cautela JR. Covert sensitization. Psychol Rep 1967;20:459–68.
49. Homme LE. Perspectives in psychology: XXIV. Control of coverants, the operants of the mind. Psychol Rec 1965;15:501–11.
50. Rush AJ, Beck AT, Kovacs M, et al. Comparative efficacy of cognitive therapy and pharmacotherapy in the treatment of depressed outpatients. Cognit Ther Res 1977;1:17–38.
51. Trexler LD, Karst TO. Rational-emotive therapy, placebo, and no treatment effects on public speaking anxiety. J Abnorm Psychol 1972;79:60–7.
52. Clark LA, Watson D. Tripartite model of anxiety and depression: psychometric evidence and taxonomic implications. J Abnorm Psychol 1991;100:316–36.
53. Barlow DH, Chorpita BF, Turovsky J. Fear, panic, anxiety, and the disorders of emotion. In: Hope DA, editor, Nebraska symposium on motivation: perspectives on anxiety, panic, and fear, vol. 43. Lincoln (NE): University of Nebraska Press; 1996. p. 251–328.
54. Chorpita BF, Albano AM, Barlow DH. The structure of negative emotions in a clinical sample of children and adolescents. J Abnorm Psychol 1998;107:74–85.
55. Hastings PD, Sullivan C, McShane KE, et al. Parental socialization, vagal regulation, and preschoolers' anxious difficulties: direct mothers and moderated fathers. Child Dev 2008;79:45–64.
56. Ollendick TH, Horsch LM. Fears in clinic-referred children: relations with child anxiety sensitivity, maternal overcontrol, and maternal phobic anxiety. Behav Ther 2007;38:402–11.
57. Kendall PC, editor. Child and adolescent therapy: cognitive-behavioral procedures. New York: Guilford Press; 1991.
58. Kendall PC, editor. Child and adolescent therapy: cognitive-behavioral procedures. 4th edition. New York: Guilford Press; 2011.
59. American Psychological Association Task Force on Promotion and Dissemination of Psychological Procedures. Training in and dissemination of empirically validated psychological treatments: report and recommendations. Clin Psychol 1995;48:3–23.
60. Chambless D, Hollon S. Defining empirically supported treatments. J Consult Clin Psychol 1998;66:5–17.
61. Barrett PM, Farrell L, Pina AA, et al. Evidence-based psychosocial treatments for child and adolescent obsessive-compulsive disorder. J Clin Child Adolesc Psychol 2008;37:131–55.
62. David-Ferdon C, Kaslow NJ. Evidence-based psychosocial treatments for child and adolescent depression. J Clin Child Adolesc Psychol 2008;37:62–104.
63. Silverman WK, Ortiz CD, Viswesvaran C, et al. Evidence-based psychosocial treatments for children and adolescents exposed to traumatic events. J Clin Child Adolesc Psychol 2008;37:156–83.
64. Silverman WK, Pina AA, Viswesvaran C. Evidence-based psychosocial treatments for phobic and anxiety disorders in children and adolescents. J Clin Child Adolesc Psychol 2008;37:105–30.

65. Cohen JA, Mannarino AP, Deblinger E. Treating trauma and traumatic grief in children & adolescents. New York: Guildford Press; 2006.
66. Kendall PC, Hedtke K. Cognitive-behavioral therapy for anxious children: therapist manual. 3rd edition. Ardmore (PA): Workbook Publishing; 2006. Available at: www.WorkbookPublishing.com.
67. Stein BD, Jaycox LH, Kataoke SH, et al. A mental health intervention for school children exposed to violence. J Am Med Assoc 2003;290:603–11.
68. Pediatric OCD Treatment Study Team. Cognitive-behavior therapy, sertraline, and their combination for children and adolescents with obsessive-compulsive disorder. JAMA 2004;292:1969–76.
69. Piacentini J, Peris T, March J, et al. Cognitive-behavioral therapy for youth with obsessive-compulsive disorder. In: Kendall PC, editor. Child and adolescent therapy: cognitive-behavioral procedures. 4th edition. New York: Guilford Press; 2011.
70. Waldron HB, Turner CW. Evidence-based psychosocial treatments for adolescent substance abuse. J Clin Child Adolesc Psychol 2008;37:238–61.
71. Lochman JE, Barry TD, Pardini DA. Anger control training for aggressive youth. In: Kazdin AE, Weisz JR, editors. Evidence-based psychotherapies for children and adolescents. New York: Guilford; 2003. p. 263–81.
72. Block J. Effects of rational-emotive mental health program on poorly achieving, disruptive high school students. J Couns Psychol 1978;25:61–5.
73. Kazdin AE, Kendall PC. Current progress and future plans for developing effective treatments: comments and perspectives. J Clin Child Psychol 1998;27:217–26.
74. Kendall PC, Ollendick T. Setting the research and practice agenda for anxiety in children and adolescents: a topic comes of age. Cognit Behav Pract 2004;11:65–74.
75. Weisz JR, Jensen AL. Child and adolescent psychotherapy in research and practice contexts: review of the evidence and suggestions for improving the field. Eur Child Adolesc Psychiatry 2001;10:I12–8.
76. Kiesler DJ. Some myths of psychotherapy research and the search for a paradigm. Psychol Bull 1966;65:110–36.
77. Shirk S, Jungbluth N, Karver M. Change processes in cognitive behavioral therapy for children and adolescents. In: Kendall PC, editor. Child and adolescent therapy: cognitive-behavioral procedures. 4th edition. New York: Guilford Press; 2011.
78. Khanna M, Kendall PC. Computer-assisted CBT for child anxiety: the coping cat DVD (camp cope-a-lot). Cognit Behav Pract 2008;15:159–65.
79. Khanna M, Kendall PC. Computer-assisted cognitive-behavioral therapy for child anxiety: results of a randomized clinical trial. J Consult Clin Psychol 2010;78(5): 737–45.
80. Beidas R, Kendall PC. Training therapists in evidence based practice: a critical review of studies from a systems-contextual perspective. Clin Psychol 2010;17:1–30.
81. Tansella M, Thornicroft G. Implementation science: understanding the translation of evidence into practice. Br J Psychiatry 2009;195:283–5.

Cognitive-Behavioral Therapy for Adolescent Depression and Suicidality

Anthony Spirito, PhD, ABPP[a],*,
Christianne Esposito-Smythers, PhD[b],
Jennifer Wolff, PhD[c], Kristen Uhl, BS[d]

KEYWORDS

• Adolescents • Suicide • Depression • CBT

Depression is one of the most common reasons adolescents seek treatment. Although there are several treatment options available, cognitive-behavioral therapy (CBT) has been the most widely researched psychotherapy approach for treating depression in adolescents. Among depressed adolescents, it is common for these youths to experience suicidal thoughts or engage in suicidal behaviors. Although it is evident that such symptoms require psychological treatment, there is some debate about the best means of targeting these distressing thoughts and behaviors. Some clinical researchers have postulated that if the underlying depressive disorder is treated adequately, suicidal ideation and behavior will remit along with the disorder. However, there has been some evidence with adults[1] that suggests this is not the case. That is, suicidal thoughts and behavior need to be directly addressed if these problems are to improve. This article first reviews the rationale underlying the use of CBT for the treatment of depression and suicidality (defined as suicidal thoughts and suicide attempts) in adolescents. The literature supporting the efficacy of CBT for depressed adolescents is then briefly reviewed. Because there are many excellent recent reviews of the efficacy of CBT for adolescent depression (see later discussion), the review of the depression literature is brief. Instead, the article focuses primarily on whether

The authors have nothing to disclose.

[a] Division of Clinical Psychology, Department of Psychiatry and Human Behavior, Warren Alpert Medical School of Brown University, Box G – BH, Providence, RI 02912, USA

[b] Department of Psychology, George Mason University, 4400 University Drive, Fairfax, VA 22030, USA

[c] Department of Psychiatry and Human Behavior, Rhode Island Hospital/Warren Alpert Medical School of Brown University, 593 Eddy Street, POB 122, Providence, RI 02903, USA

[d] Department of Psychiatry, Rhode Island Hospital, 593 Eddy Street, POB 122, Providence, RI 02903, USA

* Corresponding author.
E-mail address: Anthony_Spirito@Brown.edu

Child Adolesc Psychiatric Clin N Am 20 (2011) 191–204
doi:10.1016/j.chc.2011.01.012
1056-4993/11/$ – see front matter © 2011 Elsevier Inc. All rights reserved.

childpsych.theclinics.com

CBT for depression reduces suicidal thoughts and behavior. A description of some of the core cognitive, affective, and behavioral techniques used in CBT treatments of suicidal ideation and behavior in depressed adolescents concludes the article.

RATIONALE FOR TREATING SUICIDAL STATES WITH CBT

A developmentally sensitive cognitive-behavioral model of adolescent suicidal behavior[2] adapted from an adult model of suicidality[3] postulates that suicide attempts emerge from reciprocity among maladaptive cognition, behavior, and affective responses to stressors. This model posits that there is a predisposing vulnerability among youth who attempt suicide, which results from a significant genetic predisposition toward psychopathology[4] and/or exposure to significant negative life events, such as a history of abuse or neglect,[5] adverse parenting resulting from parental psychopathology,[6] and peer victimization and bullying.[7] These same factors also place youth at risk for a depressive episode.

Stress, most commonly from an interpersonal conflict, may initially trigger a depressive episode and/or suicidal crisis in predisposed adolescents. In the face of stress, cognitive errors (eg, catastrophizing, personalization) and negative views of self and the future may occur. Indeed, 1 study[8] that examined adolescents with a mood disorder in an inpatient setting found higher catastrophizing, personalization, selective abstraction, overgeneralization, and total cognitive errors, in those who were suicidal compared with nonsuicidal adolescents with a mood disorder. In addition to cognitively distorting the severity and consequences of the stressor, predisposed youth may also experience difficulties generating and/or viewing solutions to the stressor. Suicidal adolescents report greater difficulty generating and implementing effective alternative solutions to problems compared with nonsuicidal adolescents.[9] Suicidal youth are also more likely to view problems as irresolvable.[10] This difficulty in cognitive processing and problem solving, which is also characteristic of depressed adolescents, can result in negative affect including anger[11] and a worsening of the current mood state. Suicidal adolescents report greater difficulty regulating their internal states and using affect regulation skills compared with nonsymptomatic adolescents.[12]

In response to distorted cognitive processing, lack of perceived adaptive solutions, and heightened affective arousal related to the stressor, adolescents may engage in maladaptive behavior as a means to cope with the stressor, and may include the use of passive and/or aggressive communication styles and behavior to address stressors resulting from conflict with peers[13] and family members.[14] Self-medication with alcohol or drugs,[15] and nonsuicidal self-injury, such as superficially cutting or burning oneself,[16] may also be used as an means to reduce negative affect. The maladaptive behavior chosen may have been modeled by parents, peers, or other important figures in the life of suicidal depressed adolescents.

Adolescents may cycle through this cognitive, affective, and behavioral process numerous times, with each cycle leading to greater dysfunction and depressed mood. This cycle may last for a few days, weeks, or even months. Either way, the end result of this cycle, if not interrupted, is intolerable affect and the perception that the situation is hopeless. Adolescents may then begin to experience passive suicidal thoughts, such as "I would be better off dead" which over time may become active suicidal thoughts, and a suicide attempt, with or without prior planning, may result.

Once suicidal behavior occurs, it may sensitize adolescents to future suicide-related thoughts and behavior.[17] Suicidal behavior makes the suicidal cognitive schema more easily accessible and triggered in future stressful situations.[18] Joiner[17] suggests that suicide attempts habituate individuals to the experience of engaging in dangerous self-injurious behavior. When combined with interpersonally related cognitive distortions, this habituation increases the possibility of future suicidal behavior. Once the taboo against suicide has been broken, it becomes easier to view suicide as a viable solution to life's problems. CBT may be effective with depressed, suicidal adolescents because it is based on the premise that maladaptive cognitive, behavioral, and affective responses, such as those described in the model described earlier, can be changed.

THE EFFICACY OF CBT IN THE TREATMENT OF ADOLESCENT DEPRESSION

CBT treatments for adolescent depression place varying emphasis on the cognitive and behavioral components of care. The behavioral component of treatments for depression emphasizes various skill deficits in the domains of coping skills, interpersonal relationships, social problem solving, and participation in pleasant activities.[19] The cognitive component typically focuses on identifying and challenging schemas, automatic thoughts, and cognitive distortions that cast experiences in an overly negative manner. CBT for depressed adolescents addresses lagging cognitive and behavioral skills that are needed to create and maintain supportive relationships and to regulate emotion.

The first reviews of the efficacy of CBT for adolescent depression demonstrated strong support for the use of CBT with depressed youth.[20,21] For example, the effect sizes calculated in early meta-analytical reviews were 1.27 in one study[22] and 1.02 in another study.[23] A more recent meta-analysis of youth depression psychotherapy trials, including both CBT and non-CBT approaches to treatment,[24] concluded that the mean effect size of treatment was 0.34 (ie, somewhere between a small and medium effect). Five studies demonstrated large effects and 3 of these used CBT. Nonetheless, within the CBT category, effects were variable. In another meta-analysis using 11 randomized trials of CBT for adolescents who met diagnostic criteria for unipolar depression,[25] the investigators found a mean effect size of 0.53 (ie, a medium effect). These smaller effects might be a function of the increasing severity of the samples studied or larger methodological differences in trials, which can have a substantial influence on effect sizes.

In 2008, a review of the literature was conducted to determine what treatments for childhood depression could qualify as evidence based.[26] Given that the childhood depression treatment literature includes primarily between-group experiments, studies were rated using criteria for between-group designs. Interventions were deemed, from most to least rigorous, as well-established, probably efficacious, or experimental treatments. For a treatment to be considered well established, there had to be at least 2 well-conducted between-group design experiments, conducted by at least 2 independent researchers or research teams, that found the treatment to either be superior to pill or psychological placebo or to another treatment, or equivalent to an already established treatment in adequately powered experiments. Further, these studies had to use treatment manuals and present detailed sample characteristics. Treatments were deemed probably efficacious if they were supported by at least 2 well-conducted between-group experiments that found the treatment to be superior to a wait-list control group, or 1 or more well-conducted experiments that met the well-established treatment criteria, with the exception of the requirement that the treatment was tested by at least 2 independent researchers or research teams. Probably efficacious treatments also had to include a treatment manual and well-specified sample characteristics. Experimental treatments were defined as treatments with at least 1 well-conducted study that yielded a significant treatment effect. This review of the depression treatment literature[26] concluded that for children and adolescents, group CBT programs, with or without a parent component, are well-established treatment approaches. For adolescents, individual CBT, with or without a parent component, and individual interpersonal therapy, were deemed to be "probably efficacious" treatments. Other approaches, such as supportive group therapy and family systems-oriented treatments, were rated as experimental.

The aforementioned review included the multisite Treatment for Adolescents Depression Study (TADS),[27] the largest multisite treatment study for adolescent depression. TADS examined the efficacy of 4 interventions (CBT alone, fluoxetine alone, a combination of both medication and CBT, and placebo pill alone) for adolescents with depression. The study was a randomized, masked effectiveness trial that included 439 adolescents between the ages of 12 and 17 years. Participants could attend up to 15 sessions during the first 12 weeks of treatment, weekly or biweekly sessions during the next 6 weeks, and booster sessions every 6 weeks thereafter. Results suggest that the combined treatment was more effective (73% response rate) than either fluoxetine alone (62%), CBT alone (48%), or the pill placebo in reducing clinician-rated depressive symptoms. Fluoxetine alone was superior to CBT alone, and CBT alone was not more effective than placebo. Following 12 weeks of acute treatment, 71% of teens across groups no longer met diagnostic criteria, but 50% had residual symptoms. Follow-up results at longer time periods were more positive for CBT; at week 18, the response rates were 85% for combination therapy, 69% for fluoxetine therapy, and 65% for CBT. At week 36, response rates were 86% for combination therapy, 81% for fluoxetine therapy, and 81% for CBT.[28]

Since this review,[26] several other studies have added to the literature supporting individual CBT for adolescent depression. In the multisite Treatment of SSRI-Resistant Depression in Adolescents (TORDIA) study,[29] 334 depressed adolescents who failed to respond to a previous trial of a selective serotonin reuptake inhibitor (SSRI) were randomized to 1 of 4 conditions: change to a different SSRI (n = 85), change to a different SSRI plus CBT (n = 83), change to venlafaxine (n = 83), or change to venlafaxine plus CBT (n = 83). CBT participants attended weekly sessions for the first 3 months of treatment then biweekly sessions. Results showed that switching to either medication regimen plus CBT resulted in a higher rate of clinical response (54.8%) than a medication switch alone (40.5%). Most recently, Goodyer and colleagues[30] reported data from a study of British adolescents with moderate to severe major depressive disorder (MDD) or probable MDD who had not responded to a brief initial intervention. They were randomized to either receive SSRI plus routine care (n = 103) or an SSRI, routine care, and individual CBT (n = 75). At the end of the 12-week acute phase and 28-week maintenance phase, the addition of CBT had no benefit over treatment with the SSRI alone. These results stand in contrast to the TORDIA study, which had a similar population of more severely depressed adolescents but did find an additive effect for CBT over medication alone. However, the investigators noted that there was relatively low attendance in the CBT condition, which may have affected their outcomes. One additional study[31] randomized 46 youths aged 11 to 18 years who had responded to 12 weeks of fluoxetine to either medication management only (n = 24) or medication management with CBT (n = 22). The addition of CBT lowered the risk of relapse compared with medication management alone.

CBT for adolescent depression has received considerable support in the research literature. Individual and group CBT, with and without a parent component, seems to be well established and/or efficacious for most participants. The next section discusses the use of these treatments in addressing suicidality.

THE EFFECTS OF CBT FOR ADOLESCENT DEPRESSION ON SUICIDAL IDEATION AND ATTEMPTS

There have been several treatment studies on adolescent depression that have examined the effect of CBT on participant suicidality. This article primarily reviews studies that were conducted in the last decade. Overall, results have shown that CBT for depression in adolescents is effective in reducing suicidality. In general, these programs teach coping skills and affect regulation techniques that can be applied to suicidal ideation.

In 1 of the first studies, 107 adolescents (13–18 years old) diagnosed with MDD were randomized into 1 of 3 treatment groups: individual CBT, systematic behavior family therapy (SBFT), or individual nondirective supportive therapy (NST).[32] Each treatment condition consisted of an active phase of 12 to 16 sessions over 12 to 16 weeks, and a booster phase of 2 to 4 sessions over 12 to 16 weeks. At baseline nearly one-third of participants in each condition endorsed current suicidality, and close to 25% had a history of a suicide attempt. Participants in the CBT group showed a lower rate of MDD compared with those in the NST group at the end of the study, and a higher rate of remission than the SBFT group. There was also a significant decrease in suicidality for all 3 treatment conditions, with the greatest decrease occurring between intake and 6 weeks. These findings suggest that suicidality and depression in adolescents may be reduced through different processes, and that suicidality tends to drop in the early stages of treatment regardless of treatment modality. Similar results were found in a group CBT study[33] with a sample of 88 depressed adolescents, aged 13 to 18 years, who also had depressed parents. Adolescents exhibited comparable reductions in suicidal ideation, regardless of whether they were randomized to a 16-week group CBT program or care as usual.[33]

Suicidal ideation in depressed adolescents has also been examined in studies that evaluate the effectiveness of combined CBT therapy and medication. One study[34] evaluated combined CBT and an SSRI compared with either treatment on its own. In this study, 73 adolescents (age 12–18 years) diagnosed with MDD, dysthymic disorder, or depressive disorder not otherwise specified, were randomized to 12 weeks of CBT, CBT and sertraline, or sertraline alone. Results from the 3 treatment groups showed comparable, statistically significant improvement in suicidal ideation after acute treatment, which was maintained at the 6-month follow-up.[34]

In another study,[30] 208 depressed adolescents (ages 11–17 years) were randomized into groups that received 12 weeks of both CBT and an SSRI (primarily fluoxetine), or clinical care and SSRI. Suicidality was rated at baseline, 6, 12, and 28 weeks. At each follow-up point, the number of participants experiencing suicidal symptoms and the frequency of these symptoms (thoughts, ideation, attempts, and self-harm) was lower in both groups compared with baseline. There was no significant difference found between adolescents receiving SSRIs and clinical care or those receiving CBT plus SSRIs.[30]

Treatment with fluoxetine and CBT was also examined in a study of 13- to 19-year-old adolescents with major depression, behavior problems, and substance use disorders.[35] In this study, 126 adolescents were randomized to a fluoxetine and CBT group or a placebo and CBT group. Each group had 16 weekly therapy and medication monitoring sessions. Participant suicidality was assessed monthly and found to be comparable in both groups; however, 5 participants were hospitalized during the course of treatment for increased suicidality (4 in the fluoxetine-CBT condition). For all 5 of these participants, suicide severity ratings decreased during the first month of treatment, but worsened during weeks 8 and 12 in response to psychosocial stressors.

Thus, although suicidality showed an initial response to treatment, these adolescents did not respond well when additional psychosocial stressors arose. However, given the small number of hospitalizations in this trial, it is difficult to draw conclusions.

Rohde and colleagues[36] examined depressed adolescents, aged 13 to 17 years, with comorbid conduct disorder. Depressed adolescents with conduct disorder were randomized to a CBT intervention designed for adolescents with this comorbid symptomatology (CWD-A) or a life skills/tutoring control (LS) program. Each treatment option offered 16 group sessions over 8 weeks. Of the 93 participating adolescents, 40% had a history of suicide attempts. Results showed that CWD-A intervention was initially more effective at reducing MDD than the LS program. However, posttreatment, 6-, and 12-month assessments revealed no significant difference in the number of suicide attempts.[36]

Two large multisite studies examining combined pharmacotherapy and CBT for MDD also examined the effects of their protocols on suicidality. In TADS,[27] which was discussed earlier, 30% of participants had clinically significant suicidal ideation at baseline. At 12 weeks, reductions in suicidality were greater for youth randomized to combination therapy than fluoxetine therapy, CBT only, and the placebo condition, although suicidal ideation was lower than baseline in all conditions. Participants who received CBT (4.5%), placebo (5.4%), or combination therapy (8.4%) were less likely to experience a suicidal event during treatment than those who received fluoxetine alone (11.9%). The investigators concluded that there was a slight protective effect of CBT on both suicidal ideation and suicidal behavior. At 36 weeks of treatment, suicidal events were more common in patients treated with fluoxetine alone (14.7%), compared with 8.4% for combination therapy and 6.3% for CBT alone in the intent-to-treat analyses.[37]

In the multisite TORDIA study[29] described previously, 58.5% of participants reported clinically significant suicidal ideation and 23.7% reported a previous suicide attempt. During the trial, suicidal ideation after treatment decreased from baseline for participants across all conditions. Approximately 5% of participants attempted suicide and 20% experienced a self-harm related event (suicidal ideation, suicide attempt, self-injurious behavior) during treatment, with no differences across conditions.

In summary, most studies of CBT for depressed adolescents have found a reduction in suicidal ideation regardless of CBT format (ie, individual, group). Reductions in suicidality have also been found in response to family therapy,[32] supportive therapy[32] and pharmacotherapy.[30,34] Nonetheless, although various forms of therapy resulted in comparable reductions in adolescent suicidality, CBT has shown the most promise in concurrently reducing MDD diagnoses/symptoms and suicidal ideation.

CBT STUDIES SPECIFICALLY TREATING SUICIDALITY IN ADOLESCENTS

Only a few studies have used CBT to specifically treat suicidal ideation and behavior. One study[38] used a quasi-experimental design to compare the treatment efficacy of dialectical behavior therapy (DBT), a treatment approach that uses cognitive-behavioral techniques, to treatment as usual (TAU), for suicidal adolescents. The DBT protocol was designed to improve distress tolerance, emotional regulation, and interpersonal effectiveness. Although adolescents in the DBT condition reported more severe baseline symptomatology than those in the TAU condition, they had fewer psychiatric hospitalizations and higher rates of treatment completion than the TAU group at follow-up. No differences were found on repeat suicide attempts. About 40% of adolescents reattempted during treatment.

In another trial,[39] individual CBT was compared with an individual problem-oriented supportive therapy with adolescents immediately following a suicide attempt. More than half of the sample reported at least 1 previous suicide attempt. Adolescents were randomized to either 10 sessions of CBT (N = 15) or the problem-oriented supportive treatment (N = 16). The CBT condition focused on teaching adolescents problem-solving and affect management skills. Each session included an assessment of suicidality, instruction in a skill, and skill practice (both in-session and homework assignments). Participants were taught steps of effective problem solving and cognitive and behavioral strategies for affect management (eg, cognitive restructuring, relaxation). Homework assignments were given to assist in skill acquisition and generalization. Participants in both conditions reported significant reductions in suicidal ideation and depression at 3-month follow-up but there were no between-group differences. At 6 months, both groups retained improvement over baseline but levels of suicide ideation and depression were slightly higher (although not statistically significant) than at the 3-month follow-up. Only 5% of adolescents reattempted during the course of the study.

A more recent study (Esposito-Smythers C, Spirito A, Hunt J, et al. Treatment of co-occurring substance abuse and suicidality among adolescents: a randomized pilot trial. Manuscript submitted for publication) compared an integrated cognitive-behavioral treatment (I-CBT; N = 19) protocol for adolescents with co-occurring suicidality (suicidal ideation and/or attempt) and substance use disorders to enhanced treatment as usual (E-TAU; N = 17) in a randomized clinical trial. Approximately 77% of adolescents had a previous suicide attempt and 94% a current depressive disorder. I-CBT included a 6-month active, 3-month continuation, and 3-month maintenance treatment phase. The protocol included individual, parent training, and family therapy sessions and used a 2-therapist model. One therapist worked with the adolescent and a second therapist worked with the parents. E-TAU included psychotherapy services through community providers. However, adolescents in both treatment conditions were offered free medication management with the same child psychiatrist employed for the study. I-CBT was associated with a lower incidence of suicide attempts (5% in I-CBT vs 35% in E-TAU) as well as fewer psychiatric hospitalizations, heavy drinking days, and days of cannabis use relative to E-TAU over 18 months. There was a trend for fewer youth in I-CBT than E-TAU to have a depressive disorder (7% vs 31%) by 18 months. Comparable reductions in adolescent self-report of suicidal ideation, number of drinking days, and depressive symptoms were reported across groups.

In a multisite study, referred to as Treatment of Adolescent Suicide Attempters (TASA),[40] 124 depressed adolescents who made a suicide attempt in the previous 3 months were entered in 1 of 3 conditions: SSRI (n = 15), CBT for suicide prevention (CBT-SP; n =18), or combination therapy (n = 93). Treatment assignment could be random or chosen by study participants. Most participants (84%) chose their treatment condition. CBT-SP incorporated a risk reduction and relapse prevention approach to treatment and integrated CBT techniques, DBT techniques, and other intervention techniques for depressed youth with suicidality. Participants could attend up to 22 sessions over 6 months, including individual adolescent and conjoint parent-adolescent sessions. All participants showed a significant decrease in suicidal ideation from baseline to the end of treatment. Approximately 12% of participants reattempted suicide and 19% experienced a suicidal event (suicide attempt, suicide completion, preparatory acts toward suicidal behavior, significant suicidal ideation) during treatment. After controlling for baseline differences across treatment conditions, there was no differential effect of monotherapy versus combination therapy on suicide outcomes.[40]

Treatment studies that target adolescent suicidality suggest that CBT results in improvements in suicidal ideation and depressed mood, although results are generally comparable with active comparison treatments. Similarly, with 1 exception (Esposito-Smythers C, Spirito A, Hunt J, et al. Treatment of co-occurring substance abuse and suicidality among adolescents: a randomized pilot trial. Manuscript submitted for publication) the incidence of suicide attempts rarely differs between CBT and other active interventions. A significant percentage of adolescents reattempt suicide (5%–40%) during the course of treatment of suicidal behavior.

CBT TECHNIQUES COMMONLY USED TO ADDRESS DEPRESSION AND SUICIDALITY

In our studies and treatment manuals for suicidal adolescents[39] (Esposito-Smythers C, Spirito A, Hunt J, et al. Treatment of co-occurring substance abuse and suicidality among adolescents: a randomized pilot trial. Manuscript submitted for publication) individual CBT sessions follow a standard format. They begin with a medication adherence check, if applicable, followed by an assessment of suicidal thoughts or behavior as well as any alcohol or drug use since the last session. If the adolescent does seem to be at significant risk for suicidal behavior, we conduct an assessment of current suicidality, and either review or negotiate a safety plan, adapted from other important work in this area.[37] The safety plan includes a "personal reasons to live" list with at least 5 reasons to live (eg, "to have a family of my own and to see my little brother grow up"). A coping card is created in which the adolescent generates a list of strategies that they can use in stressful situations, as well as phone numbers to contact in an emergency. A copy of the coping card is given to the adolescent to place in their wallet for immediate access.

A typical cognitive-behavioral session that follows the format used in TADS[27] and TORDIA[29] is: the adolescent is first asked to identify an agenda item that will be discussed in the session, homework from the previous session is reviewed, a new skill is introduced or a previously taught skill reviewed, the skill is practiced, the agenda item is discussed, and whenever possible the newly taught skill or a previously taught skill is applied to the agenda item. Worksheets and handouts for each skill taught are used to assist in the learning process. All individual sessions also include a parent check-in at the end and a personalized homework assignment is created.

Cognitive and behavioral techniques that can be used to address both depression and suicidality in the skill portion of a CBT session are described in the following sections. First, the approach used by our group to teach cognitive restructuring and problem solving, 2 key cognitive interventions with this population, is described. More details on how to implement these techniques have been described elsewhere.[41] Several cognitive techniques specifically useful for suicidalilty, which are based on suggestions by Freeman and Reinecke,[42] are described. A more in-depth description of how to adapt these techniques with adolescents is also available.[43] A description of affect regulation techniques is provided.

Cognitive Restructuring

In our studies we have modified techniques based on rational emotive therapy[44] for children and adolescents[45] to teach cognitive restructuring. We call our techniques the ABCDE method and introduce this method as a skill that helps adolescents deal with negative beliefs or thoughts. Each letter of the ABCDE method stands for a different step in the cognitive restructuring process. The first step in changing negative thought is to identify the A, activating event, that is associated with negative thoughts. In teaching the ABCDE method to the adolescent, the letter C (consequences) is described next as the consequences or feelings related to the activating event. Next, the adolescent is taught that the B of the ABCDE method stands for beliefs, and that it is one's beliefs that lead to negative affect. The adolescent is then taught that, to feel better, they must confront these negative beliefs or dispute them. We explain to the adolescent that most people do not dispute their negative beliefs, are left feeling very upset, and that is when they make unsafe decisions, such as hurting themselves. The last step begins with an E and stands for effect. Effecting something is presented as trying to change something. Adolescents are taught that they may not be able to change the fact that a negative activating event happened but they can change negative beliefs and feelings surrounding the event.

When adolescents begin to use this method, the therapist helps the adolescent question the evidence that is used to support a negative view through Socratic questioning.[46] Questions that we commonly use include: Is this belief true? What is the evidence for or against this belief? Does this belief help you feel the way that you want? What would your friend say if he/she heard this belief? and Is there another explanation for this event? This technique is based on findings that suicide attempters often selectively attend to a particular set of evidence that confirms their negative interpretation. We also give the adolescent a handout on "Thinking Mistakes," for example, black/white thinking, predicting the worst, missing the positive, feelings as facts, jumping to conclusions, expecting perfection, which we simplified from a similar worksheet for adults.[47] We ask the adolescent to identify any thinking mistakes in their beliefs and then to dispute these mistakes.

Problem Solving

Deficits in problem solving include difficulty generating alternative solutions and identifying positive consequences of potential solutions. We use the acronym SOLVE,[48] to cover the basic steps in problem solving. We begin with generating a list of triggers for suicidality, typically 2 to 5 events, and then the therapist teaches the adolescent the SOLVE system. Each letter in the word SOLVE stands for a different step of the problem-solving process: S stands for "Select a problem," O for "generate Options," L for rate the "Likely outcome" of each option, V for choose the "Very best option," and E stands for "Evaluate" how well each option worked. A worksheet is used to assist in the SOLVE process. The therapist may need to model the skills necessary to progress through the problem-solving steps. The typical depressed adolescent will have difficulties generating "Options" but usually improves with practice. After each option is rated, the therapist helps the adolescent select the "Very best option" or combination of options to try out. The adolescent is then asked to evaluate how well the process works. If it seems the option will work out well, then this option is selected. If it does not seem to lead to a workable solution, then the adolescent is instructed to go back to the list of "Options," weigh them again, and pick another option to try. The adolescent does this until a solution to the problem is generated. A simpler version of problem solving is to ask the adolescent to list the pros and cons of an action such as breaking up with a boyfriend/girlfriend.

When working with adolescents who have attempted suicide, the therapist reframes the suicide attempt as a failure in problem solving. This explanation helps provide adolescents with a better sense of control over future problems that arise. The therapist points out that many teenagers who attempt suicide pick the only option that they think they have, which is to hurt themselves. The therapist emphasizes that the more adolescents practice coming up with a list of "Options," the more potential solutions they have to choose from when stressed, and the less likely they will believe that the only thing they can do is to hurt themselves.

One contentious aspect of problem solving is whether to have a suicidal individual include suicide as an option during the brainstorming portion of SOLVE. Some therapists believe that allowing suicide as an option facilitates the problem-solving discussion. Others fear that a cognitively restricted suicidal individual will not be able to generate other options beside kill oneself. Schneidman[49] described 1 way to include suicide as an option with a suicidal young adult who was pregnant. After allowing his client to list suicide as an option to her problem, Schneidman had her write a list of alternatives without regard to their feasibility (eg, have an abortion, put the child up for adoption, raise the child on her own, and so forth). Then he had her rank order the options from the least onerous to most onerous. Although she said that none of the options were good ones, this procedure helped her to see that there were other options besides suicide. Moreover, once she no longer ranked suicide as her first or second option, her suicidal ideation decreased significantly.

Other Cognitive Techniques

Many other techniques to address suicidal thinking have been outlined in detail elsewhere.[42,43] A few techniques are briefly reviewed here. First, reattribution is a technique that can be used to help the adolescent change the self-statement, "It's all my fault" to a new statement in which responsibility is attributed more appropriately, perhaps to friends or parents, or chance. The therapist may initially support the adolescent's view that it is their fault but then asks the adolescent to break down what they contribute to the situation and what other people contribute. Second, decatastrophizing helps the adolescent decide whether they are overestimating the catastrophic nature of the precipitating event. The therapist asks the adolescent, "What would be the worst thing that will arise if … occurs?" "If … does occur, how will it affect your life in 3 months? 6 months?" "What is the most likely thing to happen here?" "How will you handle it?" A third cognitive approach is scaling the severity of an event. In this technique, the therapist asks the adolescent to scale the suicidal precipitant or anticipated future stressful event on a scale from 0 to 100. Scaling the severity of an event provides a way for adolescents to view situations along a continuum rather than in a dichotomous fashion.

Affect Regulation Techniques

Affect regulation techniques, that is, training adolescents to recognize stimuli that provoke negative emotions and teaching them to reduce physiologic arousal via self-talk and relaxation, are also commonly used with suicidal adolescents. Our approach to affect management with suicidal adolescents is described in the next paragraph. Another useful approach to affect management with these adolescents is DBT,[50] a therapy designed to specifically target affect dysregulation in individuals with borderline personality disorder and self-injurious behavior. The reader is referred to the article by Klein and Miller in this issue for a review of DBT with suicidal adolescents.

In our approach to affect management, we first review the rationale for managing emotions. Specifically, we relate the notion that when negative activating events trigger negative or untrue beliefs, these beliefs can cause depressed mood and anger. These negative feelings can also cause the body to start feeling out of control, which can be experienced as muscle tightness, a faster heart rate, sweating, or shortness of breath. The more one's body feels out of control, the harder it is to use problem solving or dispute negative beliefs. Therefore, it is important to learn ways to keep negative affect under control.

The therapist then shows the adolescent a series of feelings cards and asks them to choose the card that best describes how they were feeling when a recent event resulted in upset. With suicidal adolescents, it is useful to focus on events that result in suicidal ideation or behavior. Next, the therapist presents the adolescent with a list of physiologic and behavioral symptoms associated with negative affect, referred to as "body talk," and asks the adolescent to pick out the symptoms they experienced when in the stressful situation. The adolescent is then introduced to the concept of a "feelings thermometer."[51] The bottom of the thermometer has a rating of "1" and stands for "calm and cool" and the top is "10" and stands for "extremely upset" or whatever the predominant feeling (eg, anger) was for the adolescent at the time of the stressful event. Next, the adolescent is asked to indicate their personal "danger zone" on the thermometer or the point where their body spirals so far out of control that they are at risk for unsafe or suicidal behavior. Finally, the adolescent is asked to create a "stay cool" plan to use when they begin to notice early "body talk" and negative beliefs to prevent them from reaching the point of "extreme upset" and unsafe behavior. Relaxation training is often taught to the adolescent as a means of managing physiologic arousal. There are many approaches to relaxation training including progressive muscle relaxation, guided imagery, and autogenics, which have been described elsewhere.[52]

Anger is a common emotion experienced by depressed youth who attempt suicide. There are some specific techniques for managing anger that may be useful when dealing with this population. One anger management protocol for adolescents[53] integrates cognitive restructuring and the affect regulation technique described previously. Steps in this protocol include identifying the trigger for one's anger, altering the thoughts that lead to the angry feelings, using self-statements to guide one self through angry provocations, and relaxation techniques to modulate physiologic arousal. Modeling and behavioral rehearsal are used to help teach the adolescent how to use these skills in anger-provoking situations.

SUMMARY

In summary, considerable progress has been made in the past several years in the treatment of depression and suicidality in adolescence. CBT has emerged as a well-established treatment approach for children and adolescents.[26] Although the number of efficacy studies for depression has increased, there is still little evidence-based information indicating how or why these treatments work. In addition, treatment trials for adolescents with suicidality are few in number, and their efficacy to date is limited, especially with regard to repeat suicidal behaviors. A definitive treatment of adolescent suicide attempters has yet to be established, but the limited literature suggests that suicidal thoughts and behavior should be directly addressed for optimal treatment outcome. Training adolescents in specific coping skills and affect regulation techniques that can be applied to thoughts and behaviors associated with suicidality, shows some initial promise. However, future trials are necessary to inform best practices in treating this high-risk population.

REFERENCES

1. Linehan M. Behavioral treatments of suicidal behaviors. Definitional obfuscation and treatment outcomes. Ann N Y Acad Sci 1997;836:302–28.
2. Spirito A, Esposito C, Weismore J, et al. Addressing adolescent suicidal behavior: cognitive-behavioral strategies. In: Kendall PC, editor. Child and adolescent therapy. 3rd edition. New York: Guilford Press; 2006. p. 217–42.

3. Rudd MD, Joiner TE, Rajab MH. Treating suicidal behavior: an effective, time-limited approach. New York: Guilford Press; 2001.

4. Brent D, Melhem N. Familial transmission of suicidal behavior. Psychiatr Clin North Am 2008;31(2):157–77.

5. King C, Merchant C. Social and interpersonal factors relating to adolescent suicidality: a review of the literature. Arch Suicide Res 2008;12(3):181–96.

6. Melhem N, Brent D, Ziegler M, et al. Familial pathways to early-onset suicidal behavior: familial and individual antecedents of suicidal behavior. Am J Psychiatry 2007;164(9):1364–70.

7. Kim Y, Leventhal B. Bullying and suicide. A review. Int J Adolesc Med Health 2008;20(2):133–54.

8. Brent D, Kolko D, Allan M, et al. Suicidality in affectively disordered adolescent inpatients. J Am Acad Child Adolesc Psychiatry 1990;29(4):586–93.

9. Adams J, Adams M. The association among negative life events, perceived problem solving alternatives, depression, and suicidal ideation in adolescent psychiatric patients. J Child Psychol Psychiatry 1996;37(6):715–20.

10. Orbach I, Mikulincer M, Blumenson R, et al. The subjective experience of problem irresolvability and suicidal behavior: dynamics and measurement. Suicide Life Threat Behav 1999;29(2):150–64.

11. Daniel SS, Goldston DB, Erkanli A, et al. Trait anger, anger expression, and suicide attempts among adolescents and young adults: a prospective study. J Clin Child Adolesc Psychol 2009;38(5):661–71.

12. Fritsch S, Donaldson D, Spirito A, et al. Personality characteristics of adolescent suicide attempters. Child Psychiatry Hum Dev 2000;30(4):219–35.

13. Prinstein M, Boergers J, Spirito A, et al. Peer functioning, family dysfunction, and psychological symptoms in a risk factor model for adolescent inpatients' suicidal ideation severity. J Clin Child Psychol 2000;29(3):392–405.

14. Wagner B, Silverman M, Ce M. Family factors in youth suicidal behaviors. Am Behav Sci 2003;46:1171–91.

15. Esposito-Smythers C, Spirito A. Adolescent substance use and suicidal behavior: a review with implications for treatment research. Alcohol Clin Exp Res 2004; 28(Suppl 5):77S–88S.

16. Guertin T, Lloyd-Richardson E, Spirito A, et al. Self-mutilative behavior in adolescents who attempt suicide by overdose. J Am Acad Child Adolesc Psychiatry 2001;40(9):1062–9.

17. Joiner TE. Why people die by suicide. Cambridge (MA): Harvard University Press; 2005.

18. Beck A. Beyond belief: a theory of modes, personality, and psychopathology. In: Salkovskis P, editor. Frontiers of cognitive therapy. New York: Guilford Press; 1996. p. 1–25.

19. Kazdin A, Weisz J. Identifying and developing empirically supported child and adolescent treatments. J Consult Clin Psychol 1998;66(1):19–36.

20. Curry J. Specific psychotherapies for childhood and adolescent depression. Biol Psychiatry 2001;49(12):1091–100.

21. Kaslow N, Thompson M. Applying the criteria for empirically supported treatments to studies of psychosocial interventions for child and adolescent depression. J Clin Child Psychol 1998;27(2):146–55.

22. Lewinsohn P, Clarke G. Psychosocial treatments for adolescent depression. Clin Psychol Rev 1999;19(3):329–42.

23. Reinecke M, Ryan N, DuBois D. Cognitive-behavioral therapy of depression and depressive symptoms during adolescence: a review and meta-analysis. J Am Acad Child Adolesc Psychiatry 1998;37(1):26–34.

24. Weisz J, McCarty C, Valeri S. Effects of psychotherapy for depression in children and adolescents: a meta-analysis. Psychol Bull 2006;132(1):132–49.
25. Klein J, Jacobs R, Reinecke M. Cognitive-behavioral therapy for adolescent depression: a meta-analytic investigation of changes in effect-size estimates. J Am Acad Child Adolesc Psychiatry 2007;46(11):1403–13.
26. David-Ferdon C, Kaslow N. Evidence-based psychosocial treatments for child and adolescent depression. J Clin Child Adolesc Psychol 2008;37(1): 62–104.
27. March J, Silva S, Petrycki S, et al. Fluoxetine, cognitive-behavioral therapy, and their combination for adolescents with depression: treatment for Adolescents with Depression Study (TADS) randomized controlled trial. JAMA 2004;292(7): 807–20.
28. March J, Silva S, Petrycki S, et al. The Treatment for Adolescents with Depression Study (TADS): long-term effectiveness and safety outcomes. Arch Gen Psychiatry 2007;64(10):1132–43.
29. Brent D, Emslie G, Clarke G, et al. Switching to another SSRI or to venlafaxine with or without cognitive behavioral therapy for adolescents with SSRI-resistant depression: the TORDIA randomized controlled trial. JAMA 2008;299(8):901–13.
30. Goodyer I, Dubicka B, Wilkinson P, et al. Selective serotonin reuptake inhibitors (SSRIs) and routine specialist care with and without cognitive behaviour therapy in adolescents with major depression: randomised controlled trial. BMJ 2007; 335(7611):142.
31. Kennard B, Emslie G, Mayes T, et al. Cognitive-behavioral therapy to prevent relapse in pediatric responders to pharmacotherapy for major depressive disorder. J Am Acad Child Adolesc Psychiatry 2008;47(12):1395–404.
32. Brent D, Holder D, Kolko D, et al. A clinical psychotherapy trial for adolescent depression comparing cognitive, family, and supportive therapy. Arch Gen Psychiatry 1997;54(9):877–85.
33. Clarke G, Hornbrook M, Lynch F, et al. Group cognitive-behavioral treatment for depressed adolescent offspring of depressed parents in a health maintenance organization. J Am Acad Child Adolesc Psychiatry 2002;41(3):305–13.
34. Melvin G, Tonge B, King N, et al. A comparison of cognitive-behavioral therapy, sertraline, and their combination for adolescent depression. J Am Acad Child Adolesc Psychiatry 2006;45(10):1151–61.
35. Riggs P, Mikulich-Gilbertson S, Davies R, et al. A randomized controlled trial of fluoxetine and cognitive behavioral therapy in adolescents with major depression, behavior problems, and substance use disorders. Arch Pediatr Adolesc Med 2007;161(11):1026–34.
36. Rohde P, Clarke G, Mace D, et al. An efficacy/effectiveness study of cognitive-behavioral treatment for adolescents with comorbid major depression and conduct disorder. J Am Acad Child Adolesc Psychiatry 2004;43(6):660–8.
37. Rudd MD. The assessment and management of suicidality. Sarasota (FL): Professional Resource; 2006.
38. Rathus J, Miller A. Dialectical behavior therapy adapted for suicidal adolescents. Suicide Life Threat Behav 2002;32(2):146–57.
39. Donaldson D, Spirito A, Esposito-Smythers C. Treatment for adolescents following a suicide attempt: results of a pilot trial. J Am Acad Child Adolesc Psychiatry 2005;44(2):113–20.
40. Brent D, Greenhill L, Compton S, et al. The Treatment of Adolescent Suicide Attempters Study (TASA): predictors of suicidal events in an open treatment trial. J Am Acad Child Adolesc Psychiatry 2009;48(10):987–96.

41. Spirito A, Esposito C. Evidence-based therapies for adolescent suicidal behavior. In: Steele R, Elkin D, Roberts M, editors. Handbook of evidence-based therapies for children and adolescents. New York: Springer; 2008. p. 177–96.
42. Freeman A, Reinecke M. Cognitive therapy for suicidal behavior. New York: Springer; 1993.
43. Spirito A, Esposito C. Individual therapy techniques with adolescent suicide attempters. In: Wasserman D, Wasserman C, editors. Oxford textbook of suicidology and suicide prevention. New York: Oxford; 2009. p. 677–84.
44. Ellis A. The revised ABC's of rational-emotive therapy (RET). J Ration Emot Cogn Behav Ther 1991;9(3):139–72.
45. McClung T. Rational emotive therapy adapted for adolescent psychiatric inpatients [unpublished manual]. West Virginia University School of Medicine; 2000.
46. Overholser JC. Elements of the Socratic method: I. systematic questioning. Psychotherapy 1993;30:67–74.
47. Beck AT, Rush AJ, Shaw BF, et al. Cognitive therapy of depression. New York: Guilford Press; 1979.
48. Donaldson D, Spirito A, Overholser J. Treatment of adolescent suicide attempters. In: Spirito A, Overholser J, editors. Evaluating and treating adolescent suicide attempters: from research to practice. San Diego (CA): Academic Press; 2003. p. 295–321.
49. Schneidman E. The definition of suicide. New York: John Wiley & Sons; 1985.
50. Linehan M. Cognitive behavior therapy of borderline personality disorder. New York: Guilford Press; 1993.
51. Rotheram-Borus M, Piacentini J, Miller S, et al. Brief cognitive-behavioral treatment for adolescent suicide attempters and their families. J Am Acad Child Adolesc Psychiatry 1994;33(4):508–17.
52. Powers S, Spirito A. Relaxation training. In: Noshpitz JD, Alessi NE, Coyle JT, et al, editors. Basic psychiatric science and treatment. New York: John Wiley & Sons; 1998. p. 411–7.
53. Feindler E, Ecton R. Adolescent anger control: cognitive-behavioral techniques. New York: Pergamon Press; 1986.

Dialectical Behavior Therapy for Suicidal Adolescents with Borderline Personality Disorder

Dena A. Klein, PhD*, Alec L. Miller, PsyD

KEYWORDS

- Adolescents • Suicidal • Dialectical behavior therapy
- Borderline personality disorder

Dialectical behavior therapy (DBT) was first adapted for use with multiproblem suicidal adolescents more than a decade ago in response to a dearth of empirically supported psychosocial treatments for this population.[1] Miller and colleagues[1,2] retained the core principles and strategies of Linehan's[3] original DBT for suicidal women with borderline personality disorder (BPD), and made modifications based on developmental and contextual considerations for adolescents and their families. Although research to date on DBT for adolescents has its limitations, growing evidence suggests that DBT is a promising treatment for adolescents with a range of problematic behaviors, including but not limited to suicidal and nonsuicidal self-injury.[4] The purpose of this article is to introduce dialectical behavior therapy's theoretical underpinnings, to describe its adaptation for suicidal adolescents, and to provide a brief review of the empirical literature evaluating DBT with adolescents.

DEVELOPMENT OF DIALECTICAL BEHAVIOR THERAPY FOR ADULTS
Theoretical Underpinnings

The theoretical influences of DBT include behavioral science, dialectical philosophy, Eastern contemplative practice, and the biosocial theory of personality functioning.[3] It began as an application of standard behavioral therapy for the treatment of chronically suicidal women diagnosed with BPD. These patients lacked the requisite skills for coping with life problems and considered suicide their best solution. However, in

The authors have nothing to disclose.
Child Outpatient Psychiatry Department, Montefiore Medical Center/Albert Einstein College of Medicine, 3340 Bainbridge Avenue, Bronx, NY 10467, USA
* Corresponding author.
E-mail address: dklein@montefiore.org

Child Adolesc Psychiatric Clin N Am 20 (2011) 205–216
doi:10.1016/j.chc.2011.01.001
1056-4993/11/$ – see front matter © 2011 Elsevier Inc. All rights reserved.

the process of developing the treatment, it became evident to Linehan[3] that a focus solely on change was too emotionally dysregulating for patients who were exquisitely emotionally sensitive and reactive. These patients felt as though the therapist did not understand how difficult it was for them to change their thinking and behavior. Yet, relinquishing the emphasis on change and becoming exclusively acceptance oriented was equally problematic because it often resulted in patients feeling that the therapist was not taking their pain seriously or, even worse, was thinking that they were too dysfunctional to be able to change. These clinical observations led to Linehan's discovery that by flexibly balancing and synthesizing acceptance (Eastern contemplative practice) *and* change (cognitive-behavioral strategies) in her therapeutic interactions, her suicidal patients felt better understood (validated/accepted) while also recognizing the need for them to change their own behavior. It is this synthesis of acceptance and change that is most fundamental to DBT and led to its description as dialectical behavior therapy. Dialectical refers to the notion that there is no absolute truth and that seemingly opposite constructs can both be true at the same time (eg, you are doing the best you can in the moment *and* you need to do better, try harder, and be more motivated to change). DBT therapists teach their patients to move away from either-or thinking to both-and ways of thinking to reduce thinking processes and behaviors becoming polarized.

At its core, DBT shares the same underlying assumptions as other behavioral treatments.[3] A fundamental assumption of behavioral treatments is that the causes or maintaining conditions of behavior exist in the current environment. Hence, DBT focuses on current rather than historical determinants of behavior and relies on ongoing behavioral assessment and data collection. Target behavior is specifically defined, treated, and measured. In DBT, cognitive and behavioral interventions serve as the technology of change and focus on the alteration of learned, maladaptive emotional, cognitive, and behavioral sequences. Even more than other behavioral approaches, DBT relies on collaboration between patients and therapist and emphasizes the importance of the working therapeutic relationship. As a behavioral science, DBT is informed by basic research in psychology and is described in objective terms so that replication is possible.

Dialectical philosophy is also central to DBT.[3] First, it provides a philosophic position on the fundamental nature of reality that serves as the basis for DBT. According to the dialectical perspective, reality is an interrelated system comprised of internal opposing forces that are in a continuous state of change because of the inherent tensions (polarities) of reality. The dialectical worldview assumes there is no absolute truth or indisputable fact and posits that the synthesis (or balance) of seemingly opposite positions produces wisdom and new meaning. The core dialectic in DBT is accepting patients where they are in the moment *and* working to help them change. Second, dialectical philosophy provides a framework for therapeutic interactions and interventions so that therapeutic movement can occur. Dialectical strategies elicit change by persuasion and by making use of the opposites inherent in the therapeutic relationship. They include strategies for balancing the dialectical tensions inherent in the therapeutic relationship, including change and acceptance, flexibility and stability, challenging and nurturing, and deficits and capabilities. They also include instruction for reducing behavioral extremes (ie, cognitive, emotional, and behavioral patterns) and moving toward more dialectical (ie, balanced) ways of thinking and acting. Lastly, dialectic strategies include methods for highlighting contradictions in patients' behavior and thinking by offering opposite or alternative positions (eg, entering the paradox, using metaphor, and playing devil's advocate). It is the application of these treatment strategies that produces the movement, speed, and flow characteristic of DBT.

The emphasis on acceptance as a balance to change is largely derived from Eastern (Zen) contemplative practice.[3] DBT tenets of observing, mindfulness, and avoidance of judgment flow directly from Zen meditative practice. Linehan[3] translated mindfulness practice into behavioral skills that could be taught to patients to increase self-awareness and to increase self-acceptance as well as to accept the world as it is in the moment. In contrast to cognitive and behavioral interventions, this mindfulness training and practice is part of dialectical behavior therapy's technology of acceptance.

DBT is also based on Linehan's[3] biosocial theory of personality functioning. According to this theory, BPD is primarily a dysfunction of the emotional regulation system resulting from the transaction between a biologically emotionally vulnerable individual and an environment that is a poor fit with this vulnerability (ie, invalidating). Emotional vulnerability refers to high emotional sensitivity (ie, low threshold for having an emotional reaction) and reactivity (ie, intense emotional reactions), and a slow return to emotional baseline. An invalidating environment refers to environments that communicate to individuals that their inner and outer experiences (emotional, behavioral, and cognitive) are incorrect, inaccurate, or inappropriate. An environment, which may include parents, siblings, teachers, coaches, therapists, and others, may begin as invalidating or transform over time in response to stress from the emotionally sensitive individual. In the context of the biosocial theory, dysfunctional behaviors characteristic of BPD are conceptualized as maladaptive solutions to overwhelming and intensely painful negative affect. The biosocial theory promotes empathic interpretations of patient behavior, validates individual and family experiences, and can increase commitment and treatment engagement when used as psychoeducation. Importantly, the biosocial model provides support for conceptually driven treatment interventions aimed at skill acquisition to modulate extreme emotional experiences, reduce emotional vulnerability, and reduce maladaptive mood dependent behaviors, while increasing validation of self and others' emotions, thoughts, and behaviors.

Empirical Support

DBT is the only evidence-based outpatient treatment for chronically suicidal adults diagnosed with BPD.[5] Numerous randomized controlled trials have found DBT to be superior to treatment as usual (TAU) for problems associated with BPD.[6-11] When compared with TAU, DBT participants have demonstrated greater improvements in treatment-adherence rates, reductions in the frequency and length of inpatient psychiatric hospitalization, and reductions in the frequency and severity of suicide attempts, nonsuicidal self-injury, and suicidal ideation.[6-8,10-13] DBT for adults has been widely disseminated to multiple therapeutic settings and applied to a variety of diagnoses. Research suggests that DBT can be conducted with various adult populations, including outpatient,[7-11] inpatient,[6,12,14-17] and forensic.[18-20] Research has also expanded and diversified to included adaptations of DBT for adults with comorbid BPD and substance abuse problems,[10,16,21] comorbid BPD and eating disorders,[22] eating disorders,[23,24] and geriatric outpatients with depression and mixed personality features.[13,25] For a comprehensive review of clinical outcome studies, see Lynch, Trost, Salsman, and Linehan.[5]

ADAPTATION OF DIALECTICAL BEHAVIOR THERAPY FOR ADOLESCENTS

Miller and colleagues[1,2] first adapted DBT for use with suicidal adolescents in response to an absence of empirically supported psychosocial treatments for youth. At the time, DBT was the only established treatment for chronically suicidal individuals.

Several evaluations of DBT included older adolescents, but no clinical trials examined outcomes for adolescents specifically.[2] Although the diagnosis of BPD in adolescents is controversial, growing evidence suggests that it could be validly and reliably diagnosed in adolescents.[26] Moreover, there is significant overlap between adolescent suicidal behaviors and the behavioral criteria for BPD.[2] Hence, DBT was adapted for use with multiproblem suicidal adolescents based on promising indicators and in the absence of suitable alternatives, suggesting that this treatment is appropriate for this emotionally dysregulated and impulsive population.

Treatment Modifications

In adapting DBT for adolescents, Miller and colleagues[1,2] retained the core tenets and modes of treatment of DBT while making several changes to the treatment based on developmental and contextual considerations. First, treatment length was decreased from 12 months to 16 weeks based on the rationale that teens may not require the same length of treatment as adults with BPD and may be more likely to commit to a shorter treatment. Second, family members were included in the weekly skills-training groups to enhance generalization and maintenance of skills. Teaching skills to family members helps them act as coaches to the adolescents and may improve potentially invalidating home environments. Third, offering intersession skills coaching to family members who attend the skills group was also added to foster their skills generalization. Fourth, family sessions were added to the treatment program to address any paramount familial issues. Fifth, the number of skills taught was reduced to facilitate learning the content within a shorter period of time. Sixth, age-appropriate terminology was incorporated to make skills handouts more developmentally appropriate. Lastly, a fifth skills-training module, Walking the Middle Path, was added to help adolescents and their families develop the skills needed to overcome polarized ways of thinking, feeling, and interacting, including the addition of validation skills, behavioral principles, and a set of adolescent-family–specific dialectical dilemmas and corresponding secondary treatment targets.

Treatment Modes and Stages

DBT for adolescents is a comprehensive, multimodal intervention that uses individual psychotherapy, multifamily skills-training groups, family therapy, telephone coaching for patients and family members, and therapist consultation meetings to address both suicide risk factors and the multitude of other problems simultaneously.[2] Like DBT for suicidal adults, DBT with adolescents relies on a collaborative, nonjudgmental approach to improve patient motivation to change, enhance patient capabilities, promote generalization of new behaviors, structure the environment, and enhance therapist capability and motivation. During phase I, adolescents commit to 16 weeks of twice-weekly therapy, which includes participation in all 5 treatment modes (described in greater detail later). This phase focuses on increasing safety and establishing behavioral control. Once completed, adolescents participate in phase II of treatment, which consists of 1 (or more) 16-week treatment course focused on maintenance and generalization. During this phase, patients participate in the Graduate Group, telephone consultation and family therapy as needed. Individual therapy may also continue during this phase with the goal of fading it out over time.

Treatment modes

The 5 treatment modes that comprise DBT for adolescents include individual therapy, multifamily skills-training groups, family therapy, telephone consultation, and therapist consultation meetings.[2] The individual therapist is the primary therapist and is responsible for increasing the adolescent's motivation, inhibiting maladaptive behaviors, increasing the adolescent's skillful behaviors, and generalizing newly acquired skillful behaviors outside the therapy setting. The individual therapist organizes other treatment modes to address all problem areas. Patients participate in weekly 50- to 60-minute individual therapy sessions, which may be held more often during crisis periods or at the beginning of treatment. Similar to other behavioral treatments, individual sessions typically begin with the following sequence of strategies: (1) greeting the client, (2) reviewing the diary card, (3) setting the session agenda, (4) assessing patients' current emotional state, (5) reviewing individual therapy homework assignments (if given), and (6) checking progress in other modes of therapy. The bulk of the individual therapy is conducting behavioral chain and solution analyses of patients' target behaviors. DBT therapists balance a benevolently demanding style with compassionate flexibility, irreverence with warmth, and weave in dialectical strategies to keep patients slightly off balance. This fosters movement, speed, and flow in order for the therapy to not become plodding or for patients and the therapist to become polarized.

The function of skills training is to help patients (and families) acquire, strengthen, and generalize new sets of behavioral skills. Whenever possible, skills training is conducted in a multifamily group format and follows the same didactic behavioral format as outlined in Linehan's[27] *Skills Training Manual for Treating Borderline Personality Disorder*. Five sets of skills are covered in the multifamily skills group: core mindfulness, interpersonal effectiveness, emotion regulation, distress tolerance, and Walking the Middle Path. Each skills module includes didactic presentation of skills, role plays, and other experiential components, and review of homework exercises. DBT skills trainers rely on all of the DBT principles and strategies when leading these groups. Validation, irreverence, principles of shaping, and dialectical strategies are just a few of the strategies used to help engage, teach, and elicit new behaviors from multiproblem youth and their families.

Additional family therapy sessions are conducted to address problems in the adolescent's primary support system. These sessions are conducted on an as-needed basis for the following reasons: when a family member provides a central source of conflict and an adolescent needs more intensive coaching or support to resolve this conflict, when a family crisis erupts that needs immediate attention, when treatment would be enhanced by educating/orienting a family member to a particular aspect of treatment, or when contingencies at home are too powerful to ignore and are reinforcing maladaptive behavior. Family members may attend as few as 3 or 4 sessions or as many as 12 to 14 during the first 16-week phase of treatment.

The primary therapist is responsible for providing telephone consultation on an as-needed basis to patients. The purpose of this treatment mode is to enable the therapist to provide in-vivo skills coaching to help generalize the new behavioral skills being learned in the group, to provide emergency crisis intervention, to enable patients to report good news, and to provide patients and the therapist with an opportunity to repair any ruptures in the therapeutic relationship.

Last, but not least, the therapist consultation meeting is integral to DBT and consists of weekly meetings attended by all DBT therapists. The goals of these meetings are (1) to enhance the therapists' capabilities by providing an ongoing educational component to ensure the highest level of care, and (2) to provide support to all of the DBT therapists (ie, therapy for the therapists). Given the high rates of burnout among therapists working with this high-risk population, the DBT consult team serves to prevent and protect therapists from such an unfortunate and counter-therapeutic result. Hence, DBT is a community of therapists treating a community of patients.

Treatment stages and targets

DBT is comprised of 4 treatment stages and an additional pretreatment stage, each of which matches the level of severity and complexity of the patients' problems.[2] Each stage includes a hierarchy of specific treatment targets (ie, behaviors to increase or decrease). The responsibility for meeting these behavioral targets is spread among the various treatment modes. The pretreatment stage aims to orient patients and their families to DBT; obtain their commitment to participate in treatment; and establish agreement on treatment goals, including the reduction of suicidal and nonsuicidal self-injurious behavior. Patients initiate treatment in this stage and return to it if their commitment or engagement declines.

Stage 1 of treatment, which has been the focus of treatment studies to date, aims to increase safety and establish behavioral control by addressing 4 primary behavioral targets that are prioritized in the following order: decreasing life-threatening behaviors, decreasing therapy-interfering behaviors, decreasing quality-of-life interfering behaviors, and increasing behavioral skills. During this treatment stage, the targets are addressed hierarchically and recursively as higher-priority behaviors reappear.

Within stage 1, life-threatening behaviors refer to suicide-related behaviors, including suicidal ideation, intention, plan, and nonsuicidal self-injury. These behaviors are addressed before all other treatment targets, based on the rationale that patients must be alive for therapy to be helpful. Therapy-interfering behaviors refer to behaviors that interfere with the patients (or other patients) receiving therapy (eg, problems with attendance, collaboration, and compliance) or behaviors that reduce the therapist's ability to be effective (eg, behaviors that reduce the therapist's motivation to treat or that punish effective therapist behaviors). These targets are addressed second, based on the rationale that it is impossible to address other targets if treatment is failing or is terminated prematurely. Therapy-interfering behaviors by patients, families, and therapists are monitored and addressed accordingly. Quality-of-life interfering behaviors include those behaviors that interfere with the patients building a life worth living and working toward long-term goals. These behaviors may be related to problems with relationships, school performance, impulsivity, substance use, physical health, and all Axis I and Axis II disorders. Collaboratively, the therapist and patients identify and prioritize quality-of-life interfering behavioral targets. In addition to reducing the aforementioned behavioral targets, Stage 1 simultaneously seeks to increase behavioral skills through patient participation in the multifamily skills-training group and individual therapy. The idea is to replace their old maladaptive behaviors (targets 1 and 2) with new behavioral skills.

Stages 2 through 4 are characterized by life patterns that are increasingly functional and stable. Stage 2 aims to decrease posttraumatic stress and emotionally process the past. Stage 3 focuses on increasing respect for self and achieving individual goals. Lastly, stage 4 aims to increase hedonic capacity by developing a sense of completeness and finding freedom and joy.

In addition to the primary behavioral targets specific to stage 1, secondary behavioral targets are addressed throughout all treatment stages.[2,3,28] They are functionally related to the primary target problems and are based on the extreme behavioral patterns characteristic of patients with BPD who are suicidal. Each pattern represents an aspect of the transaction between an emotionally vulnerable individual and his or her invalidating environment. Linehan[3] noted that over time, patients diagnosed with BPD learn to alternate between one extreme behavioral pattern that under-regulates their emotions and another that over-regulates their emotions. Vacillations between behavioral extremes, known as dialectical dilemmas, sustain patients' dysfunctional behaviors and are significant obstacles to therapeutic change. Among suicidal adolescents, Miller and colleagues[2] identified similar vacillations and developed a set of secondary treatment targets to assist adolescents and their parents to find a synthesis and walk the middle path to resolve many of the dialectical tensions inherent in their thoughts, feelings, and behaviors.[2] These dialectical dilemmas include (1) excessive leniency versus authoritarian control, (2) normalizing pathologic behaviors versus pathologizing normative behaviors, and (3) forcing autonomy versus fostering dependence. At each polar extreme, there are 2 secondary treatment targets: one aimed at increasing adaptive behavior and another aimed at decreasing maladaptive behavior (see Miller, Rathus, and Linehan[2] for an in-depth discussion).

Empirical Support

According to a recent literature review by Groves and colleagues,[4] 12 published studies have examined the effectiveness of DBT with adolescents using quasi-experimental and pre-post treatment designs. Although no randomized controlled trials have been published to date, 2 are in progress. Despite significant variability in populations, settings, structure, and format of treatment, the results of the review suggest that DBT is a promising treatment for adolescents with a range of problems, including suicidal and nonsuicidal self-injury and other problems associated with BPD, bipolar disorder, externalizing behavior problems, and eating disorders.

Several studies have examined the application of DBT for suicidal adolescents with features of BPD in outpatient settings. In 1 of the 2 published studies that used a quasi-experimental design, Rathus and Miller[29] compared depressed and suicidal adolescents treated with an adaptation of DBT to treatment as usual in a 12-week outpatient program. Despite more severe pretreatment symptomatology, the adolescents treated with DBT had significantly fewer psychiatric hospitalizations during the course of treatment (0% vs 13%) and significantly higher treatment completion rates (60% vs 38%). Within the DBT group, there were significant before-and-after reductions in suicidal ideation, general psychiatric symptoms, and symptoms of borderline personality. Similarly, several studies that evaluated pretreatment and posttreatment outcomes without randomization or control groups found that suicidal adolescents treated with DBT in outpatient settings exhibited significant improvements in general functioning[30] and reductions in depressive symptoms,[30–32] life threatening behaviors,[30–32] and number of psychiatric hospitalizations.[31] James and colleagues[30] found that adolescents maintained their posttreatment improvements 8 months later. Woodberry and Popenoe[32] found that improvements in depressive symptoms were not limited to adolescents but also experienced by caregivers, as evidenced by significant reductions in their scores on the Beck Depression Inventory.

Studies of DBT have also been conducted with suicidal adolescents in inpatient and residential treatment settings. In the second of 2 published studies that used a quasi-experimental design, Katz and colleagues[33] compared adolescents treated with DBT to TAU in a 2-week general child and adolescent psychiatric inpatient program. Compared with adolescents treated with TAU, those who received DBT demonstrated greater reductions in behavioral incidents (including nonsuicidal self-injury) and increases in treatment adherence (including medication compliance) during their inpatient stay. At 1-year follow-up, both groups displayed significant reductions in suicidal ideation, nonsuicidal self-injury, and depressive symptoms. Although the effect sizes at follow-up were greater for DBT than TAU for self-reported depressive symptoms and suicidal ideation, differences were not statistically significant. In an uncontrolled open trial of a comprehensive DBT program for multiproblem adolescent girls in a residential treatment facility, before-and-after results documented significant reductions in premature terminations caused by suicidality, the number of days spent in psychiatric hospitals because of self-injurious behaviors, and the length of time patients were held in restraints or seclusion.[34] Taken together, the aforementioned studies suggest that DBT may be an effective treatment for suicidal adolescents with borderline personality traits in outpatient, inpatient, and residential treatment settings.

DBT has also been expanded for use with adolescents diagnosed with bipolar disorder. Similar to BPD, bipolar disorder is associated with severe impairments in emotion regulation and impulse control. Goldstein and colleagues[35] conducted a 1-year open trial of DBT with 10 outpatient adolescents diagnosed with bipolar disorder, most of whom had a history of at least 1 suicide attempt and many of whom had intermittent suicidal ideation. The study's first author was the only DBT-trained clinic staff member and provider, and therefore a major limitation of the study is the absence of a consultation team. Nevertheless, results at posttreatment revealed a high rate of subject retention (ie, 90% completed treatment, with 1 subject moving away); significant reductions in suicidal ideation, emotion dysregulation, and depressive symptoms; and high subject-reported and parent-reported acceptability and satisfaction ratings. Although not statistically significant, nonsuicidal self-injury also decreased over the course of treatment. Additional research is needed to further evaluate the efficacy of this treatment for adolescents suffering from bipolar disorder.

Research suggests that DBT may also have utility for multiproblem adolescents who exhibit problems and symptoms other than those associated with BPD and mood disorders, including a range of externalizing behaviors. In one study, Trupin and colleagues[36] compared incarcerated female juvenile offenders treated by an intensely trained DBT team (ie, mental health unit) to those treated by a less intensely trained DBT team (ie, general population unit) and those who received treatment from clinicians with no DBT training (ie, TAU unit). Despite more severe pretreatment symptomatology, the teens in the mental health unit displayed significant reductions in aggression, classroom disruptions, and suicidal and nonsuicidal self-injury that exceeded the changes displayed by the other 2 units. In another study with less impaired adolescents, Nelson-Gray and colleagues[37] conducted a 16-week open trial of an outpatient DBT skills training group for nonsuicidal adolescents diagnosed with oppositional defiant disorder. The treatment was based on a modified version of Linehan's[27] skills-training manual that included financial incentives for homework compliance and used group therapy as the single treatment modality. Teens did not receive any individual therapy or telephone consultation. Posttreatment outcomes showed reductions in parent-rated externalizing behavior problems, oppositional defiant disorder symptoms, and depressive symptoms along with increases in positive behaviors, suggesting that the more comprehensive outpatient DBT model may not be necessary for this population of adolescents.

Lastly, several studies have examined the application of DBT for adolescents with eating disorders.[23,38,39] Two studies used modified versions of Miller and colleagues'[2] DBT treatment model for adolescents diagnosed with anorexia nervosa or bulimia nervosa. One study was conducted in an inpatient setting[39] and the other was conducted in an outpatient setting.[38] Results showed significant posttreatment improvements in eating-disorder symptoms,[38,39] general psychopathology,[38,39] and body mass index scores.[39] Promising results were also reported from a single case study of a 16-year-old adolescent with binge eating disorder.[23] The investigators used a modified version of DBT for binge eating in adults[24] based on the premise that binge eating is a behavioral attempt to modify painful emotional states. Reductions in the frequency and severity of binge eating were reported after treatment.

SUMMARY AND FUTURE DIRECTIONS

DBT with suicidal adolescents diagnosed with borderline personality disorder is a compassionate and promising multimodal treatment approach. Intensive training and supervision is critical if therapists intend to apply this comprehensive treatment to this high-risk population. Although many clinicians hesitate to apply a diagnosis of BPD to adolescents because of insufficient assessment, stigma, and reimbursement concerns, to name a few, the authors think it is imperative for clinicians to rethink this approach. Not applying the diagnosis or at least classifying the adolescent as having features of BPD when appropriate may result in the adolescent receiving inappropriate or insufficient treatment and may lead this individual down a less-effective treatment pathway.

To date, clinical research on the application of DBT with adolescents suggests that DBT may be an effective treatment for suicidal adolescents with borderline personality disorder features. Outpatient and inpatient applications for suicidal youth have been associated with reductions in suicidal and nonsuicidal self-injury, psychiatric hospitalizations, and other problem areas associated borderline personality disorder. Furthermore, preliminary findings suggest that it is a well-tolerated treatment with high-acceptability ratings and treatment retention rates, which is particularly compelling given the high rates of treatment dropout among suicidal teens.[40] Expansions of DBT to the treatment of bipolar disorder, externalizing behavior problems, and eating disorders suggest that DBT may improve functioning and reduce psychopathology across a range of problem areas and treatment settings. However, it is important to note that numerous methodological shortcomings across the aforementioned studies limit the conclusions that can be drawn about DBT.[4] Specifically, all the aforementioned studies lack randomization and it is difficult to compare findings across studies because there is significant variability in populations, settings, structure and format of treatment, and outcome measures. No other psychosocial interventions for suicidal adolescents diagnosed with BPD have been empirically evaluated and published. The authors strongly encourage researchers to develop and conduct randomized controlled trials of various psychosocial interventions for this challenging multiproblem patient population. We may discover that although DBT is effective for some patients, a different therapeutic approach may be more effective for others. In addition, component analyses may also prove useful to determine which specific DBT treatment modes (eg, skills training, individual therapy, intersession telephone coaching) are necessary and sufficient to obtain the desired therapeutic affects. Finally, researchers must employ treatment adherence and coding measures to ensure treatment fidelity.

REFERENCES

1. Miller AL, Rathus JH, Linehan MM, et al. Dialectical behavior therapy adapted for suicidal adolescents. Journal of Practical Psychiatry & Behavioral Health 1997; 3(2):67–95.
2. Miller AL, Rathus JH, Linehan MM. Dialectical behavior therapy with suicidal adolescents. New York (NY): Guilford Publications; 2007.
3. Linehan MM. Cognitive-behavioral treatment of borderline personality disorder. New York: Guilford Press; 1993.
4. Groves SS, Miller AL, Backer HS, et al. Dialectical behavior therapy with adolescents: a review. Child Adolesc Ment Health, in press.
5. Lynch TR, Trost WT, Salsman N, et al. Dialectical behavior therapy for borderline personality disorder. Annu Rev Clin Psychol 2007;3:181–205.

6. Koons CR, Robins CJ, Tweed JL, et al. Efficacy of dialectical behavior therapy in women veterans with borderline personality disorder. Behav Ther 2001;32(2): 371–90.

7. Linehan MM, Armstrong HE, Suarez A, et al. Cognitive-behavioral treatment of chronically parasuicidal borderline patients. Arch Gen Psychiatry 1991;48(12): 1060–4.

8. Linehan MM, Comtois KA, Murray AM, et al. Two-year randomized controlled trial and follow-up of dialectical behavior therapy vs therapy by experts for suicidal behaviors and borderline personality disorder. Arch Gen Psychiatry 2006;63(7): 757–66.

9. Linehan MM, Heard HL, Armstrong HE. Naturalistic follow-up of a behavioral treatment for chronically parasuicidal borderline patients. Arch Gen Psychiatry 1993;50(12):971–4.

10. van den Bosch LM, Koeter MW, Stijnen T, et al. Sustained efficacy of dialectical behaviour therapy for borderline personality disorder. Behav Res Ther 2005; 43(9):1231–41.

11. Verheul R, van den Bosch LM, Koeter MW, et al. Dialectical behaviour therapy for women with borderline personality disorder: 12-month, randomised clinical trial in The Netherlands. Br J Psychiatry 2003;182(2):135–40.

12. Bohus M, Haaf B, Simms T, et al. Effectiveness of inpatient dialectical behavioral therapy for borderline personality disorder: a controlled trial. Behav Res Ther 2004;42(5):487–99.

13. Lynch TR, Morse JQ, Mendelson T, et al. Dialectical behavior therapy for depressed older adults: a randomized pilot study. Am J Geriatr Psychiatry 2003;11(1):33–45.

14. Barley WD, Buie SE, Peterson EW, et al. Development of an inpatient cognitive-behavioral treatment program for borderline personality disorder. J Pers Disord 1993;7(3):232–40.

15. Bohus M, Haaf B, Stiglmayr C, et al. Evaluation of inpatient dialectical-behavioral therapy for borderline personality disorder–a prospective study. Behav Res Ther 2000;38(9):875–87.

16. Linehan MM, Schmidt H III, Dimeff LA, et al. Dialectical behavior therapy for patients with borderline personality disorder and drug-dependence. Am J Addict 1999;8(4):279–92.

17. Simpson EB, Pistorello J, Begin A, et al. Use of dialectical behavior therapy in a partial hospital program for women with borderline personality disorder. Psychiatr Serv 1998;49(5):669–73.

18. Berzins LG, Trestman RL. The development and implementation of dialectical behavior therapy in forensic settings. The International Journal of Forensic Mental Health 2004;3(1):93–103.

19. Evershed S, Tennant A, Boomer D, et al. Practice-based outcomes of dialectical behaviour therapy (DBT) targeting anger and violence, with male forensic patients: a pragmatic and non-contemporaneous comparison. Crim Behav Ment Health 2003;13(3):198–213.

20. Bradley RG, Follingstad DR. Group therapy for incarcerated women who experienced interpersonal violence: a pilot study. J Trauma Stress 2003;16(4): 337–40.

21. Linehan MM, Dimeff LA, Reynolds SK, et al. Dialectal behavior therapy versus comprehensive validation therapy plus 12-step for the treatment of opioid dependent women meeting criteria for borderline personality disorder. Drug Alcohol Depend 2002;67(1):13–26.

22. Palmer RL, Birchall H, Damani S, et al. A dialectical behavior therapy program for people with an eating disorder and borderline personality disorder-description and outcome. Int J Eat Disord 2003;33(3):281–6.
23. Safer DL, Lock J, Couturier JL. Dialectical behavior therapy modified for adolescent binge eating disorder: a case report. Cognit Behav Pract 2007;14(2): 157–67.
24. Telch CF, Agras WS, Linehan MM. Dialectical behavior therapy for binge eating disorder. J Consult Clin Psychol 2001;69(6):1061–5.
25. Lynch TR. Treatment of elderly depression with personality disorder comorbidity using dialectical behavior therapy. Cognit Behav Pract 2000;7(4):468–77.
26. Miller AL, Muehlenkamp JJ, Jacobson CM. Fact or fiction: diagnosing borderline personality disorder in adolescents. Clin Psychol Rev 2008;28(6):969–81.
27. Linehan MM. Skills training manual for treating borderline personality disorder. New York: Guilford Press; 1993.
28. Rathus JH, Miller AL. DBT for adolescents: dialectical dilemmas and secondary treatment targets. Cognit Behav Pract 2000;7(4):425–34.
29. Rathus JH, Miller AL. Dialectical behavior therapy adapted for suicidal adolescents. Suicide Life Threat Behav 2002;32(2):146–57.
30. James AC, Taylor A, Winmill L, et al. A preliminary community study of dialectical behaviour therapy (DBT) with adolescent females demonstrating persistent, deliberate self-harm (DSH). Child Adolesc Ment Health 2008;13(3):148–52.
31. Fleischhaker C, Munz M, Böhme R, et al. Dialektisch-behaviorale therapie für adoleszente (DBT-A)–eine pilotstudie zur therapie von suizidalität, parasuizidalität und selbstverletzenden verhaltensweisen bei patientinnen mit symptomen einer borderlinestörung [Dialectical behaviour therapy for adolescents (DBT-A)–A pilot study on the therapy of suicidal, parasuicidal, and self-injurious behaviour in female patients with a borderline disorder]. Z Kinder Jugendpsychiatr Psychother 2006;34(1):15–27 [in German].
32. Woodberry KA, Popenoe EJ. Implementing dialectical behavior therapy with adolescents and their families in a community outpatient clinic. Cognit Behav Pract 2008;15(3):277–86.
33. Katz LY, Cox BJ, Gunasekara S, et al. Feasibility of dialectical behavior therapy for suicidal adolescent inpatients. J Am Acad Child Adolesc Psychiatry 2004; 43(3):276–82.
34. Sunseri PA. Preliminary outcomes on the use of dialectical behavior therapy to reduce hospitalization among adolescents in residential care. Residential Treatment for Children & Youth 2004;21(4):59–76.
35. Goldstein TR, Axelson DA, Birmaher B, et al. Dialectical behavior therapy for adolescents with bipolar disorder: a 1-years open trial. J Am Acad Child Adolesc Psychiatry 2007;46(7):820–30.
36. Trupin EW, Stewart DG, Beach B, et al. Effectiveness of dialectical behaviour therapy program for incarcerated female juvenile offenders. Child Adolesc Ment Health 2002;7(3):121–7.
37. Nelson-Gray RO, Keane SP, Hurst RM, et al. A modified DBT skills training program for oppositional defiant adolescents: promising preliminary findings. Behav Res Ther 2006;44(12):1811–20.
38. Salbach-Andrae H, Bohnekamp I, Pfeiffer E, et al. Dialectical behavior therapy of anorexia and bulimia nervosa among adolescents: a case series. Cognit Behav Pract 2008;15(4):415–25.
39. Salbach H, Klinkowski N, Pfeiffer E, et al. Dialektisch-behaviorale Therapie für jugendliche Patientinnen mit Anorexia und Bulimia nervosa (DBT-AN/BN) – eine

pilotstudie [Dialectical behavior therapy for adolescents with anorexia and bulimia nervosa (DBT-AN/BN) – a pilot study]. Prax Kinderpsychol Kinderpsychiatr 2007;56(2):91–108 [in German].

40. Spirito A, Boergers J, Donaldson D, et al. An intervention trial to improve adherence to community treatment by adolescents after a suicide attempt. J Am Acad Child Adolesc Psychiatry 2002;41(4):435–42.

Cognitive-Behavioral Therapy for Anxiety Disorders in Youth

Laura D. Seligman, PhD[a],*, Thomas H. Ollendick, PhD[b,c]

KEYWORDS

• Anxiety • Cognitive therapy • Behavioral therapy
• Children • Adolescents

Epidemiologic studies suggest that anxiety disorders are the most frequently diagnosed class of disorders in children and adolescents and that most people who develop an anxiety disorder do so by late adolescence or early adulthood.[1,2] Although some fears and anxiety can be adaptive and developmentally appropriate,[3] clinical levels of fear and anxiety can engender significant distress in children and their families and are likely to interfere with academic and social functioning.[4–6] Moreover, the high prevalence of anxiety disorders coupled with the negative effects on functioning results in a significant economic burden on society.[7]

According to the *Diagnostic and Statistical Manual of Mental Disorders (DSM), Fourth Edition, Text Revision*,[8] children and adolescents can be diagnosed with 12 different anxiety disorders: separation anxiety disorder, panic disorder with or without agoraphobia, agoraphobia without a history of panic disorder, specific phobias, social phobia, obsessive-compulsive disorder, posttraumatic stress disorder, acute stress disorder, generalized anxiety disorder, anxiety disorder due to a medical condition, substance-induced anxiety disorder, and an anxiety disorder not otherwise specified. Although decisions regarding the status of anxiety disorders in DSM-V have not been finalized, it seems that only a few changes are proposed for the updated diagnostic manual planned for publication in 2013. Specifically, changes under consideration include specific criteria for posttraumatic stress disorder in preschool children, removal of agoraphobia without a history of panic disorder, and movement of separation anxiety disorder from "Disorders Usually First Diagnosed in Infancy, Childhood, or Adolescence" to the "Anxiety Disorders" section of the DSM.[9]

The authors have nothing to disclose. This review was funded in part by the National Institute of Mental Health Grant R01 074777 to Thomas H. Ollendick (PI).
[a] Department of Psychology, University of Toledo, Toledo, OH 43606, USA
[b] Department of Psychology, Virginia Polytechnic Institute and State University, Blacksburg, VA 24060, USA
[c] Department of Psychology, Child Study Center, Virginia Polytechnic Institute and State University, 460 Turner Street, Suite 207, Blacksburg, VA 24060, USA
* Corresponding author.
E-mail address: laura.seligman@utoledo.edu

Comorbidity is the rule rather than the exception in the clinical presentation of anxiety disorders. Epidemiologic and clinical studies show that in about 75% of cases youth are diagnosed with multiple anxiety disorders and about 50% to 60% of children and adolescents diagnosed with an anxiety disorder evidence a comorbid affective disorder.[10,11] Comorbidity of anxiety disorders with disruptive behavior disorders is also common, with some estimates suggesting that between 25% and 33% of youth diagnosed with an anxiety disorder will evidence a comorbid externalizing disorder.[12] Therefore the treatment of anxiety disorders in youth must necessarily take into account the presence of comorbid conditions. Interestingly, however, comorbidity does not seem to predict treatment outcome,[13] suggesting that cognitive-behavior therapy (CBT) for anxiety disorders can be effective regardless of the presence of comorbid conditions. Presentations of somatic complaints in anxious youth, particularly stomach complaints in younger children and headache in older children and adolescents, is common.[14]

HISTORY OF CBT FOR ANXIETY DISORDERS IN CHILDHOOD

Like CBT for anxiety disorders in adults, CBT for childhood anxiety disorders emerged from two areas of experimental psychology—learning theory and cognitive psychology. Mary Cover Jones, one of J.B. Watson's students, was among the first to apply behavioral principles to the treatment of childhood anxiety. More specifically, Jones used modeling and exposure to treat childhood fears and phobias. Although these types of treatments were considered controversial at first, by the 1960s and 1970s recognition of their success was growing and behavioral treatments became widely accepted. Also, around this time, significant developments in the clinical application of social learning theory and cognitive theory by Bandura and Beck led to an integration of cognitive and behavioral treatments.

Two pioneering books were among the first to recognize the importance of these approaches. First, Donald Meichenbaum's *Cognitive-Behavior Modification*,[15] discussed CBT for the treatment of anxiety; soon after, Ollendick and Cerny published *Clinical Behavior Therapy with Children*.[16] Today, there is a growing literature on the use of CBT for the treatment of anxiety disorders in youth and, although questions and controversies remain—including the comparative and combined efficacy of CBT and other available treatments and the active "ingredients" or mediators of CBT—CBT is used in a variety of settings including schools, outpatient clinics, inpatient or partial-hospitalization programs, and primary care practices. Moreover, research suggests that these treatments can be effective in significantly ameliorating the distress suffered by children with anxiety disorders.

EVIDENCE OF EFFICACY AND EFFECTIVENESS

Over 40 studies have been conducted to examine CBT for anxiety disorders and anxiety symptoms in youth and, taken together, these studies provide the empirical support necessary to make CBT the only psychological treatment identified to date as an evidence-based treatment **Table 1**.[17,18] contains a list of these studies. Effect sizes from randomized controlled trials are generally large,[19] and posttreatment assessments suggest that approximately two out of three children treated with CBT can expect to be free of their primary diagnosis with a course of treatment that usually lasts between 12 and 16 weeks. Maintenance of treatment gains, and in some cases, further improvement, can seen in studies that follow treated youth up to nine years posttreatment.[20] Moreover, as indicated previously, CBT for anxiety disorders in youth appears to efficacious even in the presence of comorbid conditions[13,21] and across different ethnic and cultural groups.[22–24] Although more work is needed to test the effectiveness or generalizability of CBT for youth with anxiety disorders, available evidence suggests the potential transportability of these treatments from the laboratory to a wide variety of clinical settings with little detriment to the size of treatment effects.[19,25]

CORE PROCEDURES IN THE CBT OF ANXIETY DISORDERS IN YOUTH

Given CBTs roots in learning and cognitive theory, it follows that the primary goals of CBT for child anxiety are to change maladaptive learning and thought patterns. What may be less obvious are that the implications of these foci make CBT approaches to child anxiety distinct from many other psychosocial interventions for youth. First, CBT approaches to child anxiety attempt to understand the roots of the presenting problem only to the degree that this understanding gives rise to a way to intervene in the "here and now." Treatment is much more focused on addressing the factors that maintain the child's symptoms rather than understanding what gave rise to the disorder. For example, one might want to know how a parent has reacted in the past to a child's attempts at avoidance but rather than focusing on these past interactions, this knowledge would be used to help the clinician know whether to work with parents on developing a new approach with the result of allowing for an altered learning experience for the child.

Additionally, CBT is a skills building approach. This means that clinicians are directive and sessions may appear very didactic. However, sessions are seen only as an initial step in the learning process. Meetings with the child or parents are used to introduce skills, provide initial practice, and problem-solve; however, homework assignments outside of session provide the repeated practice required for complete skill acquisition and refinement. Moreover, given the importance of the context in which the anxious behavior occurs in behavioral theory, it necessarily follows that CBT for child anxiety often introduces new skills for parents, teachers, and sometimes even siblings or peers. In fact, the child's parents often become the major agents of change and work together with the clinician to implement the treatment, especially so with younger children. Parents and teachers are often asked to change their behavior (eg, model nonanxious self-talk), change their approach to their child's anxiety (eg, reinforce approach and provide less opportunity for avoidance), and to act as a coach for the child when he or she is completing homework assignments or generalizing skills into everyday situations. This requires a commitment on the part of the child and his or her parents that extends beyond the typical one hour per week session. On the other hand, treatment is typically time-limited. Goals are set by the child and parents in collaboration with the therapist and, once adequate skills have been developed and treatment goals are reached, the termination process begins. In the case of most childhood anxiety disorders, treatment usually takes 12 to 16 weeks, rarely extending beyond 6 months of active treatment. However, spaced out "booster sessions" that may extend over 4 to 6 months, may be used as a way to provide review of difficult skills. This may be particularly helpful in that effective treatment may lead a child to encounter new situations because of an increase in the ability to engage in a full-range of activities. Booster sessions may be used to help a child generalize skills to these situations and ensure durability of treatment gains.

Although several different CBT manuals have been developed to more specifically explicate CBT treatment procedures for child anxiety, Woody and Ollendick[26] and Ollendick and Hovey[27] have identified several principles that cut across these treatments (see later discussion).

Table 1
Summary of treatment studies

Authors, Year	Sample Size	Age (y)	Diagnosis or Symptom Clusters	Treatment Conditions	Results
Kendall,[23] 1994	47	9–13	OAD, SAD, AD	CBT WL	CBT was superior to WL.
Barrett et al,[51] 1996	79	7–14	SAD, OAD, SOC	CBT CBT + family treatment WL	Both treatments were better than WL. Some measures showed marginal improvements with addition of family treatment component.
Kendall & Southam-Gerow,[50] 1996	36	11–18	OAD, SAD, AD	CBT – follow-up study	Treatment gains were generally maintained after approximately 3 y.
Kendall et al,[37] 1997	94	9–13	OAD, SAD, AD	CBT WL	CBT was superior to WL.
Kendall & Sugarman,[52] 1997	190	8–14	OAD, SAD, AD	Examined termination in CBT	Termination was more likely for ethnic minority children, children who were less anxious, and children living in a single-parent household.
Barrett,[53] 1998	60	7–14	SAD, OAD, SOC	CBT – group CBT + family treatment – group WL	Both treatments were better than WL. Some measures showed marginal improvements with addition of family treatment component.
Cobham et al,[54] 1998	67	7–14	SAD, OAD, GAD, SPEC, SOC, AG	CBT CBT + family treatment	The addition of family treatment was beneficial only in cases in which there was significant parental anxiety.
De Haan et al,[55] 1998	22	8–18	OCD	BT Clomipramine	BT was superior to clomipramine on some measures; on others the two treatments were not different.
King et al,[56] 1998	34	5–15	School refusal	CBT + parent and teacher training WL	CBT was superior to WL.

Study	N	Age	Disorder	Treatment	Results
Last et al,[57] 1998	56	6–17	School refusal	CBT Attention control treatment	Both treatments were effective; there was no differences between treatments.
Muris et al,[58] 1998	26	8–17	SPEC	EMDR - In vivo exposure Computerized exposure	In vivo-exposure was superior to computerized exposure and EMDR.
Mendlowitz et al,[59] 1999	62	7–12	Any anxiety disorder	CBT – parent only CBT – child only CET – parent + child	All treatments were effective; some benefits with parental involvement.
Silverman et al,[60] 1999	81	6–16	SPEC, SOC, AG	Exposure-based self control treatment Exposure-based contingency management treatment Education support	All groups showed improvement.
Silverman et al,[61] 1999	56	6–16	GAD, SOC, OAD	CBT – Group WL	CBT was superior to WL.
Beidel et al,[62] 2000	67	8–12	SOC	CBT Active, nonspecific treatment	CBT was superior to nonspecific treatment.
Berman et al,[63] 2000	106	6–17	SPEC, OAD, SOC, GAD, AG	CBT	Best predictors of treatment outcome were child's pretreatment levels of anxiety and depression and parental depression, hostility, and paranoia; however, effects of parental psychopathology were weaker for older children.
Flannery-Schroeder & Kendall,[64] 2000	37	8–14	GAD, SAD, SOC	CBT – Individual CBT – Group WL	Most measures suggested that both CBT treatments were better than WL but not different than each other.

(continued on next page)

Table 1
(*continued*)

Authors, Year	Sample Size	Age (y)	Diagnosis or Symptom Clusters	Treatment Conditions	Results
Hayward et al,[65] 2000	35	13–17	SOC	CBT – Group No treatment control	CBT was more effective than no treatment at posttreatment but not at 1 y follow-up. CBT did seem to decrease risk of relapse of depression for those who had already experienced a major depressive episode
King et al,[66] 2000	36	5–17	PTSD	CBT CBT + family treatment WL	Both treatments were superior to WL but the additional family treatment did not add significant benefit.
Spence et al,[67] 2000	50	7–14	SOC	CBT CBT + family treatment WL	Both treatments were superior to WL but the additional family treatment did not add significant benefit. Treatment gains were generally maintained after approximately 1 y.
Barrett et al,[68] 2001	52	13–21	SAD, OAD, SOC	CBT CBT + family treatment – follow-up study	Treatment gains were generally maintained after approximately 6 y. Most measures did not show differences between the two treatments.
Kendall et al,[69] 2001	173	8–13	GAD, SOC, SAD	Examined comorbidity in CBT and WL	Comorbidity did not predict treatment outcome or interact with treatment group.
Muris et al,[70] 2001	36	8–13	GAD, SAD, SOC, OCD	CBT CBT – Group	Treatments were about equally effective.
Ost et al,[71] 2001	60	7–17	SPEC	CBT CBT + Parent WL	Both treatments were effective but not different than one another; treatment gains maintained at approximately 1 y.

Study	N	Age	Disorders	Treatment	Outcome
Shortt et al,[38] 2001	71	6–10	SAD, SOC, GAD	CBT + family treatment – group WL	CBT was superior to WL
Southam-Gerow et al,[72] 2001	135	7–15	SAD, GAD, SOC, AD	Examined correlates of outcome in CBT	Poorer treatment outcome was related to older age at treatment, more internalizing symptoms at pretreatment, and higher levels of maternal depression. Most demographic variables did not predict outcome.
Waters et al,[73] 2001	7	10–14	OCD	CBT + family treatment	Six of the seven youth were diagnosis-free at posttreatment.
Ginsburg & Drake,[22] 2002	9	14–17	Any anxiety disorder except PTSD or OCD	CBT Attention Control Placebo	CBT was superior to placebo.
Heyne et al,[74] 2002	61	7–14	Anxiety-based school refusal	CBT Parent and teacher training CBT⁻ + Parent and teacher training	All treatments were effective but CBT for the child only was not as good at increasing school attendance in the short-term. The combined treatment did not result in a significant benefit.
Manassis et al,[75] 2002	78	8–12	GAD, SAD, SPEC, SOC, PD	CBT CBT – Group	Few differences between the two treatments.
Muris et al,[76] 2002	30	9–12	SAD, GAD, SOC	CBT – Group Emotional disclosure WL	CBT superior to emotional disclosure and WL; emotional disclosure and WL did not result in significant improvements.
Nauta et al,[77] 2003	79	7–18	SAD, SOC, GAD, PD	CBT CBT + family treatment WL	CBT treatments were both superior to WL.
Pina et al,[78] 2003	131	6–16	SPEC, SOC, AG, GAD, OAD	Examined ethnicity as a predictor of treatment outcome in CBT	Treatment outcomes and maintenance of treatment gains were similar for Latino and European-American youth.

(continued on next page)

Table 1
(continued)

Authors, Year	Sample Size	Age (y)	Diagnosis or Symptom Clusters	Treatment Conditions	Results
Rapee,[79] 2003	165	7–16	SAD, GAD, SOC, SPEC, OCD, PD	CBT + family treatment – Group	Treatment was about equally effective for youth with or without comorbid disorders.
Barrett et al,[80] 2004	77	7–17	OCD	CBT + family treatment – Individual CBT + family treatment – Group WL	Both treatments were effective but not different than one another.
Flannery-Schroder et al,[81] 2004	38	15–22	GAD, SAD, AD either with or without a comorbid externalizing disorder	CBT – follow-up study	Treatment was about equally effective for both those with and without an externalizing disorder at approximately 7 ½ y.
Gallagher et al,[82] 2004	23	8–11	SOC	CBT – Group WL	Treatment was effective even through it was abbreviated (3 wk).
Kendall et al,[83] 2004	86	15–22	OAD, SAD, AD	CBT – follow-up study	Treatment gains were generally maintained after approximately 7 ½ y.
Manassis et al,[84] 2004	43	Mean = 16.5	Any anxiety disorder	CBT – follow-up study	Males, youth diagnosed with GAD, and those with less severe anxiety at pretreatment had better outcomes at 6–7 y follow-up.
POTS Team,[85] 2004	112	7–17	OCD	CBT Sertraline, CBT + sertraline Pill placebo	All active treatments better than placebo, combined treatments better than CBT or sertraline alone; CBT and sertraline did not differ.
Asbahr et al,[86] 2005	40	9–17	OCD	CBT – Group Sertraline	Both treatments were effective but CBT resulted in lower relapse rates.

	N	Age	Diagnosis	Treatment	Results
Baer & Garland,[87] 2005	12	13–18	SOC	CBT – Group WL	CBT was superior to WL
Beidel et al,[88] 2005	29	11–18	SOC	CET – follow-up study	Treatment gains were generally maintained after approximately 3 y.
Berstein et al,[89] 2005	61	7–11	SAD, GAD, or SOC	CBT – Group CBT + Parent training – Group No treatment control	Both treatments were effective, some benefit with addition of parent training.
Flannery-Schroder et al,[90] 2005	30	9–15	SAD, GAD, or SOC	CBT CBT – Group	Treatment was about equally effective for both groups at approximately 1 y.
Masia-Warner et al,[91] 2005	35	13–17	SOC	CBT – Group WL	CBT was superior to WL.
Beidel et al,[92] 2006	31	13–20	SOC	CBT – follow-up study	Treatment gains were generally maintained after approximately 5 y. Treated group was not different on a number of measures than youth who had never had social phobia.
Lyneham & Rapee,[93] 2006	100	6–12	GAD, SAD, SOC, OCD, SPEC, PD	CBT – Bibliotherapy + email contact CBT – Bibliotherapy + telephone contact CBT – Bibliotherapy + client initiated contacts WL	Bibliotherapy with therapist-initiated telephone contact produced the best outcomes.
Rapee et al,[94] 2006	267	6–12	GAD, SOC, SAD, SPEC, OCD, PD	CBT – Group CBT – Bibliotherapy WL	Both treatments superior to WL but bibliotherapy not as effective as standard CBT.
Spence et al,[95] 2006	72	7–14	GAD, SAD, SOC, SPEC	CBT CBT delivered through Internet WL	Both treatments were superior to WL but not different than one another; gains maintained at approximately 1 y.

(continued on next page)

Table 1
(continued)

Authors, Year	Sample Size	Age (y)	Diagnosis or Symptom Clusters	Treatment Conditions	Results
Wood et al,[96] 2006	40	6–13	SAD, GAD, SOC	CBT CBT + family treatment	Both treatments were effective; some evidence of additional benefit of family treatment.
Beidel et al,[97] 2007	60	7–17	SOC	CBT Fluoxetine Placebo	Both treatments were superior to placebo but CBT was superior to fluoxetine and the only treatment better than placebo for improving social skills.
Chalfant et al,[98] 2007	47	8–13	High-functioning Autism Spectrum Disorders + an anxiety disorder	Family based CBT – Group WL	CBT was effective in treating anxiety disorders in youth comorbid with high-functioning autism spectrum disorders.
de Groot et al,[99] 2007	29	7–12	Any anxiety disorder	CBT CBT – Group	Treatments were about equally effective.
Levy et al,[100] 2007	69	8–14	Aggression comorbid with SAD, GAD, SOC, SPEC, or PD	CBT – for anxiety only CBT – for anxiety and aggression	Both treatments were effective; no significant benefit with the combined treatment.
March et al,[101] 2007	112	7–17	OCD with or without comorbid tics	CBT Sertraline CBT + sertraline Placebo	Medication alone was less effective for youth with tics; comorbid tics did not negatively affect outcomes for CBT. In general the combination treatment resulted in the best outcome for youth with or without tics.
Masia-Warner et al,[102] 2007	36	14–16	SOC	CBT – Group Attention control	CBT was superior to attention control treatment.
Smith et al,[103] 2007	24	8–18	PTSD WL	CBT	CBT superior to WL; outcome partially mediated by cognitive change.

Study	N	Age	Disorder	Treatment	Results
Storch et al,[104] 2007	40	7–17	OCD	CBT – Intensive CBT – Weekly	Some short-term advantage for the intensive treatment but both treatments about equal at 3 mo posttreatment.
Victor et al,[105] 2007	61	7–11	SAD, GAD, or SOC	CBT – Group No treatment control	Higher family cohesion was related to better outcome in CBT group.
Berstein et al,[25] 2008	61	7–11	SAD, GAD, or SOC	CBT – Group CBT + Parent training – Group No treatment control	Treatment gains were generally maintained after approximately 1 y; some evidence of added benefit with addition of parent training.
Kendall et al,[106] 2008	161	7–14	SAD, SOC, GAD	CBT Family-based CBT Family-based education support	CBT groups were superior to family-based support in reducing principal anxiety disorder. Individual CBT was superior to family-based CBT on some measures, but family based CBT was superior to individual CBT if both parents had an anxiety disorder.
Warner et al,[107] 2009	7	8–15	Anxiety disorder + somatic complaints	CBT	All children responded to treatment.
Waters et al,[108] 2009	60	4–8	SPEC, SOC, GAD, SAD	CBT – Parent only CBT – Parent + child WL	Both treatments were superior to WL but not significantly different than one another; gains were generally maintained after approximately 1 y.
Cobham et al,[109] 2010	60	10–17	SAD, OAD, GAD, SPEC, SOC, AG	CBT CBT + family treatment – follow-up study	Children were more likely to be diagnosis-free at 3 y follow-up if they had been in the CBT + family treatment condition, regardless of parents' level of anxiety at pretreatment.
Garcia et al,[110] 2010	112	7–17	OCD	CBT Sertraline CBT + Sertraline Placebo	Less severe OCD, fewer externalizing symptoms, less family accommodation, and more insight was predictive of better treatment outcome.

Abbreviations: AD, avoidant disorder; AG, agoraphobia; BT, behavior therapy; EMDR, eye movement desensitization and reprocessing therapy; GAD, generalized anxiety disorder; OAD, overanxious disorder; OCD, obsessive-compulsive disorder; PD, panic disorder; PTSD, posttraumatic stress disorder; SAD, separation anxiety disorder; SOC, social phobia; SPEC, specific phobia; WL, waitlist.

EMPIRICALLY SOUND ASSESSMENT OF ANXIETY DISORDERS IN CHILDREN

A thorough assessment is necessary before beginning a successful course of CBT to address an anxiety disorder with a child or adolescent and his or her family. The assessment should begin with a complete diagnostic evaluation including determining whether the presenting symptoms are clinically significant and, if so, conducting a thorough differential diagnosis to discriminate amongst the anxiety disorders and between anxiety disorders and those disorders with similar presentations, including medical conditions such as hyperthyroidism and asthma. Given the high rate of comorbidity in children seeking treatment for anxiety disorders, it is also necessary to determine if comorbid psychiatric conditions exist and, if so, which symptoms should be the primary targets of early treatment. In addition, specific examples of functional impairment, along with indicators of severity, should be identified to aide the child and therapist in establishing treatment goals and monitoring treatment progress. Cognitive appraisals of feared stimuli, attempts at approach, and environmental reactions to the child's avoidance should also be thoroughly assessed to develop a thorough case conceptualization.

Although a thorough review of the available measures and approaches to assessment of anxiety in youth is beyond the scope of this article, recent reviews suggest that numerous standardized measures, including diagnostic interviews and questionnaires, are available for collecting information from children, parents, and teachers.[28] In addition, individually tailored behavioral avoidance–approach tests and monitoring forms can be particularly helpful in assessing functional impairment and monitoring treatment progress. However, much work remains to be done in this area, including understanding discrepancies between parent and child reports of symptoms and the discordance in the assessment of the tripartite features of anxiety (ie, physiologic arousal, subjective anxiety, and behavioral avoidance).[29–31] Moreover, additional work is needed to establish the clinical utility of laboratory measures of anxiety[32] (eg, computerized measures of attentional biases) and in efficiently assessing potential mediators of change and meaningful quality of life indicators. Further, in order for CBT to be considered as a first-line treatment, and for clinicians and patients to make informed choices about treatment options, better measures of the costs (financial and otherwise) associated with CBT for anxious youth are needed to allow for cost-benefit analysis at the individual and societal scale.

ESTABLISHING RAPPORT AND WORKING WITH THE PARENTS OF CHILDREN WITH ANXIETY DISORDERS

The importance of the therapeutic relationship has long been recognized by clinicians working with children and adolescents. However, cognitive-behavioral theory clearly hypothesizes specific factors in addition to the therapeutic relationship that are thought to be necessary for a full treatment response. Moreover, much of the CBT research has focused on treatment procedures given the relationship of these procedures to the core hypothesized mechanisms of change implicated in cognitive and behavioral theory. This is in contrast to humanistic therapies in which the therapeutic relationship is hypothesized to be the key mechanism for change. Perhaps because of this contrast, CBT has sometimes been characterized as sterile or mechanistic and practitioners of CBT have been criticized for their lack of attention to the importance of the therapeutic relationship. The authors would submit, however, that this is far from the truth.[33,34] In fact, even a cursory examination of most CBT treatment manuals for anxiety disorders in youth reveals that CBT treatments require development of a therapeutic relationship and working alliance in addition to an active, relatively prolonged effort on the part of the child and his or her family. Exposure sessions, discussed later and widely recognized as a core component of effective CBT treatments for anxiety in youth, are inherently distressing and compliance would seem unlikely without a strong relationship with both the parents and the child and agreement on both the tasks and goals of treatment.[35] However, in addition to the empathic listening skills, genuineness, and positive regard often thought to be primary means of establishing the therapeutic relationship, CBT therapists may rely more heavily on the collaborative relationship inherent in CBT and the provision of a theoretical rationale and treatment plan to enable the child to experience the therapist as someone who can be of help. To date, though we know that a positive therapeutic relationship is related to better outcomes in CBT for childhood anxiety disorders,[33] little is known about what constitutes a positive relationship or whether the therapist behaviors contributing to the therapeutic relationship vary across different therapeutic approaches.

COGNITIVE RESTRUCTURING

Given the theoretical link posited by cognitive theory between erroneous or maladaptive cognitions, the subjective experience of anxiety, and anxious behavior, one of the core components of CBT for child anxiety is cognitive restructuring of anxious cognitions. This requires the child to first explicitly recognize their self-talk and then to understand the links between self-talk and their symptoms. Monitoring in anxiety-provoking situations is often used to help a child identify specific maladaptive cognitions. Restructuring may take the form of direct discussion or guided discovery to question the validity of a thought or belief. This discussion can take several forms. One basic approach is summarized in four steps recommended by Padesky,[36] these include (1) asking informational questions to identify the thought and find data to test the veracity of the thought, (2) empathic listening, (3) summarizing, and (4) using synthesizing or analytical questions to help the child come to a new understanding. Of course, a purely cognitive exercise may be difficult to accomplish depending on the age and cognitive development of the child. Behavioral experiments may be particularly effective methods of cognitive restructuring in such cases.

Behavioral experiments can be used to target a specific cognition such as "if I ask a child to play with me, he will laugh at me." In this case the child and therapist would design an experiment asking a peer to play with the explicit goal of testing the veracity of the child's belief. The child is asked to engage in the experiment with the explicit goal of "data collection." Almost all of the CBT treatments for anxiety disorders in youth use some form of cognitive restructuring. Most programs will have a component in which the child first monitors thoughts to identify those giving rise to symptoms, then actively disputes those thoughts first with the therapist and then with increasing independence, and then develops new more adaptive, coping thoughts.[23,37,38]

REPEATED EXPOSURE AND REDUCTION OF AVOIDANCE

Exposure to feared stimuli is arguably the central component in most CBTs for child anxiety. In fact, Chorpita and colleagues[19] found exposure-based treatments for anxiety disorders in youth to be associated with the largest effect sizes. Early exposure therapies guided by a reciprocal inhibition hypothesis paired feared stimuli (eg, dogs, social situations, germs) with a response incompatible with anxiety—often muscle relaxation.[39] In such an approach the child would be trained in relaxation techniques and a hierarchy of feared stimuli would be developed. Systematic exposure to the feared stimuli would proceed with the child engaging in relaxation procedures. Any symptoms of anxiety would be countered with relaxation, as the goal would be to avoid the experience of anxiety to condition an association between the once-feared stimuli and relaxation. However, such an approach has largely fallen out of favor, in part because it has been found that the relaxation training component of the treatment was often not necessary and in part because of updated theories regarding the mechanisms responsible for change In exposure therapies.[40–42] Today exposure-based treatments generally have four basic phases (1) instruction, (2) hierarchy development, (3) exposure proper, and (4) generalization and maintenance.

Instruction

In the instruction phase, the parent and child are presented with the rationale for exposure treatment. This often includes a learning-based rationale; that is, that past avoidance has been negatively reinforced with the reduction of anxiety thereby increasing the likelihood of future avoidance and escape during the peak of their fear. As such, there is little opportunity to learn the feared stimulus is in fact innocuous. A cognitive rationale emphasizing the role of increased self-efficacy and the development of more accurate and adaptive cognitions may also be included, helping the child and parent to understand that exposure without avoidance will show the child that he or she has the skills to cope with the feared situation. It is also important that the instruction phase include basic information on the understanding of fear and anxiety as many anxious children, and perhaps their parents, at least implicitly expect the anxiety to increase interminably and to spiral out of control with prolonged exposure. For this reason, the child and parents need to understand the nature of anxiety and that it will peak and then decrease with prolonged exposure.

Development of a Hierarchy

Once the child and parents understand the rationale for exposure therapy the next step is typically to develop a graded hierarchy of feared situations that can realistically be used for exposure sessions. More specially, an exposure hierarchy consists of a series of anxiety provoking situations arranged from the least anxiety provoking to the most. It is important to make sure that enough steps are included in the hierarchy so that each step represents a gradual progression from the previous step and that the hierarchy as a whole captures all the components necessary to illicit the fear response in the child. For example, a child experiencing social anxiety may need to include steps in his or her hierarchy that include overt criticism to evoke an anxiety response and allow for habituation and the development of an increased perception of self-efficacy. Importantly, it may be necessary to include steps in the hierarchy that are more anxiety provoking than those the child may ever realistically be expected to face.

Exposure Proper

In this step the child is exposed to each of the situations in the hierarchy until the anxiety dissipates. Modeling by the therapist, in which the therapist first engages in the anxiety provoking task allowing the child to watch, may precede direct engagement by the child. Attention should be paid to both within-session habituation (eg, decrease in subjective distress or indicators of physiologic arousal) and between-session habituation, as these have been found to be predictive of outcome.[42–44] Exposure may be in vivo or imaginary, although in most cases in vivo exposure is generally preferred and more effective. When circumstances do not allow for in vivo exposures (eg, repeated flights for a child with a fear of flying), virtual-reality based exposures may prove to be a useful alternative when available. During this phase, elimination of avoidance or escape behaviors is emphasized to facilitate exposure and allow the child a return to normal activities.[27]

Generalization and Maintenance

To generalize treatment gains across situations the child is usually given homework assignments to repeat exposures that are mastered in session across similar situations outside of the therapy room. In addition to allowing for generalization, these activities allow for solidification of the skills learned in session, and ensure that the child does not see the presence of the therapist as necessary to the control of the anxiety. Once the child has progressed through the entire hierarchy and anxiety has significantly dissipated, planning for termination and maintenance begins. Given that anxiety and stressful situations are a normal part of life, termination should be considered when treatment goals are achieved and anxiety appears to be within normal levels for the child's developmental level. Depending on the age of the child, this phase includes giving the child or parent increasing responsibility for planning exposure or cognitive restructuring exercises when new challenges present themselves. Planning for stressful situations and providing the child with written materials that can be used to reinforce and review skills after the termination of therapy can be helpful.[45] Moreover, current research on the mechanisms involved in the extinction of anxious responses suggests several important avenues for planning for relapse prevention. This may include increasingly conducting exposure sessions outside of the typical therapy context (ie, in real life situations in which the client might expect a relapse) and providing the child with a physical or cognitive cue of the exposure sessions to facilitate retrieval of the nonanxious learning that took place during treatment sessions (Wuyek LA, Seligman LD. *Reducing the renewal effect: cognitive retrieval cues in maintaining extinction.* Manuscript submitted for publication, 2010).[46–49]

SKILLS TRAINING AND BEHAVIORAL REHEARSAL

There is some debate about whether children with anxiety disorders evidence true skills deficits (eg, social skills deficits, lack of test-taking skills, emotion regulation skill deficits) or whether they possess these skills but are unable to effectively use them because of the interference engendered by their anxiety. However, because the research is equivocal, many CBT treatments for child anxiety include a skills training component. In early phases, this training may be very didactic and psychoeducational but learning is often reinforced with modeling by the therapist and behavioral rehearsal. Behavioral rehearsal is coupled with reinforcement by the therapist, oftentimes social reinforcement in the form of praise and positive feedback that is gradually phased out in favor of self-reinforcement.

SUMMARY AND FUTURE DIRECTIONS

CBT for child anxiety disorders has a rich history dating back to the beginnings of the behavioral movement in the 1920s. These treatments were unique in their strong ties to both theory and empiricism. Today, over 40 randomized clinical trials support the efficacy of CBT for the treatment of anxiety disorders in children and adolescents. These studies find that the majority of youth with anxiety disorders treated with CBT will see substantial benefits. Moreover, the effects seen in these studies suggest that changes are clinically significant as well as statistically significant. Further, CBT is a time-limited skills building treatment and this has important implications for families. This means that children can expect relief from symptoms within a relatively brief period (ie, 3 to 4 months) and that the need for a therapist can be phased out as the child and family master the requisite skills. Continued improvement does not depend on regular meetings with the therapist. In fact, follow-up studies suggest that many children who see benefits from CBT will maintain their treatment gains and continue to improve even after treatment has formally terminated.[20,50] These characteristic have the potential to make CBT for child anxiety stand-out amongst other treatment options for its high potential benefit and relatively low costs.

Given the preponderance of evidence in support of CBT as an evidence-based treatment for child anxiety, future research needs to move beyond the basic question of whether CBT works. Although clinicians in practice must adapt traditional CBT methods to a child or adolescent's developmental level and other contextual factors, little systematic research is available to guide these decisions. Moreover, additional work is needed to establish the mediators and moderators of treatment outcome— essentially for whom is CBT more or less effective and why does CBT for child anxiety work. Further, although some work has been done to guide clinicians in treatment-resistant cases, additional studies are needed to guide clinician decision-making when first-line CBT treatments do not work. Finally, although studies suggest that CBT should represent a first-line treatment for children presenting with an anxiety disorder, it is rarely the case that these children receive CBT at any point in their treatment. This seems to be the case even when families see a clinician claiming to use CBT. Therefore, additional empirical work is needed to guide the training and supervision of student clinicians and to investigate effective means of disseminating knowledge of CBT treatments and treatment advances to those already in clinical practice.

REFERENCES

1. Kessler RC, Berglund P, Demler O, et al. Lifetime prevalence and age-of-onset distributions of DSM-IV disorders in the national comorbidity survey replication. Arch Gen Psychiatry 2005;62(6):593–602.
2. Cartwright-Hatton S, McNicol K, Doubleday E. Anxiety in a neglected population: prevalence of anxiety disorders in pre-adolescent children [Special Issue: Anxiety of childhood and adolescence: challenges and opportunities]. Clin Psychol Rev 2006;26(7):817–33.
3. Gullone E. The development of normal fear: a century of research. Clin Psychol Rev 2000;20(4):429–51.
4. Strauss CC, Frame CL, Forehand R. Psychosocial impairment associated with anxiety in children. J Clin Child Psychol 1987;16(3):235–9.
5. Ginsburg GS, La Greca AM, Silverman WK. Social anxiety in children with anxiety disorders: relation with social and emotional functioning. J Abnorm Child Psychol 1998;26(3):175–85.
6. Ialongo N, Edelsohn G, Werthamer-Larsson L, et al. Social and cognitive impairment in first-grade children with anxious and depressive symptoms. J Clin Child Psychol 1996;25(1):15–24.
7. Greenberg PE, Sisitsky T, Kessler RC, et al. The economic burden of anxiety disorders in the 1990s. J Clin Psychiatry 1999;60(7):427–35.
8. American Psychiatric Association. Diagnostic and statistical manual of mental disorders. Revised. 4th edition. Washington, DC: American Psychiatric Assocation; 2000.
9. American Psychiatric Assocation. DSM-5: the future of psychiatric diagnosis. Washington, DC: American Psychiatric Association; 2010.
10. Brady EU, Kendall PC. Comorbidity of anxiety and depression in children and adolescents. Psychol Bull 1992;111(2):244–55.

11. Seligman LD, Ollendick TH. Comorbidity of anxiety and depression in children and adolescents: an integrative review. Clin Child Fam Psychol Rev 1998;1(2): 125–44.

12. Russo MF, Beidel DC. Comorbidity of childhood anxiety and externalizing disorders: prevalence, associated characteristics, and validation issues. Clin Psychol Rev 1994;14(3):199–221.

13. Ollendick TH, Jarrett MA, Grills-Taquechel AE, et al. Comorbidity as a predictor and moderator of treatment outcome in youth with anxiety, affective, attention deficit/hyperactivity disorder, and oppositional/conduct disorders. Clin Psychol Rev 2008;28(8):1447–71.

14. Masi G, Favilla L, Millepiedi S, et al. Somatic symptoms in children and adolescents referred for emotional and behavioral disorders. Psychiatry 2000;63(2):140–9.

15. Meichenbaum D. Cognitive behavior modification. New York: Plenum Press; 1977.

16. Ollendick TH, Cerny JA. Clinical behavior therapy with children. New York: Plenum Press; 1981.

17. Ollendick TH, King NJ. Empirically supported treatments for children with phobic and anxiety disorders: current status. J Clin Child Psychol 1998;27(2):156–67.

18. Ollendick TH, King NJ, Chorpita BF. Empirically supported treatments for children and adolescents. In: Kendall PC, editor. Child and adolescent therapy: cognitive-behavioral procedures. 3rd edition. New York: Guilford Press; 2006. p. 492–520.

19. Chorpita BF, Yim LM, Donkervoet JC, et al. Toward large-scale implementation of empirically supported treatments for children: a review and observations by the Hawaii Empirical Basis to Services Task Force. Clin Psychol Sci Pract 2002;9(2):165–90.

20. Nevo GA, Manassis K. Outcomes for treated anxious children: a critical review of long-term follow-up studies. Depress Anxiety 2009;26(7):650–60.

21. Ollendick TH, Öst L-G, Reuterskild L, et al. Comorbidity in youth with specific phobias: impact of comorbidity on treatment outcome and the impact of treatment on comorbid disorders. Behav Res Ther 2010;48:827–31.

22. Ginsburg GS, Drake KL. School-based treatment for anxious African-American adolescents: a controlled pilot study. J Am Acad Child Adolesc Psychiatry 2002; 41(7):768–75.

23. Kendall PC. Treating anxiety disorders in children: results of a randomized clinical trial. J Consult Clin Psychol 1994;62(1):100–10.

24. Toren P, Eldar S, Cendorf D, et al. The prevalence of mitral valve prolapse in children with anxiety disorders. J Psychiatr Res 1999;33(4):357–61.

25. Bernstein GA, Bernat DH, Victor AM, et al. School-based interventions for anxious children: 3-, 6-, and 12-month follow-ups. J Am Acad Child Adolesc Psychiatry 2008;47(9):1039–47.

26. Woody SR, Ollendick TH. Technique factors in treating anxiety disorders. In: Castonguay L, Beutler LE, editors. Principles of therapeutic change that work. New York: Oxford University Press; 2006. p. 167–86.

27. Ollendick TH, Hovey LD. Competencies for treating phobic and anxiety disorders in children and adolescents. In: Thomas J, Hersen M, editors. Handbook of clinical psychology competencies. New York: Springer Verlag; 2009. p. 1219–44.

28. Silverman WK, Ginsburg GS. Anxiety disorders. In: Ollendick TH, Hersen M, editors. Handbook of child psychopathology. 3rd edition. New York: Plenum Press; 1998. p. 239–68.

29. Silverman WK, Ollendick TH. Evidence-based assessment of anxiety and its disorders in children and adolescents. J Clin Child Adolesc Psychol 2005; 34(3):380–411.
30. Grills AE, Ollendick TH. Multiple informant agreement and the anxiety disorders interview schedule for parents and children. J Am Acad Child Adolesc Psychiatry 2003;42(1):30–40.
31. Reuterskiold L, Ost L-G, Ollendick T. Exploring child and parent factors in the diagnostic agreement on the anxiety disorders interview schedule. J Psychopathol Behav Assess 2008;30(4):279–90.
32. Egloff B, Schmukle SC. Predictive validity of an implicit association test for assessing anxiety. J Pers Soc Psychol 2002;83(6):1441–55.
33. Hughes AA, Kendall PC. Prediction of cognitive behavior treatment outcome for children with anxiety disorders: therapeutic relationship and homework compliance. Behav Cogn Psychother 2007;35(4):487–94.
34. Leahy RL. The therapeutic relationship in cognitive-behavioral therapy [Special Issue: Developments in the theory and practice of cognitive and behavioural therapies]. Behav Cogn Psychother 2008;36(6):769–77.
35. Hayes SA, Hope DA, VanDyke MM, et al. Working alliance for clients with social anxiety disorder: relationship with session helpfulness and within-session habituation. Cogn Behav Ther 2007;36(1):34–42.
36. Padesky CA. Guided discovery using Socratic dialogue [compact disc]. Huntington Beach (CA): Center for Cognitive Therapy; 1996.
37. Kendall PC, Flannery-Schroeder E, Panichelli-Mindel SM, et al. Therapy for youths with anxiety disorders: a second randomized clinical trial. J Consult Clin Psychol 1997;65(3):366–80.
38. Shortt AL, Barrett PM, Fox TL. Evaluating the FRIENDS program: a cognitive-behavioral group treatment for anxious children and their parents. J Clin Child Psychol 2001;30(4):525–35.
39. Wolpe J. Psychotherapy by reciprocal inhibition. Oxford (England): Stanford University Press; 1958.
40. Stewart SH, Watt MC. Introduction to the special issue on interoceptive exposure in the treatment of anxiety and related disorders: novel applications and mechanisms of action. J Cognit Psychother 2008;22(4):291–302.
41. Foa EB, Kozak MJ. Emotional processing of fear: exposure to corrective information. Psychol Bull 1986;99(1):20–35.
42. Foa EB, Huppert JD, Cahill SP. Emotional processing theory: an update. In: Rothbaum BO, editor. Pathological anxiety: emotional processing in etiology and treatment. New York: Guilford Press; 2006. p. 3–24.
43. Jaycox LH, Foa EB, Morral AR. Influence of emotional engagement and habituation on exposure therapy for PTSD. J Consult Clin Psychol 1998;66(1):185–92.
44. van Minnen A, Hagenaars M. Fear activation and habituation patterns as early process predictors of response to prolonged exposure treatment in PTSD. J Trauma Stress 2002;15(5):359–67.
45. Linares Scott TJ, Feeny NC. Relapse prevention techniques in the treatment of childhood anxiety disorders: a case example. J Contemp Psychother 2006; 36(4):151–7.
46. Bouton ME, Woods AM, Moody EW, et al. Counteracting the context-dependence of extinction: relapse and tests of some relapse prevention methods. In: Craske MG, Hermans D, Vansteenwegen D, editors. Fear and learning: from basic processes to clinical implications. Washington, DC: American Psychological Association; 2006. p. 175–96.

47. Hermans D, Craske MG, Mineka S, et al. Extinction in human fear conditioning. Biol Psychiatry 2006;60(4):361–8.
48. Vansteenwegen D, Dirikx T, Hermans D, et al. Renewal and reinstatement of fear: evidence from human conditioning research. In: Craske MG, Hermans D, Vansteenwegen D, editors. Fear and learning: from basic processes to clinical implications. Washington, DC: American Psychological Association; 2006. p. 197–215.
49. Bouton ME, Frohardt RJ, Sunsay C, et al. Contextual control of inhibition with reinforcement: adaptation and timing mechanisms. J Exp Psychol Anim Behav Process 2008;34(2):223–36.
50. Kendall PC, Southam-Gerow MA. Long-term follow-up of a cognitive-behavioral therapy for anxiety-disordered youth. J Consult Clin Psychol 1996;64(4): 724–30.
51. Barrett PM, Dadds MR, Rapee RM. Family treatment of childhood anxiety: a controlled trial. J Consult Clin Psychol 1996;64(2):333–42.
52. Kendall PC, Sugarman A. Attrition in the treatment of childhood anxiety disorders. J Consult Clin Psychol 1997;65(5):883–8.
53. Barrett PM. Evaluation of cognitive-behavioral group treatments for childhood anxiety disorders. J Clin Child Psychol 1998;27(4):459–68.
54. Cobham VE, Dadds MR, Spence SH. The role of parental anxiety in the treatment of childhood anxiety. J Consult Clin Psychol 1998;66(6):893–905.
55. De Haan E, Hoogduin Kees AL, Buitelaar Jan K, et al. Behavior therapy versus clomipramine for the treatment of obsessive-compulsive disorder in children and adolescents. J Am Acad Child Adolesc Psychiatry 1998;37(10):1022–9.
56. King NJ, Tonge BJ, Heyne D, et al. Cognitive-behavioral treatment of school-refusing children: a controlled evaluation. J Am Acad Child Adolesc Psychiatry 1998;37(4):395–403.
57. Last CG, Hansen C, Franco N. Cognitive-behavioral treatment of school phobia. J Am Acad Child Adolesc Psychiatry 1998;37(4):404–11.
58. Muris P, Merckelbach H, Holdrinet I, et al. Treating phobic children: effects of EMDR versus exposure. J Consult Clin Psychol 1998;66(1):193–8.
59. Mendlowitz SL, Manassis K, Bradley S, et al. Cognitive-behavioral group treatments in childhood anxiety disorders: the role of parental involvement. J Am Acad Child Adolesc Psychiatry 1999;38(10):1223–9.
60. Silverman WK, Kurtines WM, Ginsburg GS, et al. Contingency management, self-control, and education support in the treatment of childhood phobic disorders: a randomized clinical trial. J Consult Clin Psychol 1999;67(5):675–87.
61. Silverman WK, Kurtines WM, Ginsburg GS, et al. Treating anxiety disorders in children with group cognitive-behavioral therapy: a randomized clinical trial. J Consult Clin Psychol 1999;67(6):995–1003.
62. Beidel DC, Turner SM, Morris TL. Behavioral treatment of childhood social phobia. J Consult Clin Psychol 2000;68(6):1072–80.
63. Berman SL, Weems CF, Silverman WK, et al. Predictors of outcome in exposure-based cognitive and behavioral treatments for phobic and anxiety disorders in children. Behav Ther 2000;31(4):713–31.
64. Flannery-Schroeder EC, Kendall PC. Group and individual cognitive-behavioral treatments for youth with anxiety disorders: a randomized clinical trial. Cognit Ther Res 2000;24(3):251–78.
65. Hayward C, Varady S, Albano AM, et al. Cognitive-behavioral group therapy for social phobia in female adolescents: results of a pilot study. J Am Acad Child Adolesc Psychiatry 2000;39(6):721–6.

66. King NJ, Tonge BJ, Mullen P, et al. Treating sexually abused children with post-traumatic stress symptoms: a randomized clinical trial. J Am Acad Child Adolesc Psychiatry 2000;39(11):1347–55.
67. Spence SH, Donovan C, Brechman-Toussaint M. The treatment of childhood social phobia: the effectiveness of a social skills training-based, cognitive-behavioural intervention, with and without parental involvement. J Child Psychol Psychiatry 2000;41(6):713–26.
68. Barrett PM, Duffy AL, Dadds MR, et al. Cognitive-behavioral treatment of anxiety disorders in children: Long-term (6-year) follow-up. J Consult Clin Psychol 2001; 69(1):135–41.
69. Kendall PC, Brady EU, Verduin TL. Comorbidity in childhood anxiety disorders and treatment outcome. J Am Acad Child Adolesc Psychiatry 2001;40(7): 787–94.
70. Muris P, Mayer B, Bartelds E, et al. The revised version of the screen for child anxiety related emotional disorders (SCARED-R): treatment sensitivity in an early intervention trial for childhood anxiety disorders. Br J Clin Psychol 2001; 40(3):323–36.
71. Ost L-G, Svensson L, Hellstrom K, et al. One-session treatment of specific phobias in youths: a randomized clinical trial. J Consult Clin Psychol 2001; 69(5):814–24.
72. Southam-Gerow MA, Kendall PC, Weersing VR. Examining outcome variability: correlates of treatment response in a child and adolescent anxiety clinic. J Clin Child Psychol 2001;30(3):422–36.
73. Waters TL, Barrett PM, March JS. Cognitive-behavioral family treatment of childhood obsessive-compulsive disorder: preliminary findings. Am J Psychother 2001;55(3):372–87.
74. Heyne D, King NJ, Tonge BJ, et al. Evaluation of child therapy and caregiver training in the treatment of school refusal. J Am Acad Child Adolesc Psychiatry 2002;41(6):687–95.
75. Manassis K, Mendlowitz SL, Scapillato D, et al. Group and individual cognitive-behavioral therapy for childhood anxiety disorders. A randomized trial. J Am Acad Child Adolesc Psychiatry 2002;41(12):1423–30.
76. Muris P, Meesters C, Gobel M. Cognitive coping versus emotional disclosure in the treatment of anxious children: a pilot-study. Cogn Behav Ther 2002;31(2): 59–67.
77. Nauta MH, Scholing A, Emmelkamp PMG, et al. Cognitive-behavioral therapy for children with anxiety disorders in a clinical setting: no additional effect of a cognitive parent training. J Am Acad Child Adolesc Psychiatry 2003;42(11): 1270–8.
78. Pina AA, Silverman WK, Fuentes RM, et al. Exposure-based cognitive-behavioral treatment for phobic and anxiety disorders: treatment effects and maintenance for Hispanic/Latino relative to European-American youths. J Am Acad Child Adolesc Psychiatry 2003;42(10):1179–87.
79. Rapee RM. The influence of comorbidity on treatment outcome for children and adolescents with anxiety disorders. Behav Res Ther 2003;41(1):105–12.
80. Barrett P, Healy-Farrell L, March JS. Cognitive-behavioral family treatment of childhood obsessive-compulsive disorder: a controlled trial. J Am Acad Child Adolesc Psychiatry 2004;43(1):46–62.
81. Flannery-Schroeder E, Suveg C, Safford S, et al. Comorbid externalising disorders and child anxiety treatment outcomes. Behaviour Change 2004;21(1):14–25.

82. Gallagher HM, Rabian BA, McCloskey MS. A brief group cognitive-behavioral intervention for social phobia in childhood. J Anxiety Disord 2004;18(4): 459–79.
83. Kendall PC, Safford S, Flannery-Schroeder E, et al. Child anxiety treatment: outcomes in adolescence and impact on substance use and depression at 7.4-year follow-up. J Consult Clin Psychol 2004;72(2):276–87.
84. Manassis K, Avery D, Butalia S, et al. Cognitive-behavioral therapy with childhood anxiety disorders: functioning in adolescence. Depress Anxiety 2004; 19(4):209–16.
85. Pediatric OCD Treatment study team. Cognitive-behavior therapy, sertraline, and their combination for children and adolescents with obsessive-compulsive disorder: the pediatric OCD treatment study (POTS) randomized controlled trial. JAMA 2004;292(16):1969–76.
86. Asbahr FR, Castillo AR, Ito LM, et al. Group cognitive-behavioral therapy versus sertraline for the treatment of children and adolescents with obsessive-compulsive disorder. J Am Acad Child Adolesc Psychiatry 2005;44(11): 1128–36.
87. Baer S, Garland EJ. Pilot study of community-based cognitive behavioral group therapy for adolescents with social phobia. J Am Acad Child Adolesc Psychiatry 2005;44(3):258–64.
88. Beidel DC, Turner SM, Young B, et al. Social effectiveness therapy for children: three-year follow-up. J Consult Clin Psychol 2005;73(4):721–5.
89. Bernstein GA, Layne AE, Egan EA, et al. School-based interventions for anxious children. J Am Acad Child Adolesc Psychiatry 2005;44(11):1118–27.
90. Flannery-Schroeder E, Choudhury MS, Kendall PC, et al. Group and treatments for youth with anxiety disorders: 1-year follow-up. Cognit Ther Res 2005;29(2): 253–9.
91. Masia-Warner C, Klein RG, Dent HC, et al. School-based intervention for adolescents with social anxiety disorder: results of a controlled study. An official publication of the International Society for Research in Child and Adolescent Psychopathology. J Abnorm Child Psychol 2005;33(6):707–22.
92. Beidel DC, Turner SM, Young BJ. Social effectiveness therapy for children: five years later. Behav Ther 2006;37(4):416–25.
93. Lyneham HJ, Rapee RM. Evaluation of therapist-supported parent-implemented CBT for anxiety disorders in rural children. Behav Res Ther 2006;44(9):1287–300.
94. Rapee RM, Abbott MJ, Lyneham HJ. Bibliotherapy for children with anxiety disorders using written materials for parents: a randomized controlled trial. J Consult Clin Psychol 2006;74(3):436–44.
95. Spence SH, Holmes JM, March S, et al. The feasibility and outcome of clinic plus Internet delivery of cognitive-behavior therapy for childhood anxiety. J Consult Clin Psychol 2006;74(3):614–21.
96. Wood JJ, Piacentini JC, Southam-Gerow M, et al. Family cognitive behavioral therapy for child anxiety disorders. J Am Acad Child Adolesc Psychiatry 2006;45(3):314–21.
97. Beidel DC, Turner SM, Sallee FR, et al. SET-C versus fluoxetine in the treatment of childhood social phobia. J Am Acad Child Adolesc Psychiatry 2007;46(12): 1622–32.
98. Chalfant AM, Rapee R, Carroll L. Treating anxiety disorders in children with high functioning autism spectrum disorders: a controlled trial. J Autism Dev Disord 2007;37(10):1842–57.

99. de Groot J, Cobham V, Leong J, et al. Individual versus group family-focused cognitive-behaviour therapy for childhood anxiety: pilot randomized controlled trial. Aust N Z J Psychiatry 2007;41(12):990–7.

100. Levy K, Hunt C, Heriot S. Treating comorbid anxiety and aggression in children. J Am Acad Child Adolesc Psychiatry 2007;46(9):1111–8.

101. March JS, Franklin ME, Leonard H, et al. Tics moderate treatment outcome with sertraline but not cognitive-behavior therapy in pediatric obsessive-compulsive disorder. Biol Psychiatry 2007;61(3):344–7.

102. Masia Warner C, Fisher PH, Shrout PE, et al. Treating adolescents with social anxiety disorder in school: an attention control trial. J Child Psychol Psychiatry 2007;48(7):676–86.

103. Smith P, Yule W, Perrin S, et al. Cognitive-behavioral therapy for PTSD in children and adolescents: a preliminary randomized controlled trial. J Am Acad Child Adolesc Psychiatry 2007;46(8):1051–61.

104. Storch EA, Geffken GR, Merlo LJ, et al. Family-based cognitive-behavioral therapy for pediatric obsessive-compulsive disorder: comparison of intensive and weekly approaches. J Am Acad Child Adolesc Psychiatry 2007;46(4):469–78.

105. Victor AM, Bernat DH, Bernstein GA, et al. Effects of parent and family characteristics on treatment outcome of anxious children. J Anxiety Disord 2007;21(6):835–48.

106. Kendall PC, Hudson JL, Gosch E, et al. Cognitive-behavioral therapy for anxiety disordered youth: a randomized clinical trial evaluating child and family modalities. J Consult Clin Psychol 2008;76(2):282–97.

107. Warner CM, Reigada LC, Fisher PH, et al. CBT for anxiety and associated somatic complaints in pediatric medical settings: an open pilot study. J Clin Psychol Med Settings 2009;16(2):169–77.

108. Waters AM, Ford LA, Wharton TA, et al. Cognitive-behavioural therapy for young children with anxiety disorders: comparison of a child + parent condition versus a parent only condition. Behav Res Ther 2009;47(8):654–62.

109. Cobham VE, Dadds MR, Spence SH, et al. Parental anxiety in the treatment of childhood anxiety: a different story three years later. J Clin Child Adolesc Psychol 2010;39(3):410–20.

110. Garcia AM, Sapyta JJ, Moore PS, et al. Predictors and moderators of treatment outcome in the pediatric obsessive compulsive treatment study (POTS I). J Am Acad Child Adolesc Psychiatry 2010;49(10):1024–33.

Cognitive-Behavioral Therapy for Obsessive-Compulsive Disorder in Children and Adolescents

Katharina Kircanski, MA, CPhil*, Tara S. Peris, PhD,
John C. Piacentini, PhD, ABPP

KEYWORDS

- Obsessive-compulsive disorder • Cognitive-behavior therapy
- Exposure • Response prevention • Children/adolescents

Obsessive-compulsive disorder (OCD) is relatively common in children and adolescents, with a prevalence rate of 0.5% to 2% in community samples.[1–4] As defined by the *Diagnostic and Statistical Manual of Mental Disorders*, Fourth Edition, Text Revised (DSM-IV), OCD is characterized by obsessions and/or compulsions that are distressing, time-consuming (take more than 1 hour per day), or cause clinically significant impairment.[5] Obsessions are recurrent, persistent, and distressing thoughts, images, or impulses. Compulsions are repetitive behaviors or mental acts performed in response to obsessions in order to reduce distress or avoid perceived harm.

A growing body of research has demonstrated the efficacy of cognitive-behavioral therapy (CBT) for childhood OCD, both as a monotherapy and when combined with psychopharmacological interventions.[6–8] Based on a review of the literature and expert consensus, CBT is regarded as the initial treatment of choice for OCD in children and adolescents in terms of efficacy, safety, and durability of response.[9,10] This article reviews the clinical presentation and assessment of childhood OCD, cognitive-behavioral conceptualization of OCD, implementation of CBT for childhood OCD, and the body of evidence supporting this treatment approach.

Disclosures: See last page of article.

Division of Child and Adolescent Psychiatry, UCLA-Semel Institute for Neuroscience and Human Behavior, University of California-Los Angeles, 760 Westwood Plaza, Los Angeles, CA 90024, USA

* Corresponding author. Division of Child and Adolescent Psychiatry, UCLA-NPI, Room 68–218A, 760 Westwood Plaza, Los Angeles, CA 90024.

E-mail address: kkircanski@mednet.ucla.edu

Child Adolesc Psychiatric Clin N Am 20 (2011) 239–254
doi:10.1016/j.chc.2011.01.014
1056-4993/11/$ – see front matter © 2011 Elsevier Inc. All rights reserved.

CLINICAL PRESENTATION OF CHILDHOOD OCD

Most youth with OCD experience both obsessions and compulsions. Common obsessions involve excessive concern about germs, contamination, and illness, fear of harm to self or others, preoccupations with symmetry, moral and religious obsessions, intrusive sexual thoughts, and superstitious obsessions.[2,11,12] Common compulsions involve excessive and/or ritualized washing, checking, counting, touching, ordering, arranging, confessing, seeking reassurance, and mental rituals such as praying,[5,12] Compulsions may be performed to alleviate anxiety, discomfort, disgust, or the sense that something is "not right."[13]

Typical age of onset is from 8 to 11 years, although onset can occur as young as 2 to 3 years with emerging interest in early-onset childhood OCD.[14–17] Gender distribution tends to follow a 3:2 male to female ratio until adolescence, when this distribution evens out.[12] OCD in youth may be associated with significant functional impairment in home, daily living, school, and social domains.[18–23] Psychiatric comorbidities are highly common and include other anxiety disorders, mood disorders, attention-deficit hyperactivity disorder (ADHD), and tic disorders.[6,23–26] Of interest, comorbidity has been linked to greater OCD symptom severity and poorer response to CBT.[26–28] Pediatric OCD is a typically chronic condition, with 40% of youth meeting diagnostic criteria up to 15 years after initial identification and 20% exhibiting subclinical symptoms.[29,30] When untreated or inadequately treated, associated impairment tends to increase over time.[31]

ASSESSMENT OF CHILDHOOD OCD

A comprehensive diagnostic assessment is recommended for youth presenting with OCD. Initial evaluation should include assessment of current and past OCD symptoms, current symptom severity, associated functional impairment, and psychiatric comorbidity.[32] Evaluation should include information from multiple informants, as parent-child symptom agreement has been shown to be low.[33] In addition, one must distinguish OCD from normative ritualistic behavior in early childhood, and understand that youth may not recognize their symptoms as inappropriate or impairing or may be guarded about their symptoms because of fear of punishment or embarrassment.[2,11,34,35]

Several standardized measures exist for the assessment of childhood OCD, with the most commonly used presented here. The Anxiety Disorders Interview Schedule for DSM-IV—Parent and Child Version (ADIS-IV: PC) is a semi-structured clinician-administered diagnostic interview that is most commonly used in treatment studies to establish an OCD diagnosis, rule out phenomenologically similar conditions, and identify comorbidities.[36,37] The Children's Yale-Brown Obsessive Compulsive Scale (CY-BOCS) is a clinician-administered rating scale used to rate the severity of OCD symptoms.[37] The Children's Florida Obsessive-Compulsive Inventory (C-FOCI) is a brief screening instrument for pediatric OCD, and the Obsessive-Compulsive Inventory—Revised (OCI-R) measures distress associated with obsessions and compulsions.[38,39] The Child OCD Impact Scale-Revised (COIS-R) assesses OCD-related functional impairment via both parent and child self-report versions.[40] More detailed reviews of assessment strategies and instruments are provided by Merlo and colleagues[41] and Lewin and Piacentini.[37]

COGNITIVE AND BEHAVIORAL CONCEPTUALIZATIONS OF CHILDHOOD OCD
Behavioral Conceptualization

The behavioral model of OCD conceptualizes obsessions as intrusive and unwanted thoughts, images, or impulses that generate a significant and rapid increase in anxiety, distress, or discomfort, with compulsions as behaviors or cognitions that serve to reduce these negative feelings.[42] From the perspective of learning theory, compulsions become negatively reinforced over time by their ability to reduce obsession-triggered distress. In other words, the more successful compulsions are at reducing distress, the more powerful they become (the obsessive-compulsive cycle). For example, a child with fears of germs and illness may feel anxious or disgusted when confronted with the need to touch a doorknob (obsession). This distress triggers a strong desire to wash his or her hands repeatedly until they feel germ-free (compulsion). Further, each time the child engages in the compulsion (ie, hand-washing), the resultant decrease in distress strengthens the ritual (**Fig. 1**).

Cognitive Conceptualization

Cognitive models of OCD view beliefs as influential to the etiology and maintenance of OCD. Cognitive factors that have been associated with OCD in adults include exaggerated appraisals of risk, elevated responsibility for harm, and pathological self-doubt.[43–46] OCD in adults has also been associated with thought-action fusion (TAF), or the tendency to view negative thoughts and actions as equivalent.[47] Extant cognitive theories may not be fully adaptable to OCD in youth, due to children's more limited level of cognitive development.[48] Two studies comparing youth with OCD versus nonanxious controls found elevated responsibility for harm and TAF in the OCD group.[49,50] One study found the same pattern of cognitive distortions in children with OCD as in adults; however, these youths were largely similar to children with non-OCD anxiety.[51] Coles and colleagues[52] recently developed the Obsessive Belief Questionnaire—Child Version (OBQ-CV), a standardized measure of OCD-related beliefs in children, and found positive correlations between OCD symptom severity and elevated appraisals of risk and responsibility for harm, among other factors. The potential role of cognitive factors in childhood OCD warrants further investigation.[53]

FOUNDATIONS OF COGNITIVE-BEHAVIORAL TREATMENT FOR CHILDHOOD OCD
Exposure Plus Response Prevention

Exposure plus response prevention, or ERP, was developed several decades ago by Meyer[54] and remains the most effective form of behavior therapy for OCD. Originating

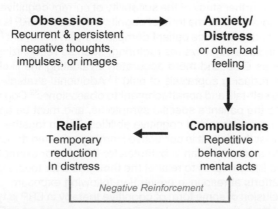

Fig. 1. The obsessive-compulsive cycle. (*Adapted from* Piacentini J, Langley A, Roblek T, et al. Treatment for childhood OCD: a combined individual child and family treatment manual. 3rd revision. Los Angeles (CA): UCLA Department of Psychiatry; 2003; with permission.)

from the behavioral model described earlier, ERP involves triggering the patient's obsessions (exposure) and assisting the patient in resisting his or her compulsions (response prevention), that is, breaking the cycle of negative reinforcement. Studies of adult OCD samples have found that both exposure and response prevention are necessary for clinical improvement.[55] Treatment traditionally proceeds in a gradual fashion according to a hierarchy of obsessive-compulsive symptoms arranged from the least distressing to the most distressing. In this manner, milder symptoms are first exposed, and exposures gradually become more difficult as treatment progresses. Treatment typically involves in vivo and/or imaginal exposure in session, followed by repeated practice in the patient's natural environment. Imaginal exposures are often useful for symptoms that are difficult to recreate in the therapy setting, symptoms that are initially too difficult for in vivo exposure, or pure obsessional symptoms.[31] It is postulated that over the course of repeated exposures, the distress associated with the triggering of obsessions gradually decreases through a process of autonomic habituation, and response prevention leads to the extinction of the negative reinforcement properties of the associated compulsion. In addition, successful completion of exposures is believed to facilitate the development and storage of corrective learning about the feared situation.[56,57] For example, the child with fears of germs and illness learns after repeatedly touching a doorknob and not washing hands that the feared consequences (eg, becoming sick) do not occur.

Although habituation is a purported mechanism of clinical improvement in exposure therapy, a recent review of the adult exposure therapy literature found no reliable evidence that the degree of habituation within session predicts clinical improvement, and only some evidence that the degree of habituation between sessions predicts improvement.[56–58] The emphasis on distress reduction in traditional models and methods of exposure therapy assumes that fear expression in session is commensurate with learning, although this is inconsistent with basic science research on learning.[59–61] Therefore, revised models of exposure therapy with adults emphasize the importance of fear or distress toleration in addition to reduction, which may be relevant to youth, as many children and adolescents with OCD do not experience immediate reduction in distress during ERP.[58] Further research is needed within the child exposure therapy literature to determine whether these adult findings translate to youth.

Cognitive Interventions

Despite the need for further study of the suitability of current cognitive models to OCD in youth, the incorporation of some form of cognitive therapy in ERP is somewhat standard and may be used to enhance patient compliance with treatment.[62] Typical cognitive interventions include cognitive restructuring, such as recognizing and relabeling intrusive thoughts as OCD and more accurately evaluating the likelihood of feared consequences (ie, reducing appraisals of risk).[48] Additional strategies include developing constructive self-talk and nonattachment to obsessions.[32] Cognitive techniques must be tailored to the patient's specific symptoms, and must be appropriate to the patient's developmental stage and cognitive abilities. Taken together, cognitive interventions aim to assist the patient in corrective learning achieved through ERP, and are viewed as facilitators of rather than substitutes for ERP.[63] For example, the child with fears of germs and illness learns to relabel the thoughts after touching a doorknob as OCD, facilitating efforts at response prevention following exposure.

Although the inclusion of some form of cognitive therapy in ERP is typical, the incremental efficacy of its inclusion is unclear. Several studies of adult OCD have found cognitive interventions to be efficacious, although more recent research comparing ERP plus cognitive therapy with ERP plus relaxation training found no differential benefit.[64–66] To date no studies have examined the incremental efficacy of cognitive interventions to ERP for childhood OCD.

DEVELOPMENTAL CONSIDERATIONS IN THE TREATMENT OF CHILDHOOD OCD

As stated earlier, CBT for youth with OCD has largely been adapted from adult models of treatment; however, several developmental factors have been noted to complicate treatment in children and adolescents. For example, many young children have difficulty describing specific obsessions or recognizing the role of obsessions in triggering rituals. Young children also tend to have a present-orientation that, relative to adults, may decrease their willingness to engage in difficult therapeutic exercises despite the potential for future symptom relief. Youths with OCD may also have less insight than adults and may be less likely to describe their symptoms as unrealistic and/or excessive, which may similarly decrease motivation for treatment. In addition to high levels of psychiatric comorbidity, low frustration tolerance and poor coping abilities can complicate treatment. As each of these developmental factors will apply differentially to different cases, optimal treatment planning entails careful evaluation of these variables.

The most successful CBT packages for youth with OCD have included elements to address these developmental considerations intrinsic to working with children and adolescents.[32,48,67] For instance, many CBT protocols include psychoeducation tailored to the child's level of cognitive development, the use of age-appropriate metaphors to facilitate cognitive restructuring, behavioral reward systems to enhance treatment compliance, and as described in the next section, greater parent involvement in treatment.[24,67–69] A detailed description of treatment tailored to OCD in early childhood is presented by Hirschfeld-Becker and colleagues elsewhere in this issue.

FAMILY FACTORS IN THE TREATMENT OF CHILDHOOD OCD

Given the developmental considerations intrinsic to treating child and adolescent OCD, family involvement in treatment is particularly important. Virtually all protocols for individual child OCD treatment call for some degree of family participation, with treatments that more directly target the family becoming increasingly more popular.[9,24,67,70,71] At the most basic level, work with families has been aimed at providing them with psychoeducation about OCD and general behavior management strategies to help them support the child's exposure-based exercises. However, there has been growing emphasis on examining family factors associated with childhood OCD more fully, to see how these features might interact with the treatment process and, in turn, what can be done to address them.

Families of youth with OCD contend with a unique set of difficulties in that they are often actively involved in symptoms. Parents may provide frequent reassurance to distressed youngsters or provide items needed to complete rituals (eg, soap, clean towels). Siblings may assume responsibility for chores that are too difficult for the affected child to complete or may facilitate avoidance of triggering stimuli. This involvement in symptoms, labeled accommodation, can take many forms, and is exceedingly common among families of youth with OCD. Indeed, recent research suggests that more than half of all families with a child with OCD participate in rituals in some form or another on a daily basis.[19] Accommodation of symptoms is problematic because it is likely to interfere directly with the key tasks of exposure-based treatment by reinforcing fear and avoidance behaviors. Indeed, there is evidence that family accommodation may mediate the link between OCD symptom severity and parent-reporting of child functional impairment, and that decreases in accommodation predict treatment outcome for youth receiving CBT for OCD.[70–72]

Beyond accommodation, however, rates of distress and disrupted family functioning are also notably high, underscoring the burden with which these families contend.[73] High rates of blame, hostility, and criticism are also common correlates of childhood OCD.[74,75] These family features, although less studied in child and adolescent OCD, are likely to be relevant for treatment in that they create an emotionally charged home environment that may complicate successful completion of exposure exercises. Given this fact, an important component of assessment and case conceptualization rests with a careful consideration of family functioning, including areas of accommodation, attributions about OCD, and emotional reactions to the issues raised by the disorder.

SPECIFIC COGNITIVE-BEHAVIORAL TREATMENT STRATEGIES
Psychoeducation

Following a comprehensive diagnostic assessment, the initial phase of CBT, typically the first session, centers on educating the patient and family about OCD, introducing the cognitive-behavioral conceptualization of OCD, and explaining what the treatment will entail. The involvement of parents during this phase may vary with the age and developmental level of the child, and can be negotiated up-front with the therapist. Psychoeducation aims to reduce stigma in the child, address a range of negative feelings (eg, anger, blame, hopelessness) in the family, and give the child and parents a sense of confidence in the therapy and therapist.

OCD and anxiety are presented as relatively common problems, and to help reduce stigma the therapist may describe prevalence rates of OCD in the context of the child's school (eg, in a school with 1000 students, between 10 and 20 children will be affected).[48] The concept of OCD as a neurobehavioral disorder, albeit with a role for environmental influences, may also help to reduce family members' negative reactions to the child's symptoms, such as the view that the behaviors are intentional.[20,68] The nature and chronicity of OCD may also be likened to another medical condition (eg, asthma, diabetes) for this purpose. It is important to describe CBT as a psychological treatment that can be very effective in improving the child's control over fears and compulsions. In addition, as some OCD symptoms may return in the future, particularly during times of change or stress, the child can use skills learned in CBT to help control them again. The metaphor of OCD as a "false fire alarm" in the brain (eg, feeling nervous and thinking something bad is going to happen, even though there is no real danger) further assists as a framework for understanding OCD.[20] Treatment may be described as a way for the child to learn that OCD fears are false alarms and that if the child ignores them nothing bad will happen. The cognitive-behavioral conceptualization of OCD illustrates the manner in which ritualizing in response to obsessions actually reinforces the OCD cycle, and that treatment will involve resisting rituals to make OCD weaker. Lastly, with regard to the concepts of repeated exposure and autonomic habituation, the metaphor of slowly entering a swimming pool (eg, at first it feels cold, however after a few minutes the body becomes accustomed to it and it does not feel so cold anymore) may be helpful in reducing anticipatory anxiety. However, as noted earlier, habituation is not the immediate goal of ERP, and distress toleration may also be a useful skill for the child to learn in treatment. Underscoring the importance of psychoeducation, patient and family understanding, and acceptance of the treatment rationale may affect compliance and ultimate success of the interventions.

Creation of Symptom Hierarchy

The next step in treatment, following from the discussion of habituation described earlier, involves creation of the graduated OCD symptom hierarchy. The symptom hierarchy guides the design of individual ERP tasks, described in the next section, and determines the order in which they will be attempted. The CY-BOCS includes a symptom checklist that may provide a useful starting point for this purpose. The therapist asks the child, and/or parents if necessary, to rank the distress associated with each obsession and compulsion using a fear thermometer (**Fig. 2**). For some symptoms, it may be useful to describe specific exposure tasks (eg, resisting hand-washing for 5 minutes) and obtain rankings of distress associated with each of these tasks. Each symptom or task is given a ranking from 1 (least distressing) to 10 (most distressing).

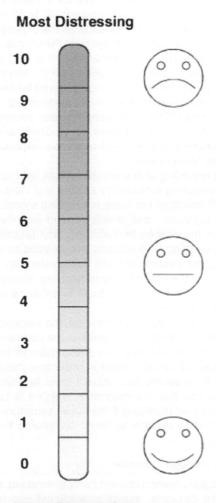

Fig. 2. OCD fear thermometer. (*Adapted from* Piacentini J, Langley A, Roblek T, et al. Treatment for childhood OCD: a combined individual child and family treatment manual. 3rd revision. Los Angeles (CA): UCLA Department of Psychiatry; 2003; with permission.)

Once the hierarchy is completed, the therapist and patient select an initial ERP task. The starting task should be a concrete behavior that is associated with relatively low distress and is easily able to be recreated in the therapy session. That is, the therapist should consider a task for which the child is likely to be successful, in order to engender feelings of self-efficacy and enhance the child's motivation for further ERP.

Exposure Plus Response Prevention

ERP comprises the largest portion of cognitive-behavioral treatment. For in-session ERP tasks, in general the therapist encourages the child to have contact with the feared stimulus (eg, doorknob) and resist all associated rituals or other distress-reduction actions (eg, distraction) over the entire exposure period. It is important that in-session ERP tasks be as realistic as possible in order to trigger the patient's distress and lead to generalization to the natural environments in which the symptoms occur.[76] Distress ratings are typically assessed every 30 to 60 seconds at the onset of the exposure trial and may occur less frequently as the exposure trial proceeds. The therapist may graph the child's distress ratings over the course of the exposure trial to monitor the pattern of habituation. In traditional models of CBT for OCD, the exposure trial is conducted until distress ratings decrease by 50%. However, as noted earlier in the adult exposure therapy literature, habituation may not be necessary for learning to occur, and reducing distress to very low levels or "overlearning" does not seem to lead to improved clinical outcomes.[58] Graphing can, however, provide a visual demonstration to the child of any habituation that does occur, and help to identify more distressing aspects of the exposure that may need additional exposure or other treatment techniques (eg, cognitive restructuring).

In addition, therapist modeling of the exposure task and coping strategies to be employed can assist in reducing anticipatory anxiety and increasing use of constructive self-talk during ERP practice. For more distressing symptoms (eg, touching the doorknob of a public bathroom and resisting hand-washing), the therapist may need to gradually shape the desired behavior (eg, first touching the doorknob with one finger and resisting washing for 5 minutes, progressing to touching the doorknob with the entire hand and not washing entirely). ERP tasks may also progress beyond what would be expected in the natural environment (eg, touching the doorknob with the hand, and then putting the hand to the face) to enhance corrective learning that the feared outcome will not occur.

Once an ERP task has been practiced in session, the therapist instructs the child to practice the task at least several times per week in the natural environments in which the symptom occurs. The therapist and child and/or parents negotiate locations and times in which exposures will be completed in order to enhance homework compliance. An ERP practice form serves as a visual trigger for the child to complete the task out of session and specifies the manner in which it is to be completed. Also, the child is instructed to resist ritualizing if the target symptom arises naturalistically. The child is not expected to be able to resist symptoms that have not yet been addressed in treatment.

Addressing Obsessions Through Exposure

Obsessions occurring in the absence of overt compulsions (eg, fears of harm to self or others, violent or horrific thoughts, sexual obsessions) can be addressed through behavioral and imaginal exposure as well. Exposure similarly proceeds in a gradual fashion, and may involve imagining the feared stimuli, writing about the feared stimuli, drawing the feared stimuli, describing the thoughts or images aloud, having the therapist describe the feared scenario to the child, and recording the child describing the scenario and listening to it repeatedly. Children and adolescents may deny associated compulsions; however, it is common for intrusive obsessions to give rise to cognitive compulsions (eg, thought suppression, ritualistic neutralizing thoughts) and/or behavioral compulsions (eg, avoiding contact with triggering stimuli). In such cases, these avoidance behaviors can be added to the symptom hierarchy and resisted in subsequent exposure tasks. An adaptation of exposure procedures for youth with OCD entails changing the emotional valence of the obsessional thought or image using age-appropriate strategies. For example, the child may sing, rap, or rhyme the content of the obsession, or change the image to a benign or humorous one (eg, imagining a water pistol instead of a real gun).

Cognitive Restructuring

Although further research is needed regarding the role of cognitive factors in childhood OCD, as described earlier, cognitive interventions can facilitate the course of ERP. As stated, recognizing and relabeling intrusive thoughts as OCD and developing constructive self-talk may help to enhance child understanding and motivation, and help to manage extreme anxiety.[32,40,62] More accurate estimation of the probability of feared events may be achieved through questions about the number of other people or specific people (eg, parents) who have come in contact with the feared stimulus and have not experienced the feared event (eg, the number of people who have touched a doorknob and have not become sick). The child may also be taught certain self-statements to use during ERP to increase the likelihood of ERP completion in the face of distress (eg, OCD is "playing a trick" on the brain, and through exposure the child is becoming "stronger" than the OCD).[20,32]

Contingency Management

A structured reward program is typically incorporated into CBT for childhood OCD to increase treatment compliance.[32,77] Of importance, the child or adolescent is rewarded for the effort involved in completing CBT tasks in and out of session, and not for habituation of distress. The specific rewards used may depend on the age of the child, as younger children tend to prefer concrete external rewards and adolescents tend to report less need for such rewards. The use of a reward program is explained by the therapist at treatment outset, and nature and type of rewards are negotiated among the child, parents, and therapist. Social reinforcement (eg, praise) is given by the therapist, parents, and others who are close to the child.

EMPIRICAL SUPPORT

Evidence in support of CBT for childhood OCD continues to mount. A recent meta-analysis of randomized controlled trials for pediatric OCD yielded a large effect size of 1.45 (95% confidence interval [CI] = 0.68–2.22).[8] This level of response, coupled with a growing number of studies documenting its efficacy, tolerability, and durability of response, has led to its designation as the first-line treatment for mild to moderate OCD in children and adolescents.[7–9,78] However, further research is needed to establish and optimize CBT for childhood OCD, especially relative to other pediatric disorders. In fact, no treatments for pediatric OCD currently meet criteria for a well-established evidence-based psychosocial treatment.[79]

A series of early single-case studies and open clinical trials of CBT for childhood OCD (eg, single case studies, open clinical trials) documented the acceptability and feasibility of CBT for childhood OCD and provided preliminary data regarding the efficacy and durability of this treatment.[69,80,81]

To date, 4 published controlled trials have assessed outcomes of individual CBT for OCD in children and adolescents.[7,24,70,71,82] Only 3 of these trials meet criteria for a Type I study (most methodologically rigorous) based on the Nathan and Gorman criteria.[9] Barrett and colleagues[24] compared individual cognitive-behavioral family-based therapy (CBFT), group CBFT, and wait-list control. At posttreatment (14 weeks), both active conditions were associated with significant improvement in OCD symptoms, and gains were largely maintained at 6-month follow-up. The Pediatric OCD Treatment Study, the largest controlled trial for childhood OCD to date, compared CBT, a selective serotonin reuptake inhibitor (SSRI) (sertraline [Zoloft; SER]), their combination (COMB), and pill placebo (PBO), over a 12-week treatment period followed by an additional 4 weeks of treatment for those who responded, with multiple follow-up assessment periods.[7] Using an intent-to-treat analytical strategy, COMB was found to outperform CBT and SER, which did not differ from one another, and all 3 conditions outperformed PBO. Of interest, further analyses based on CY-BOCS scores revealed that the 2 groups receiving CBT included greater proportions of "excellent responders" than the SER group. Finally, Piacentini and colleagues[70] (under review) tested the efficacy of a family-focused CBT protocol for childhood CBT (FCBT) against a credible psychosocial treatment involving psychoeducation and relaxation training (PRT). Results demonstrated greater reduction in CY-BOCS scores and OCD-related functional impairment in the FCBT group than in the PRT group. FCBT was also associated with greater decreases in family accommodation relative to PRT, and changes in family accommodation were found to precede improvement in the CY-BOCS and mediate reductions in child-reported functional impairment. Treatment gains were largely durable over a 6-month follow-up period.

Both of the non–Type I studies compared 2 established interventions for OCD. de Haan and colleagues[82] found CBT to be more efficacious than clomipramine (Anafranil) with regard to response rate and symptom reduction, although this study did not include a no-treatment control group. Storch and colleagues[71] compared intensive versus weekly individual CBT, which also included a structured family component, and demonstrated a 75% response rate (CY-BOCS total score of 10 or lower) in the intensive treatment condition and 50% in the weekly condition.

Predictors of Treatment Response

Several potentially important findings have emerged regarding predictors of response to treatment for childhood OCD. Greater symptom severity and poorer academic and social functioning at baseline has been associated with poorer outcome of CBT.[69,83] As stated earlier, psychiatric comorbidity has also been associated with poorer response to CBT.[28] In a recent review, poorer family functioning and greater symptom severity predicted poorer response to CBT, whereas comorbid tics and externalizing disorders predicted poorer response to medication.[84] Secondary analyses of the Pediatrics OCD Treatment Study (POTS) data similarly indicate that comorbid tics may affect outcome of medication treatment but not CBT.[7,85]

Psychopharmacology

The existing treatment literature also supports the efficacy and tolerability of pharmacological intervention for OCD in youth, specifically with the SSRIs.[9,78,86,87] Large-scaled controlled trials have indicated efficacy and tolerability of clomipramine (Anafranil), fluoxetine (Prozac), sertraline (Zoloft), and fluvoxamine (Luvox) for OCD in children and adolescents. In their meta-analysis of published psychopharmacology trials for pediatric OCD, Geller and colleagues[86] reported an overall effect size of 0.48 (95% CI = 0.36–0.61). Although methodological differences complicate direct comparison of the psychopharmacological and CBT treatment literature, the relatively modest effect size reported by Geller and colleagues is considerably smaller than that reported for CBT (eg, 1.45).[8] In the POTS study, the effect size for CBT-alone was larger than that for sertraline-alone (0.97 vs 0.67, respectively).[7] In addition, a higher proportion of children receiving CBT-alone achieved remission as compared with those in the sertraline-alone condition (39.3% vs 21.4%, respectively). However, neither of these group differences were statistically significant. Although, as noted earlier, CBT is generally considered the first-line treatment for pediatric OCD in most cases, SSRI medication can play an important role in the treatment of youth who do not fully respond to CBT, whose symptoms are too severe to allow for exposure-based treatment, and who exhibit multiple comorbidities, or in situations in which quality CBT is unavailable.

SUMMARY

Although ERP emerged as a treatment modality several decades ago, its optimal adaptation for child and adolescent OCD continues to evolve. The past two decades have seen the advancement of developmentally sensitive, multimodal treatment protocols for use across childhood and adolescence, along with an increase in methodologically rigorous, randomized controlled outcome trials of these treatments. However, further research is greatly needed. For example, as psychiatric comorbidity, which remains the norm in childhood OCD, has been shown to complicate treatment, optimal intervention is dependent on a clearer understanding of this complication and how best to address it in treatment. In addition, while ERP continues to be viewed as the primary component of treatment, cognitive and family-based interventions are areas of growing interest. In particular, evidence that family factors such as accommodation may mediate treatment outcome underscores the need for targeted family interventions that move beyond traditional psychoeducation and behavior management approaches to address family-level variables.[70,72] Future research will also need to address predictors and mechanisms of outcome across different treatment conditions, and bridge the gap between the basic science of learning and the models and methods of exposure therapy through increasingly translational methodologies.

DISCLOSURES

Drs Kircanski, Peris, and Piacentini have received grant support from the National Institute of Mental Health. In addition, Dr Piacentini has received grant support from the Tourette Syndrome Association, the Obsessive Compulsive Foundation, and the Eisner Family Foundation. He has also received royalties from Oxford University Press for the OCD treatment manuals described in this article and for treatment manuals on tic disorders, and from Guilford Press and from the American Psychological Association Press for books on child mental health. In addition, he has received a consultancy fee from Bayer Schering Pharma and speaking honoraria for CME presentations from the Tourette Syndrome Association.

REFERENCES

1. Apter A, Pauls DL, Bleich A, et al. An epidemiologic study of Gilles de la Tourette's syndrome in Israel. Arch Gen Psychiatry 1993;50(9):734–8.
2. Moore PS, Mariaskin A, March J, et al. Obsessive-compulsive disorder in children and adolescents: diagnosis, comorbidity, and developmental factors. In: Storch EA, Geffken GR, Murphy TK, editors. Handbook of child and adolescent

obsessive-compulsive disorder. Mahwah (NJ): Lawrence Erlbaum Associates Publishers; 2007. p. 17–45.

3. Rapoport J, Inoff-Germain G, Weissman MM, et al. Childhood obsessive-compulsive disorder in the NIMH MECA Study: parent versus child identification of cases. J Anxiety Disord 2000;14(6):535–48.

4. Valleni-Basile L, Garrison C, Jackson K, et al. Frequency of obsessive-compulsive disorder in a community sample of young adolescents. J Am Acad Child Adolesc Psychiatry 1994;33(6):782–91.

5. American Psychiatric Association. Diagnostic and statistical manual of mental disorders, text revision. 4th edition. Washington, DC: American Psychiatric Association; 2000.

6. Barrett P, Healy L, Piacentini J, et al. Treatment of OCD in children and adolescents. In: Barrett P, Ollendick T, editors. Handbook of interventions that work with children and adolescents. West Sussex (UK): Wiley; 2004. p. 187–216.

7. Pediatric OCD Treatment Study Team. Cognitive-behavioral therapy, sertraline, and their combination for children and adolescents with obsessive-compulsive disorder: the Pediatric OCD Treatment Study (POTS) randomized controlled trial. JAMA 2004;292(16):1969–76.

8. Watson HJ, Rees CS. Meta-analysis of randomized, controlled treatment trials for pediatric obsessive-compulsive disorder. J Child Psychol Psychiatry 2008;49(5): 489–98.

9. Barrett P, Farrell L, Pina A, et al. Evidence-based psychosocial treatments for child and adolescent OCD. J Clin Child Adolesc Psychol 2008;37:131–55.

10. March J, Frances A, Carpenter D, et al. Expert consensus guidelines: treatment of obsessive-compulsive disorder. J Clin Psychiatry 1997;58(4):1–72.

11. Geller DA, Hoog SL, Heiligenstein JH, et al. The fluoxetine treatment for obsessive-compulsive disorder in children and adolescents: a placebo-controlled clinical trial. J Am Acad Child Adolesc Psychiatry 2001;40(7):773–9.

12. Swedo S, Rapoport J, Leonard H, et al. Obsessive-compulsive disorder in children and adolescents: clinical phenomenology of 70 consecutive cases. Arch Gen Psychiatry 1989;46(4):335–41.

13. Leckman JF, Grice DE, Barr LC, et al. Tic-related vs. non-tic-related obsessive compulsive disorder. Anxiety 1994;1(5):208–15.

14. Hanna G. Demographic and clinical features of obsessive-compulsive disorder in children and adolescents. J Am Acad Child Adolesc Psychiatry 1995;34:19–27.

15. Chabane N, Delome R, Millet B, et al. Early-onset obsessive compulsive disorder: a subgroup with a specific clinical and familial pattern. J Child Psychol Psychiatry 2005;46(8):881–7.

16. Rapoport J, Swedo SE, Leonard HL. Childhood obsessive-compulsive disorder. J Clin Psychiatry 1992;53:S11–6.

17. Garcia AM, Freeman JB, Himle MB, et al. Phenomenology of early childhood onset obsessive compulsive disorder. J Psychopathol Behav Assess 2009; 31(2):104–11.

18. Markarian Y, Larson MJ, Aldea MA, et al. Multiple pathways to functional impairment in obsessive compulsive disorder. Clin Psychol Rev 2009;30: 78–88.

19. Peris TS, Bergman RL, Langley A, et al. Correlates of family accommodation of childhood obsessive compulsive disorder: parent, child, and family characteristics. J Am Acad Child Adolesc Psychiatry 2008;47(10):1173–81.

20. Piacentini J, Langley A, Roblek T. Cognitive-behavioral treatment of childhood OCD. New York: Oxford University Press; 2007.

21. Piacentini J, Bergman RL, Keller M, et al. Functional impairment in children and adolescents with obsessive compulsive disorder. J Child Adolsec Psychopharmacol 2003;13:S61–9.

22. Storch EA, Larson MJ, Muroff J, et al. Predictors of functional impairment in pediatric obsessive-compulsive disorder. J Anxiety Disord 2010;24(2):275–83.

23. Valderhaug R, Ivarsson T. Functional impairment in clinical samples of Norwegian and Swedish children and adolescents with obsessive-compulsive disorder. Eur Child Adolesc Psychiatry 2005;14(3):164–73.

24. Barrett P, Healy-Farrell L, March J. Cognitive-behavioral family treatment of childhood obsessive-compulsive disorder: a controlled trial. J Am Acad Child Adolesc Psychiatry 2004;43:46–62.

25. Ivarsson T, Melin K, Wallin L. Categorical and dimensional aspects of comorbidity in obsessive-compulsive disorder (OCD). Eur Child Adolesc Psychiatry 2008;17:20–31.

26. Langley A, Bergman RL, Lewin A, et al. Correlates of comorbid anxiety and externalizing disorders in childhood obsessive compulsive disorder. Eur Child Adolesc Psychiatry 2010;19(8):637–45.

27. Storch EA, Larson MJ, Merlo MJ, et al. Cormorbidity of pediatric obsessive compulsive disorder and anxiety disorders: impact on symptom severity and impairment. J Psychopathol Behav Assess 2008;30(2):111–20.

28. Storch EA, Merlo LJ, Larson MJ, et al. Impact of comorbidity on cognitive-behavioral therapy response in pediatric obsessive-compulsive disorder. J Am Acad Child Adolesc Psychiatry 2008;47(5):583–92.

29. Leonard H, Swedo S, Lenane M, et al. A two- to seven-year follow-up study of 54 obsessive-compulsive children and adolescents. Arch Gen Psychiatry 1993; 50(6):429–39.

30. Stewart S, Geller D, Jenike M, et al. Long-term outcome of pediatric obsessive-compulsive disorder: a meta-analysis and qualitative review of the literature. Acta Psychiatr Scand 2004;110:4–13.

31. Piacentini J, Peris T, March J, et al. Cognitive-behavioral therapy for youngsters with obsessive-compulsive disorder. In: Kendall P, editor. Child and adolescent therapy: cognitive-behavioral procedures. 4th edition. New York: Guilford, in press.

32. March J, Franklin ME. Cognitive-behavioral therapy for pediatric OCD. In: Rothbaum BO, editor. Pathological anxiety: emotional processing in etiology and treatment. New York: Guilford Press; 2006. p. 147–65.

33. Canavera KE, Wilkins KC, Pincus DB, et al. Parent-child agreement in the assessment of obsessive-compulsive disorder. J Clin Child Adolesc Psychol 2009;38(6): 909–15.

34. Evans DW, Leckman JF, Carter A, et al. Ritual, habit, and perfectionism: the prevalence and development of compulsive-like behavior in normal young children. Child Dev 1997;68:58–68.

35. Snider LA, Swedo SE. Pediatric obsessive compulsive disorder. JAMA 2001; 284(24):3104–6.

36. Silverman W, Albano AM. Anxiety disorders interview schedule for DSM-IV: parent version. San Antonio (TX): Graywing; 1996.

37. Lewin A, Piacentini J. Evidence-based assessment of child obsessive compulsive disorder: recommendations for clinical practice and treatment research. Child Youth Care Forum 2010;39(2):73–89.

38. Storch EA, Khanna M, Merlo LJ, et al. Children's Florida obsessive compulsive inventory: psychometric properties and feasibility of a self-report measure of

obsessive-compulsive symptoms in youth. Child Psychiatry Hum Dev 2009;40(3): 467–83.

39. Foa EB, Huppert JD, Leiberg S, et al. The Obsessive-Compulsive Inventory: development and validation of a short version. Psychol Assess 2002;14(4): 485–96.

40. Piacentini J, Peris TS, Bergman RL, et al. The Child Obsessive Compulsive Impact Scale-Revised (COIS-R): development and psychometric properties. J Clin Child Adolesc Psychol 2007;36(4):645–53.

41. Merlo LJ, Storch EA, Adkins JW, et al. Assessment of pediatric obsessive-compulsive disorder. In: Storch EA, Geffken GR, Murphy TK, editors. Handbook of child and adolescent obsessive-compulsive disorder. Mahwah (NJ): Lawrence Erlbaum Associates Publishers; 2007. p. 67–107.

42. Albano AM, March JS, Piacentini JC. Cognitive behavioral treatment of obsessive-compulsive disorder. In: Ammerman RT, editor. Handbook of prescriptive treatments for children and adolescents. Boston: Allyn & Bacon; 1999. p. 193–213.

43. Freeston MH, Ladouceur R. Appraisals of cognitive intrusions and response style: replication and extension. Behav Res Ther 1993;31(2):185–91.

44. Salkovskis PM. Obsessional compulsive problems: a cognitive-behavioural analysis. Behav Res Ther 1985;23(5):571–83.

45. Salkovskis PM. Cognitive behavioural factors and the persistence of intrusive thoughts in obsessional problems. Behav Res Ther 1989;27(6):677–82.

46. Shafran R. The manipulation of responsibility in obsessive-compulsive disorder. Br J Clin Psychol 1997;36(3):397–407.

47. Rachman S. Obsessions, responsibility, and guilt. Behav Res Ther 1993;31: 149–54.

48. Piacentini J, Langley A. Cognitive-behavioral therapy for children who have obsessive-compulsive disorder. J Clin Psychol 2004;60(11):1181–94.

49. Scahill L, Riddle MA, McSwiggan-Hardin MT, et al. Children's Yale-Brown obsessive compulsive scale: reliability and validity. J Am Acad Child Adolesc Psychiatry 1997;36(6):844–52.

50. Salkovskis P, Shafran R, Rachman S, et al. Multiple pathways to inflated responsibility beliefs in obsessional problems: possible origins and implications for therapy and research. Behav Res Ther 1999;37(11):1055–72.

51. Barrett P, Healy L. An examination of the cognitive processes involved in childhood obsessive-compulsive disorder. Behav Res Ther 2003;41(3):285–99.

52. Coles ME, Wolters LH, Sochting I, et al. Development and initial validation of the obsessive belief questionnaire—child version (OBQ-CV). Depress Anxiety 2010; 27(10):982–91.

53. Comer J, Kendall PC, Franklin M, et al. Obsessing/worrying about the overlap between obsessive-compulsive disorder and generalized anxiety disorder in youth. Clin Psychol Rev 2004;24(6):663–83.

54. Meyer V. Modification of expectations in cases with obsessive rituals. Behav Res Ther 1966;4(4):273–80.

55. Foa E, Steketee G, Grayson J, et al. Deliberate exposure and blocking of obsessive compulsive rituals: Immediate and long-term effects. Behav Ther 1984;15(5): 450–72.

56. Foa E, Kozak M. Emotional processing of fear: exposure to corrective information. Psychol Bull 1986;99:450–72.

57. Foa EB, McNally RJ. Mechanisms of change in exposure therapy. In: Rapee R, editor. Current controversies in the anxiety disorders. New York: Guilford; 1996. p. 329–43.

58. Craske MG, Kircanski K, Zelikowski M, et al. Optimizing inhibitory learning during exposure therapy. Behav Res Ther 2008;46:5–27.
59. Bjork RA, Bjork EL. Optimizing treatment and instruction: implications of a new theory of disuse. In: Nilsson LJ, Ohta N, editors. Memory and society: psychological perspectives. New York: Psychology Press; 2006. p. 116–40.
60. Bouton ME, Garcia-Gutierrez A, Zilski J, et al. Extinction in multiple contexts does not necessarily make extinction less vulnerable to relapse. Behav Res Ther 2006; 44(7):983–4.
61. Rescorla RA. Deepened extinction from compound stimulus presentation. J Exp Psychol Anim Behav Process 2006;32:135–44.
62. Soechting I, March J. Cognitive aspects of obsessive compulsive disorder in children. In: Frost R, Steketee G, editors. Cognitive approaches to obsessions and compulsions: theory, assessment, and treatment. Amsterdam: Pergamon/Elsevier Science; 2002. p. 299–314.
63. Franklin ME, Foa EB. Cognitive-behavioral treatment of obsessive compulsive disorder. In: Nathan P, Gorman J, editors. A guide to treatments that work. 2nd edition. Oxford (UK): Oxford University Press; 2002. p. 367–86.
64. Abramowitz JS. Effectiveness of psychological and pharmacological treatments for obsessive-compulsive disorder: a quantitative review. J Consult Clin Psychol 1997;65:44–52.
65. van Balkom A, de Haan E, van Oppen P, et al. Cognitive and behavioral therapies alone versus in combination with fluvoxamine in the treatment of obsessive compulsive disorder. J Nerv Ment Dis 1998;186(8):492–9.
66. Vogel PA, Stiles TC, Gotestam KG. Adding cognitive therapy elements to exposure therapy for obsessive compulsive disorder: a controlled study. Behav Cogn Psychother 2004;32:275–90.
67. Freeman J, Garcia AM, Coyne L. Early childhood OCD: preliminary findings from a family-based cognitive behavioral approach. J Am Acad Child Adolesc Psychiatry 2008;47(5):593–602.
68. March JS, Mulle K. OCD in children and adolescents: a cognitive-behavioral treatment manual. New York: Guilford Press; 1998.
69. Piacentini J, Bergman RL, Jacobs C, et al. Open trial of cognitive behavior therapy for childhood obsessive-compulsive disorder. J Anxiety Disord 2002; 16(2):207–19.
70. Piacentini J, Bergman LB, Chang S, et al. Controlled comparison of family cognitive behavioral therapy and psychoeducation/relaxation-training for child OCD, in press.
71. Storch EA, Geffken GR, Merlo LJ, et al. Family-based cognitive-behavioral therapy for pediatric obsessive-compulsive disorder: comparisons of intensive and weekly approaches. J Am Acad Child Adolesc Psychiatry 2007;46(4):469–78.
72. Merlo LJ, Lehmkuhl HD, Geffken GR, et al. Decreased family accommodation associated with improved therapy outcome in pediatric obsessive-compulsive disorder. J Consult Clin Psychol 2009;77(2):355–60.
73. Piacentini J, Langley A, Roblek T, et al. Multimodal CBT treatment for childhood OCD: a combined individual child and family treatment manual. 3rd revision. Los Angeles (CA): UCLA Department of Psychiatry; 2003.
74. Hibbs E, Hamburger S, Lenane M. Determinants of expressed emotion in families of disturbed and normal children. J Child Psychol Psychiatry 1991;32(5):757–70.
75. Peris TS, Roblek T, Langley A, et al. Parental responses to obsessive compulsive disorder: development and validation of the parental attitudes and behaviors scale (PABS). Child Fam Behav Ther 2008;30(3):199–214.

76. Kendall PC, Robin J, Hedtke K, et al. Considering CBT with anxious youth? Think exposures. Cogn Behav Pract 2005;12:136–48.
77. Owens E, Piacentini J. Behavioral treatment of obsessive-compulsive disorder in a boy with comorbid disruptive behavior problems. J Am Acad Child Adolesc Psychiatry 1998;37(4):443–6.
78. Brown R, Antonuccio D, DuPaul G, et al. Childhood mental health disorders: evidence base and contextual factors for psychosocial, psychopharmacological, and combined interventions. Washington, DC: American Psychological Association Press; 2008.
79. Chambless DL, Hollon SD. Defining empirically supported therapies. J Consult Clin Psychol 1998;66:7–18.
80. Franklin ME, Kozak MJ, Cashman LA, et al. Cognitive-behavioral treatment of pediatric obsessive-compulsive disorder: an open clinical trial. J Am Acad Child Adolesc Psychiatry 1998;37(4):412–9.
81. March J, Mulle K, Herbel B. Behavioral psychotherapy for children and adolescents with OCD. J Am Acad Child Adolesc Psychiatry 1994;33(3):333–41.
82. de Haan E, Hoodgum KA, Buitelaar JK, et al. Behavior therapy versus clomipramine in obsessive-compulsive disorders in children and adolescents. J Am Acad Child Adolesc Psychiatry 1998;37(10):1022–9.
83. Barrett P, Farrell L, Dadds M, et al. Cognitive-behavioral family treatment of childhood obsessive-compulsive disorder: long-term follow-up and predictors of outcome. J Am Acad Child Adolesc Psychiatry 2005;44(10):1005–14.
84. Ginsburg GS, Kingery JN, Drake KL, et al. Predictors of treatment response in pediatric obsessive-compulsive disorder. J Am Acad Child Adolesc Psychiatry 2008;47(8):868–78.
85. March JS, Franklin ME, Leonard H. Tics moderate treatment outcome with sertraline but not cognitive-behavior therapy in pediatric obsessive-compulsive disorder. Biol Psychiatry 2007;61(3):344–7.
86. Geller DA, Biederman J, Stewart SE, et al. Which SSRI? A meta-analysis of pharmacotherapy trials in pediatric obsessive-compulsive disorder. Am J Psychiatry 2003;160(11):1919–28.
87. O'Kearney RT, Anstey KJ, von Sanden C. Behavioral and cognitive behavioral therapy for obsessive compulsive disorder in children and adolescents. Cochrane Database Syst Rev 2006;4:CD004856.

Cognitive-Behavioral Treatment for Posttraumatic Stress Disorder in Children and Adolescents

Shannon Dorsey, PhD[a],*, Ernestine C. Briggs, PhD[b],
Briana A. Woods, PhD[c]

KEYWORDS

- PTSD • Children • Adolescents • Cognitive-behavioral
- Treatment

Rates of exposure to violence and traumatic events for children and adolescents are exceedingly high. In a nationally representative sample of children and adolescents in the United States, 60.4% reported exposure in the past year, with lifetime rates nearly a half to one-third higher, depending on exposure type.[1] Many children and adolescents experience repeated exposure or multiple types of events over their lifetime.[1,2] Rates of trauma exposure for youth in war-involved or high-conflict countries are even higher.[3–5] The range of potentially traumatic events includes exposure to domestic violence, child abuse and neglect, and community violence, and experiencing the violent death of a loved one, among others.

A significant number of children and adolescents exposed to traumatic events develop posttraumatic stress (PTS) symptoms, posttraumatic stress disorder (PTSD), and other common trauma-related sequelae, including depressive disorders, anxiety disorders, and externalizing behavioral disorders. Rates of PTSD among children and adolescents vary, depending on the study population of focus (eg, traumatized sample vs community sample) and particular type of trauma examined (eg, sexual abuse and extreme interpersonal trauma are associated with higher rates of PTSD). According to

This work was supported by a grant R34-MH079910 (SD) from the National Institutes of Health.
[a] Division of Public Behavioral Health and Justice Policy, University of Washington School of Medicine, 2815 Eastlake Avenue East, Suite 200, Seattle, WA 98102, USA
[b] Department of Psychiatry and the Behavioral Sciences, Duke University School of Medicine, 411 West Chapel Hill Street, Suite 200, Durham, NC 27701, USA
[c] Health Behavior Health Education, Gillings School of Global Public Health, University of North Carolina, 323-C Rosenau Hall, CB#7440, Chapel Hill, NC 27599, USA
* Corresponding author.
E-mail address: dorsey2@uw.edu

recent studies, however, even subclinical symptoms of PTSD place children at risk for other psychiatric disorders.[2] Therefore, children and adolescents must receive effective treatment for PTS, PTSD, and co-occurring conditions.[6]

Treatments are available that show effectiveness for child and adolescent PTSD, most of which are cognitive-behavioral therapies (CBT).[7,8] In a meta-analysis examining an array of treatment approaches for treating child and adolescent PTSD, Wetherington and colleagues[8] reviewed CBT, play therapy, art therapy, psychodynamic therapy, and pharmacologic therapy. The results were robust for CBT, whereas insufficient evidence was found for the other approaches. Silverman and colleagues[9] provide further evidence for CBT approaches. Their review of psychosocial treatments for trauma exposure that have evidence for improving child and adolescent outcomes (eg, post-traumatic stress, depressive symptoms, anxiety symptoms, and externalizing behavior problems) showed that the only two that met the *well-established* and *probably efficacious* criteria[10,11] were CBT approaches, namely trauma-focused cognitive-behavioral therapy (TF-CBT) and cognitive behavioral intervention for trauma in schools (CBITS).

The available CBT approaches for PTSD have several common elements, many of which are also prevalent in most CBT treatments for other internalizing disorders (eg, other anxiety, depression).[12,13] These elements include (1) psychoeducation about PTSD, anxiety, and the prevalence and impact of trauma; (2) relaxation and affective modulation skills for managing physiologic and emotional stress; (3) exposure or gradual desensitization to memories of the traumatic event and to innocuous reminders of the traumatic event; and (4) cognitive restructuring of inaccurate or maladaptive/unhelpful cognitions. In a study identifying core components in the treatment of anxiety disorders, Chorpita and colleagues[14] showed that exposure seems to be the only "universal" component. Exposure is explicitly included in the two trauma-specific CBT approaches with the most evidence (ie, TF-CBT, CBITS), but is not always an explicit component of some of the promising practices described in this article.

In addition to these common clinical elements, CBT treatment approaches to PTSD also include common structural or delivery components, including agenda setting, modeling and coached practice of new skills in session, and assignment of weekly practice of skills in real-world settings (eg, home, school), to occur in between sessions. Additional aspects of trauma-specific CBT include use of assessment measures to guide treatment, ongoing use of feedback, and progressive building on mastered skills. As in all CBT approaches, the therapist takes an active and directive role in session. In trauma-specific CBT, this role is particularly important, given that avoidance is one of the primary symptom areas of PTSD.

This article provides a detailed overview of two CBT approaches with the strongest evidence of effectiveness: TF-CBT[15] and CBITS.[16] In addition to reviewing these two approaches, a section on promising practices reviews several promising CBT approaches that contain many of the common elements listed earlier. Most of these approaches are currently under investigation and merit attention, but currently have comparatively less evidence of effectiveness.

Several investigators have reviewed psychosocial treatments for PTSD and trauma exposure.[7–9,17,18] This article provides an update to these reviews, focusing specifically on CBT approaches and highlighting selected promising practices. Moreover, evidence from the included promising practices both bolsters the evidence for CBT approaches to treating PTSD in children and adolescents in general and shows the versatility and potential of CBT in varied settings and with diverse youth and families. In addition, many of the promising practices show that trauma-specific CBT approaches can be combined with other CBT interventions for treating PTSD and co-occurring disorders.

TF-CBT
Evidence

Among the CBT approaches for trauma exposure, PTSD and co-occurring sequelae, TF-CBT has the most evidence of effectiveness[15,19,20] (http://tfcbt.musc.edu). Six published randomized controlled trials support its effectiveness in reducing PTS symptoms and PTSD, depressive symptoms, shame, and trauma-related and general behavior problems compared with non-CBT interventions (eg, supportive or client-centered therapies, waitlist control, usual care).[21–26] All randomized controlled trials except one[25] involved individual TF-CBT delivery. An additional small randomized controlled trial comparing TF-CBT alone with TF-CBT plus sertraline[27] showed little perceived benefit of added pharmacologic intervention.

Results from two additional randomized controlled trials are forthcoming, one of which focuses specifically on youth exposed to domestic violence[28] and one that examines variation in the number of sessions and aspects of gradual exposure.[29] Follow-up studies provide evidence of sustained benefit at 6 months, 1 year, and 2 years posttreatment.[30–33] Trials have focused predominantly on school-aged and preschool aged youth who have been sexually abused or multiply traumatized.

In the most recently published multisite randomized controlled trial involving 229 children ages 8 to 14 years, all youth were sexually abused, with 90% of these youth experiencing a mean of 3.7 different types of traumatic events, including sexual abuse.[21,34] Children who received TF-CBT were half as likely as those in the client-centered comparison condition to meet full *Diagnostic and Statistical Manual of Mental Disorders, Fourth Edition (DSM-IV)* PTSD criteria at the end of treatment. Children in the TF-CBT condition also had significantly lower levels of depression and behavior problems, higher levels of interpersonal trust and perceived credibility, and lower levels of shame. Parents of children who received TF-CBT also experienced improvement in depressive symptoms, parenting ability, and their own abuse-related distress.

In addition to these randomized controlled trials, the evidence for TF-CBT is supplemented by several quasi-experimental[35–37] and open trials.[19,34,38,39] Two open trials have focused specifically on childhood traumatic grief.[15,19,21,34] One open trial provides additional evidence for group delivery of TF-CBT with sexually abused youth.[39]

Model Description

The TF-CBT model includes nine components, described using the acronym PRACTICE. The PRACTICE components include *p*sychoeducation, *p*arenting skills, *r*elaxation skills, *a*ffective modulation skills, *c*ognitive coping skills, *t*rauma narrative and processing, *i*n vivo exposure, *c*onjoint child–parent sessions, and *e*nhancing safety. TF-CBT is typically delivered in 12 to 20 sessions and is appropriate for children and adolescents ages 3 to 18 years.[15,19] In TF-CBT, the clinician works with both the child and the child's nonoffending caregiver, usually a biological parent. In the beginning of treatment, the sessions typically involve meeting individually with the child and the parent. The PRACTICE skills are taught to both, with the exception of parenting, which is only taught to the parent. The goal of each component is to help the child and the parent achieve mastery over avoidance of trauma-related thoughts, feelings, reminders, and memories. The components are ordered in such a way that each component builds on the previous component, and therefore the components are typically provided in the PRACTICE order, with early PRAC skill-building components being delivered first.

A crucial part of providing TF-CBT involves the inclusion of exposure, or gradual exposure, to feared stimuli. Exposure has been identified as one of the common elements in CBT approaches for treating PTSD and other anxiety disorders. In the area of trauma, feared stimuli may include memories and physical reminders of the trauma (eg, sights, sounds, people, smells, other cues that serve as trauma reminders). Gradual exposure is integrated into all of the PRACTICE components, because it is a critical part of achieving mastery over avoidance. In each PRACTICE component, gradual exposure involves incrementally increasing the duration at which the child and the parent face feelings, thoughts, reminders, and memories of the child's traumatic experiences. The child can then habituate to the physical and psychological arousal that accompanies reminders of traumatic events so that avoidance and other symptoms are decreased. In addition to being included in all PRACTICE components, the trauma narrative portion of TF-CBT involves helping the child gradually develop a narrative of the traumatic experiences that can be reviewed during subsequent sessions. During the trauma narrative component, which occurs over several sessions (eg, three to four), the child describes details of what happened before, during, and after the traumatic events, and shares thoughts, feelings, and physiologic reactions.

When the traumatic event involves death and loss, grief-specific components are available (CTGweb: http://ctg.musc.edu), including grief-specific psychoeducation and guidance with grieving the loss, resolving ambivalent feelings, redefining the relationship (from interaction to memory), and committing to present relationships. Each of these components builds systematically on the PRACTICE skills and can be tailored to meet the unique circumstances of children and adolescents.

Implementation Considerations

Several recent efforts show success in delivering TF-CBT to special populations of youth, including those in foster care, residential settings, and international settings. Evidence of effectiveness with youth in foster care is accumulating, including from the Weiner and colleagues[37] study in Illinois and an ongoing National Institute for Mental Health (NIMH)–funded, randomized, effectiveness trial of TF-CBT in Washington State, focused on foster parent involvement and engagement (MH079910, PI: Dorsey, S).

Providing evidence for effectiveness in community-based settings, clinicians in many of the quasi-experimental and open trials of TF-CBT were masters-level clinicians employed in community mental health settings, and included youth who presented at mental health centers for treatment.[35–37] Ongoing research is evaluating TF-CBT in a range of settings with varying implementation conditions.[40] Among these, several statewide implementation projects include relatively rigorous evaluation plans (eg, Project BEST in South Carolina, www.musc.edu/projectbest; North Carolina Child Treatment Program in North Carolina, http://www.cfar.unc.edu/). Two NIMH-funded open trials of TF-CBT are currently underway in low-resource countries, one focused on HIV-infected children and adolescents who were sexually abused (from Zambia) and one focused on orphaned children and adolescents, many of whom were orphaned as a result of the AIDS epidemic and have traumatic grief symptoms (from Tanzania).

Cultural Considerations

In the United States, applications of TF-CBT have been developed for Latino[41] and Native American families.[42] These applications maintain all of the TF-CBT components but include culturally specific aspects of each (eg, cuento therapy involving story-telling for Latino families) to better engage families and ensure that the treatment is as culturally relevant as possible. In addition to these specific applications, all TF-CBT trainings, resources, and materials (eg, TF-CBTWeb, http://tfcbt.musc.edu)[15,19]

specify the need for providing the model components with fidelity, but in a manner that is flexible and engaging with regard to family and child background, ethnicity, and culture. Internationally, TF-CBT is currently being implemented in a range of settings in Zambia, Tanzania, China, Japan, Norway, Cambodia, Indonesia, Germany, the Netherlands, and other countries.

CBITS
Evidence

Current evidence for CBITS consists of one randomized controlled trial,[16] one quasi-experimental trial,[43] and one field trial.[36] In the randomized controlled trial with sixth and seventh grade students (N = 126), Stein and colleagues[16] compared CBITS with a waitlist control group. The intervention included 10 weekly 45- to 60-minute group sessions, one to three individual sessions focused on imaginal exposure to the traumatic events, two to four optional sessions with parents, and one teacher education session. After the 10-week CBITS intervention, the intervention group reported significantly lower PTSD symptoms than did the waitlist control group, with 86% of students in the CBITS condition reporting lower PTSD symptom scores than would have been expected without treatment. In addition, the CBITS group reported lower depression scores, with 67% of students reporting lower depression scores than would have been expected without treatment. For both PTSD and depression scores, differences between the groups disappeared after the waitlist delayed-intervention group received CBITS. Furthermore, 78% of parents whose children received CBITS reported reduced psychosocial problems post-treatment; however, teachers did not report a significant reduction in classroom behavioral problems. The improvements in PTSD and depression symptoms, and parent-reported behavioral problems, were sustained at 6-month follow-up.

In their quasi-experimental study, Kataoka and colleagues[43] evaluated CBITS, with Spanish-speaking, recent immigrant students (N = 113), also using a waitlist comparison condition. Students recently immigrated (ie, within the past 3 years) from Mexico (57%), El Salvador (18%), Guatemala (11%), and other Latin American countries (13%).[43] Bilingual clinicians conducted eight weekly 45- to 60-minute group sessions, one to three individual sessions with students, two to four optional sessions with parents, and one teacher education session. Specific emphasis was placed on culturally competent implementation. For example, support was provided for immigration-related loss and separation during parent sessions. Students in the CBITS condition with baseline PTSD symptoms in the clinical range showed a significant reduction in both PTSD and depression symptoms compared with those in the waitlist condition.

In the field trial for Project Fleur-de-Lis,[36] children who screened positive for PTSD symptoms 15 months after Hurricane Katrina were randomized to either a school-based group intervention (CBITS) or an individual intervention (TF-CBT) delivered at a mental health clinic. Overall, children in both intervention groups showed reductions in PTSD symptoms, although several children continued to have elevated symptoms posttreatment. CBITS seemed to be more accessible, however, with considerably more children beginning (98%) and completing (91%) treatment than in the TF-CBT condition, in which treatment was provided in a mental health clinic (23% and 15%, respectively).

Model Description

CBITS was originally designed for trauma-impacted, recently immigrated students from Latino, Korean, Armenian, and Russian backgrounds, to be delivered in inner-city school mental health clinics.[16] The developers used a participatory research framework that involved providers and family members in model design. CBITS targets youth between 10 and 15 years of age, and originally focused on exposure to community violence but also has been found effective for youth with a range of trauma histories. Although developed for the school setting, CBITS has also been implemented in other settings (eg, community mental health clinics).

CBITS, in a manner similar to TF-CBT, includes the common elements for trauma-specific CBT interventions for PTSD. CBITS incorporates psychoeducation, relaxation training, cognitive coping skills, gradual exposure to trauma memories through trauma narrative, in vivo exposure, affective modulation skills, cognitive restructuring, and social problem solving.[16] CBITS is delivered in a group setting (six to eight children per group), and typically includes 10 weekly sessions that are approximately 1 hour in length. In addition to the group sessions, one to three individual sessions focus on imaginal exposure to the traumatic event that occur before the gradual exposure exercises. CBITS also includes two parent education sessions in which parents learn about the effects of trauma on youth and the skills the youth are learning in treatment. Lastly, CBITS includes one teacher education session in which teachers learn about the effects of trauma on youth and the ways trauma-related symptoms may present in the classroom.[16]

An adaptation of CBITS, *support for students exposed to trauma* (SSET), was developed for delivery by school personnel.[44] The adaption involved using a lesson plan format, eliminating individual break-out sessions and parent sessions, and using a more curricular format for imaginal exposure. A randomized trial of SSET ($N = 76$) showed reductions in PTSD and depressive symptoms, particularly for youth with high levels of symptoms pretreatment.[44,45] Compared with CBITS effects, smaller reductions in symptoms were seen with SSET.

Implementation Considerations

CBITS has the goal of increasing intervention "reach"[46] through addressing common barriers to treatment such as stigma and access through providing treatment in the school setting. CBITS has been implemented in various communities in the United States (eg, immigrant, urban ethnic minority, low socioeconomic status, middle class) and internationally (ie, Australia, Japan; for more information, see www.nctsn.org[47]; *Treatments that Work*). CBITS has been specifically adapted for the Latino immigrant faith community[48] and to be delivered by nonclinical school staff (ie, SSET).[44,45]

TRAUMA AND GRIEF COMPONENT THERAPY
Evidence

Trauma and grief component therapy (TGCT) is a CBT-based treatment for youth (12–20 years of age) who have been exposed to trauma or are traumatically bereaved. TGCT has been primarily provided in schools, although it can be delivered in community mental health or other service settings. Evidence for TGCT comes from one randomized controlled trial,[49,50] two quasi-experimental studies,[35,51] and two open trials.[52,53] Three of these studies were conducted in a low-resource, international setting, namely Bosnia.

In the randomized controlled trial,[49] 127 war-exposed Bosnian youth (13–19 years of age) in 10 secondary schools were randomized to receive only a classroom-based psychoeducation and skills intervention (modules one and four of TGCT) or the classroom-based intervention and the 17-session group TGCT intervention. Both groups had significant reductions in PTSD symptoms at the end of treatment and at a 4-month follow-up. For youth who experienced at least one bereavement, a subgroup of those enrolled in both conditions, only those in the TGCT group had reductions in grief symptoms (at end of treatment, grief symptoms were not assessed at the 4-month follow-up). A significant decrease in depressive symptoms was seen in both groups at the 4-month follow-up, but only for the TGCT group at the end of treatment. Improvements in PTSD and depression were greater for those in the TGCT group than for those in the classroom-based intervention.

In the most recent quasi-experimental study, the Child and Adolescent Treatment Services (CATS)[35] project, which provided trauma-treatment services to children and adolescents in New York City post-9/11, more than half of the youth who received TGCT showed reduced PTSD symptoms at the end of treatment, with an even greater percentage showing improvement at 4-month follow up. In a quasi-experimental study of TGCT in Armenia (N = 64),[51] receipt of TGCT was associated with reduced PTSD symptoms and stabilization of depressive symptoms, compared with youth who did not receive TGCT (and for whom depressive symptoms worsened). In the open trial conducted in the United States (N = 26),[53] youth who received TGCT had decreased symptoms of PTSD and traumatic grief, if traumatically bereaved. In a open trial conducted in Bosnia (N = 55),[52] similar outcomes were seen for PTSD and traumatic grief, in addition to decreased depressive symptoms. However, nearly half of the 55 youth (n = 27) received only the first two of four modules (ie, did not receive the third grief-specific module; see later discussion), yet evidenced similar reductions in PTSD and traumatic grief.

Model Description

TGCT is typically group-based and includes approximately 10 to 24 sessions corresponding with four modules. The goal of the first module is to reduce acute distress and build group cohesion. Module one includes common CBT elements of psychoeducation, relaxation, and other skills for dealing with distress. Module two involves gradual exposure and cognitive processing. Module three involves providing grief-specific components (eg, psychoeducation about grief, adaptive remembering of the deceased). In the fourth module, the focus is on moving forward, and includes problem-solving of current difficulties, additional restructuring of maladaptive cognitions (eg, core beliefs), and taking steps toward restoring normal developmental progression.

Implementation Considerations

TGCT has been delivered in the United States in diverse populations and in a low-resource setting, and has been delivered by "real-world" providers, both in the domestic and international studies, indicating feasibility in community-based settings with community providers. In addition, two of the studies[49,52] showed improvement in PTSD symptoms despite groups receiving only part of TGCT, suggesting further research is warranted regarding the potential benefit of more limited duration or complexity of interventions for traumatized youth.

PROMISING PRACTICES

Several promising practices in CBT for treating PTSD are available and merit review. Many of these treatments are being evaluated and, as research continues to accumulate, may supplement the menu of options and understanding of how to effectively treat children and adolescents with PTSD. Many of these practices combine common elements of CBT approaches to treating trauma with other CBT interventions, or aspects of other interventions, to explicitly address system-related issues or common comorbid conditions (eg, substance use, emotion dysregulation, depression). The developers of many of these practices have received additional resources and support as part of the congressionally mandated National Child Traumatic Stress Network (NCTSN; www.nctsn.org) that is administered through the Substance Abuse Mental Health Services Administration (SAMHSA). The NCTSN is a science-to-practice collaborative of more than 50 currently funded centers that combines resources from hospitals, universities, community-based organizations, schools, child welfare organizations, and other entities committed to increasing access to and raising the standard of care for children, adolescents, and their families affected by trauma. Therefore, the NCTSN has been a major catalyst for the development, implementation, and dissemination of various evidence-based and promising practices. The next section reviews a few of these promising practices. Many specifically target youth with chronic trauma exposure and high levels of emotional dysregulation.

Trauma Systems Therapy

Inspired by Bronfenbrenner's[54] socio-ecological model, trauma systems therapy (TST) is a systems-oriented, CBT-informed treatment for trauma-exposed youth that focuses on both PTSD and other trauma-related symptoms, and on explicitly attempting to remediate factors in the social environment that perpetuate symptoms.[55] Evidence to support the efficacy of TST comes from an open trial of 110 youth, aged 5 to 20 years.[55,56] Participants showed significant improvements in PTSD symptoms and family and school-related problems over a 3-month follow-up period.

TST uses a multidisciplinary team to implement an array of interventions, within multiple systems, that target two key dimensions: (1) enhancing individuals' ability to regulate emotions and cope with considerable adversity, and (2) promoting change in the social environment (eg, increasing safety in the home, obtaining adequate housing) to decrease ongoing stress and threats that the child experiences. TST includes five phases (surviving, stabilizing, enduring, understanding, and transcending), which include many of the common CBT elements (eg, affective modulation, cognitive restructuring) and interventions in the broader systems designed to stabilize the child, family, or distressed and threatening social environments. For example, TST may include legal advocacy, case management, care coordination, and psychopharmacological interventions. TST uses structured assessments to determine which phase of treatment is indicated. This phase-based treatment is particularly useful for families who encounter a range of barriers to treatment engagement, multiple traumas, and a host of social environment issues.

Combined Parent–Child Cognitive-Behavioral Approach for Children and Families At-Risk for Child Physical Abuse

Combined parent–child (CPC)-CBT is a multifamily group intervention designed for families at risk for, or who have committed, child physical abuse. Compared with Kolko's[57,58] Alternatives for Families model (AF-CBT), an existing evidence-based practice (EBP) for physically abusive families, CPC-CBT specifically includes child PTSD as one of its primary treatment targets. Evidence for CPC-CBT comes from one randomized controlled trial and one small open trial. Runyon and colleagues[59] conducted a small randomized controlled trial comparing CPC-CBT with parent-only CBT among 44 parents and their 60 children (aged 7–13 years). Children and families who participated in the CPC-CBT showed significant improvements in PTS symptoms, and parents showed greater improvements in positive parenting practices. The parent-only CBT treatment group, however, showed greater reductions in the use of corporal punishment. In an open trial of CPC-CBT involving 12 families and their 21 children (aged 4–14 years) that preceded the randomized controlled trial, child PTS symptoms improved and child- and parent-reported physically abusive behavior decreased.[60] Improvements were also seen in parenting consistency and parental anger toward the children.

CPC-CBT specifically targets PTSD, depression, abuse-related attributions, and externalizing behavioral problems in children and adolescents with a history of harsh physical discipline or coercive parenting strategies. CPC-CBT includes a treatment protocol for children and families at risk for child physical abuse that is built on TF-CBT, motivational interviewing, ancillary support services (eg, babysitting, transportation), case management, and relationship enhancement skills that specifically target family violence (eg, domestic violence). Parents and children attend 16 weeks of 2-hour sessions. Parent and child interventions are conducted concurrently for the first 75 minutes of the session by two group therapists in each group. The second 45 minutes involves the integrated joint parent–child sessions.

Structured Psychotherapy for Adolescents Responding to Chronic Stress

Structured Psychotherapy for Adolescents Responding to Chronic Stress (SPARCS) is a 16-session group intervention designed specifically to address the needs of chronically traumatized adolescents aged 12 to 19 years, living in or returning to chaotic environments and who may also be experiencing PTSD and problems in several domains of functioning (eg, interpersonal problems, affect regulation and impulsivity, self-perception[61]). Evidence for SPARCS comes from a recent quasi-experimental trial implemented with 33 culturally diverse 13 to 21 year olds who had experienced a moderate or severe discrete traumatic experience.[37] Most participants were female (63.6%) and of ethnic minority (67% African American, 12% Latino, 21% White). In this study, SPARCS was found to be effective in improving traumatic stress symptoms, life domain functioning, and risk behaviors, but only for African American participants, perhaps because of insufficient sample size of the other two racial groups.

Given that chronic trauma exposure disrupts the progression of many basic developmental tasks, the overarching goals of SPARCS include helping youth deal with more complex forms of PTSD through coping more effectively with trauma and related sequelae; enhancing self-efficacy; connecting with others and establishing supportive relationships; cultivating awareness; and creating meaning. The theoretical basis for SPARCS is predominantly CBT and includes many of the common elements (eg, psychoeducation, relaxation and affective modulation, cognitive processing). SPARCS also includes modules and interventions from Dialectical Behavior Therapy for Adolescents (eg, mindfulness),[62] Trauma Affect Regulation Guide for Education and Therapy-Adolescents (TARGET-A), and TGCT. Although SPARCS does not include a formal exposure component, participants may discuss and process traumatic experiences in the group with the guidance of the group facilitator.

Trauma-Focused Coping (Multimodality Trauma Treatment)

Delivered in schools and considered a precursor to CBITS, trauma-focused coping (TFC) is a group-based CBT approach for children and adolescents exposed to single-incident traumatic stressors (eg, disaster, exposure to violence, murder, suicide, fire, accidents[63]). Evidence to support the effectiveness of TFC comes from a single-case, cross-setting design involving 17 participants[64] and a small clinic-based open trial involving seven youth.[63] In the March and colleagues[64] study, students who received TFC reported reduced PTSD symptoms at the end of treatment and at follow-up, and improved depression, anxiety, and anger. Youth with complex trauma presentations participated in the clinic-based open trial,[63] which included both individual (n = 4) and group (n = 3) provision of TFC. Youth had reduced PTSD symptoms posttreatment, but reductions were less robust than those found in the study by March and colleagues.[64]

TFC targets PTSD and collateral symptoms of depression, anxiety, anger, and external locus of control. It was designed as a peer-mediating and skill-building group intervention for youth in late elementary through middle school. TFC includes 14 to 18 group sessions delivered during one class period each week. An individual pullout session is done mid-protocol to introduce narrative exposure in a controlled way.

Risk Reduction Through Family Therapy

Risk Reduction Through Family Therapy (RRFT) is a family-focused, integrated treatment that combines TF-CBT, multisystemic therapy,[65] and other approaches to reduce risky behavior (eg, substance use, sexual risk behavior) and trauma-related symptoms among sexually assaulted youth.[66] The seven primary targets of RRFT include psychoeducation, coping, family communication, substance abuse, PTSD, healthy dating and sexual decision making, and revictimization risk reduction. In general, sessions are 60 to 90 minutes once a week with phone check-ins as needed, and the number of sessions depends on the youth's symptom level. A small open trial of RRFT (N = 10) with adolescent women (aged 14–17 years) showed reductions in PTSD and depression symptoms, reductions in substance use, slight improvements in family conflict and cohesion, and improvements in ecological functioning (eg, spending time with prosocial peers, engaging in positive family activities, attending school/work). Treatment gains were maintained at 6-month follow-up.

TARGET-A

TARGET-A is an intervention for youth between ages 12 and 19 years who have experienced interpersonal trauma (eg, maltreatment), an array of chronic trauma (eg, domestic violence, community violence), and other stressors. TARGET-A uses some CBT skills (eg, affective modulation skills, cognitive processing) in addition to other interventions. TARGET-A is usually delivered in 12 approximately 50-minute individual sessions. TARGET-A includes sequential skill-development modules designed to help adolescents in manage and prevent current PTSD symptoms.[67,68] As in SPARCS, youth may choose to talk about past traumatic events (a part of gradual exposure, one of the common elements of trauma-specific CBT), but gradual exposure is not a core component of TARGET-A. The set of seven TARGET-A skills (ie, Focusing on the present moment, Recognizing stress triggers, identifying primary Emotions, Evaluating primary thoughts, Defining primary goals, identifying positive Options, and Making an ethical and spiritual contribution (FREEDOM) skills) was specifically designed to address complex presentations of PTSD and to focus on, and be delivered to, delinquent and juvenile justice-involved youth. Findings are forthcoming from a recently completed randomized controlled trial focused on girls (ages 13–17 years; N = 59) involved in delinquency.[65] (Ford JD, Steinberg KL, Hawke J, et al, unpublished manuscript, 2010). Evidence for TARGET-A also comes from a randomized controlled trial (N = 213) of TARGET with substance-using adults in an outpatient setting.[69,70] TARGET was more effective in improving sobriety and PTSD-related outcomes, but differences in effectiveness varied by ethnicity of the participants.

CULTURAL CONSIDERATIONS

In the area of child and adolescent PTSD treatment, as in other areas, the relevance of EBPs, many of which were CBT approaches, to culturally diverse populations has been the subject of much debate. This controversy is largely because of the disproportionate use of European American, middle-class families in early treatment studies. Moreover, many questioned the validity of the use of EBPs given the absence of data supporting use with ethnically diverse populations. However, because of the relatively recent development of many of these treatments, studies of trauma-specific CBT have included diverse samples in the randomized controlled trials, quasi-experimental studies, and open trials (TF-CBT, CPC-CBT,TGCT) were developed specifically to target multicultural/multilingual populations (CBITS, TST, TARGET-A, SPARCS), and have cultural-specific applications (TF-CBT).

In addition, a growing number of studies have shown that EBPs for many disorders, including PTSD, may be more efficacious than usual care for ethnic minority youth,[71–73] and that EBPs and cultural competence and sensitivity may be more complementary than disparate.[74] Despite these advances, many questions remain regarding treatment effects and outcomes with ethnically diverse youth, both for PTSD and other disorders. Do culturally specific applications, for example, enhance treatment outcomes for ethnically diverse youth? Have these treatments been tested with diverse populations within the community-based settings in which they are typically provided? As a result of these and other questions, the field is beginning to increase its focus on the impact of cultural influences on client engagement, the therapeutic relationship, symptom expression, and improvement. In the area of trauma-specific CBT approaches, researchers and treatment developers are examining culturally specific aspects of common elements such as cognitive processing and exposure, and highlighting ways in which culture maybe a source of mastery, strength, and resilience.[41] The field is advancing and researchers in the area of PTSD treatment are at the forefront, given that the role of culture in the treatment of trauma and traumatic stress is crucial. Specifically, culture often plays a role in treatment-seeking behavior, preferences about treatment, engagement in treatment, and beliefs about why traumatic experiences happened and what is necessary for recovery and improvement.[75]

SUMMARY AND FUTURE DIRECTIONS

Trauma-specific CBT interventions for treating child and adolescent PTSD are available, and research both on existing and relatively new CBT approaches to treating PTSD continues to accumulate. CBT treatments for PTSD include individual and group approaches; interventions included in this review showed improvements in PTSD symptoms with treatment, and many of these gains were sustained over time (ie, TF-CBT, CBITS, TGCT). Most studies of CBT approaches to treating trauma also showed improvements in other commonly co-occurring difficulties (eg, depression, anxiety, behavior problems). These improvements are likely partly because of the differential developmental manifestations of PTSD and the overlap in common elements across CBT treatments that also address these co-occurring difficulties. Future directions for the field include continuing to conduct research on promising practices and their ability to remediate PTSD; examining issues related to cultural applicability and responsiveness; ensuring effective implementation and dissemination (eg, treatment reach); and sustaining treatment gains over time. Additional next steps may also include the examination of the core elements of treatments and their relevance to workforce development as increasingly more clinicians begin to embrace evidence-based treatments.

REFERENCES

1. Finkelhor D, Turner H, Omrod R, et al. Violence, abuse, and crime exposure in a national sample of children and youth. Pediatrics 2009;124:1–13.

2. Copeland WE, Keeler G, Angold A, et al. Traumatic events and posttraumatic stress in childhood. Arch Gen Psychiatry 2007;64:577–84.

3. Derluyn I, Broekaert E, Schuyten G, et al. Post-traumatic stress in former Ugandan child soldiers. Lancet 2004;363:861–3.

4. DeRosa R, Habib M, Pelcovitz D, et al. Structured Psychotherapy for Adolescents Responding to Chronic Stress (SPARCS): a trauma-focused guide for groups. Manhasset (NY): North Shore University Hospital; 2006.

5. DeRosa R, Pelcovitz D. Treating traumatized adolescent mothers: a structured approach. In: Webb N, editor. Working with traumatized youth in child welfare. New York: Guilford Press; 2006. p. 219–45.

6. American Academy of Child and Adolescent Psychiatry. Practice parameter for the assessment and treatment of children and adolescent with posttraumatic stress disorder. J Am Acad Child Adolesc Psychiatry 2010;49:414–30.

7. Chaffin M, Friedrich B. Evidence-based treatments in child abuse and neglect. Child Youth Serv Rev 2004;26(11):1097–113.

8. Wetherington HR, Hahn RA, Fuqua-Whitley DS, et al. The effectiveness of interventions to reduce psychological harm from traumatic events among children and adolescents. Am J Prev Med 2008;35(3):287–313.

9. Silverman WK, Ortiz CD, Viswesvaran C, et al. Evidence-based psychosocial treatments for children and adolescents exposed to traumatic events. J Clin Child Adolesc Psychol 2008;37(1):156–83.

10. Chambless D, Gillis M. Cognitive therapy of anxiety disorders. Advances in cognitive-behavioral therapy, vol. 2. Thousand Oaks (CA): Sage Publications, Inc; 1996. p. 116–44.

11. Chambless D, Hollon S. Defining empirically supported therapies. J Consult Clin Psychol 1998;66(1):7–18.

12. Chorpita BF. Modular cognitive behavioral therapy for childhood anxiety disorders. New York: Guilford Press; 2006.

13. Chorpita BF, Bernstein A, Daleiden EL. Driving with roadmaps and dashboards: using information resources to structure the decision models in service organizations. Adm Policy Ment Health 2008;35(1–2):114–23.

14. Chorpita BF, Daleiden EL, Weisz JR. Modularity in the design and application of therapeutic interventions. Appl Prev Psychol 2005;11(3):141–56.

15. Cohen JA, Mannarino AP, Deblinger E. Treating trauma and traumatic grief in children and adolescents. New York: Guilford Press; 2006.

16. Stein BD, Jaycox LH, Kataoka SH, et al. A mental health intervention for schoolchildren exposed to violence: a randomized controlled trial. JAMA 2003;290:603–11.

17. Feeny N, Foa E, Treadwell K, et al. Posttraumatic stress disorder in youth: a critical review of the cognitive and behavioral treatment outcome literature. Prof Psychol Res Pract 2004;35(5):466–76.

18. Taylor TL, Chemtob CM. Efficacy of treatment for child and adolescent traumatic stress. Arch Pediatr Adolesc Med 2004;158(8):786–91.

19. Cohen JA, Mannarino AP, Staron VR. A pilot study of modified cognitive-behavioral therapy for childhood traumatic grief (CBT-CTG). J Am Acad Child Adolesc Psychiatry 2006;45:1465–73.

20. Deblinger E, Heflin AH. Treating sexually abused children and their nonoffending parents: a cognitive behavioral approach. Thousand Oaks (CA): Sage Publications; 1996.

21. Cohen JA, Deblinger E, Mannarino AP, et al. A multisite, randomized controlled trial for children with sexual abuse-related PTSD symptoms. J Am Acad Child Adolesc Psychiatry 2004;43:393–403.

22. Cohen JA, Mannarino AP. A treatment outcome study for sexually abused preschool children: initial findings. J Am Acad Child Adolesc Psychiatry 1996;35:42–50.
23. Cohen JA, Mannarino AP. Factors that mediate treatment outcome of sexually abused preschool children: six- and 12-month follow-up. J Am Acad Child Adolesc Psychiatry 1998;37:44–51.
24. Deblinger E, Lippmann J, Steer RA. Sexually abused children suffering posttraumatic stress symptoms: initial treatment outcome findings. Child Maltreat 1996;1: 310–21.
25. Deblinger E, Stauffer LB, Steer RA. Comparative efficacies of supportive and cognitive behavioral group therapies for young children who have been sexually abused and their nonoffending mothers. Child Maltreat 2001;6:332–43.
26. King NJ, Tong BJ, Mullen P, et al. Treating sexually abused children with posttraumatic stress symptoms: a randomized clinical trial. J Am Acad Child Adolesc Psychiatry 2000;39:1347–55.
27. Cohen JA, Mannarino AP, Perel JM, et al. A pilot randomized controlled trial of combined Trauma-Focused CBT and sertraline for childhood PTSD symptoms. J Am Acad Child Adolesc Psychiatry 2007;46(7):811–9.
28. Cohen JA, Mannarino AP, Iyengar S. Community treatment of PTSD in children exposed to intimate partner violence: a randomized controlled trial. Arch Pediatr Adolesc Med 2011;165(1):16–21.
29. Deblinger E, Mannarino AP, Cohen JA, et al. Trauma focused cognitive behavioral therapy for children: impact of the trauma narrative and treatment length. Depress Anxiety, in press.
30. Cohen JA, Mannarino AP. A treatment study for sexually abused preschool children: outcome during a one-year follow-up. J Am Acad Child Adolesc Psychiatry 1997;36:1228–35.
31. Cohen JA, Mannarino AP, Knudsen K. Treating sexually abused children: 1 year follow-up of a randomized controlled trial. Child Abuse Negl 2005;29:135–45.
32. Deblinger E, Mannarino AP, Cohen JA, et al. A follow-up study of a multisite, randomized, controlled trial for children with sexual abuse-related PTSD symptoms. J Am Acad Child Adolesc Psychiatry 2006;45:1474–84.
33. Deblinger E, Steer RA, Lippman J. Two year follow-up study of cognitive behavioral therapy for sexually abused children suffering post-traumatic stress symptoms. Child Abuse Negl 1999;23:1371–8.
34. Cohen JA, Mannarino AP, Knudsen K. Treating childhood traumatic grief: a pilot study. J Am Acad Child Adolesc Psychiatry 2004;43:1225–33.
35. Hoagwood KE, CATS Consortium. Impact of CBT for traumatized children and adolescents affected by the World Trade Center disaster. J Clin Child Adolesc Psychol, in press.
36. Jaycox LH, Cohen JA, Mannarino AP, et al. Children's mental health care following Hurricane Katrina: a field trial of trauma-focused psychotherapies. J Trauma Stress 2010;23:223–31.
37. Weiner DA, Schneider A, Lyons JS. Evidence-based treatments for trauma among culturally diverse foster care youth: treatment retention and outcomes. Child Youth Serv Rev 2009;31:1199–205.
38. Deblinger E, McLeer S, Henry D. Cognitive behavioral treatment for sexually abused children suffering post-traumatic stress: preliminary findings. J Am Acad Child Adolesc Psychiatry 1990;29:747–52.
39. Stauffer LB, Deblinger E. Cognitive behavioral groups for nonoffending mothers and their young sexually abused children: a preliminary treatment outcome study. Child Maltreat 1996;1(1):65–76.

40. Dorsey S, Cohen J. Trauma-focused cognitive behavioral therapy. In: Clements P, Seedat S, editors. Mental health issues of child maltreatment. Saint Louis (MO): GW Medical Publishing, in press.

41. de Arellano MA, Ko SJ, Danielson CK, et al. Trauma-informed interventions: clinical and research evidence and culture-specific information project. Los Angeles (CA); Durham (NC): National Center for Child Traumatic Stress; 2008.

42. BigFoot DS, Braden J. Adapting evidence-based treatments for use with American Indian and Native Alaska children and youth. Focal Point 2007;21(1):19–22.

43. Kataoka SH, Stein BD, Jaycox LH, et al. A school-based mental health program for traumatized Latino immigrant children. J Am Acad Child Adolesc Psychiatry 2003;42:311–8.

44. Jaycox LH, Langley AK, Dean KL. Support for students exposed to trauma: the SSET program: group leader training manual, lesson plans, and lesson materials and worksheets. Santa Monica (CA): RAND Health; 2009.

45. Jaycox LH, Langley AK, Stein BD, et al. Support for students exposed to trauma: a pilot study. School Ment Health 2009;1:49–60.

46. Zatzick D, Koepsell T, Rivara F. Using target population specification, effect size, and reach to estimate and compare the population impact of two PTSD preventive interventions. Psychiatry 2009;72(4):346–59.

47. Available at: www.nctsn.org. Acessed January 6, 2011.

48. Kataoka SH, Fuentes S, O'Donoghue VP, et al. A community participatory research partnership: the development of a faith-based intervention for children exposed to violence. Ethn Dis 2006;16:89–97.

49. Layne CM, Saltzman WR, Poppleton L, et al. Effectiveness of a school-based group psychotherapy program for war-exposed adolescents: a randomized controlled trial. J Am Acad Child Adolesc Psychiatry 2008;47:1048–62.

50. Layne CM, Saltzman WR, Pynoos RS, et al. Trauma and grief component therapy. New York: New York State Office of Mental Health; 2002.

51. Goenjian AK, Karayan I, Pynoos RS, et al. Outcomes of psychotherapy among early adolescents after trauma. Am J Psychiatry 1997;154(4):536–42.

52. Layne CM, Pynoos RS, Saltzman WR, et al. Trauma/grief-focused group psychotherapy: school-based postwar intervention with traumatized Bosnian adolescents. Group Dynam 2001;5(4):277–90.

53. Saltzman W, Pynoos R, Layne C, et al. Trauma- and grief-focused intervention for adolescents exposed to community violence: results of a school-based screening and group treatment protocol. Group Dynam 2001;5(4):291–303.

54. Bronfenbrenner U. Contexts of child rearing: problems and prospects. Am Psychol 1979;34:844–50.

55. Saxe GN, Ellis BH, Kaplow J. Collaborative treatment for traumatized children and teens: a trauma systems therapy approach. New York: Guilford Press; 2007.

56. Saxe GN, Ellis BH, Fogler J. Comprehensive care for traumatized children: an open trial examines trauma systems therapy. Psychiatr Ann 2005;35(5):443–8.

57. Kolko D. Individual cognitive behavioral treatment and family therapy for physically abused children and their offending parents: a comparison of clinical outcomes. Child Maltreat 1996;1(4):322–42.

58. Kolko DJ, Swenson CC. Assessing and treating physically abused children and their families: a cognitive behavioral approach. Thousand Oaks (CA): Sage Publications; 2002.

59. Runyon MK, Deblinger D, Steer R. Comparison of combined parent-child and parent-only cognitive-behavioral treatments for offending parents and children in cases of child physical abuse. Child Fam Behav Ther 2010;32:196–218.

60. Runyon MK, Deblinger D, Schroeder CM. Pilot evaluation of outcomes of combined parent-child cognitive-behavioral group therapy for families at-risk for child physical abuse. Cognit Behav Pract 2009;16:101–18.
61. DeRosa R, Pelcovitz D. Group treatment for chronically traumatized adolescents: igniting SPARCS of change. Treating traumatized children: risk, resilience and recovery. New York: Routledge/Taylor & Francis Group; 2009. p. 225–39.
62. Miller AL, Rathus JH, Linehan MM. Dialectical behavior therapy with suicidal adolescents. New York: Guilford Press; 2007.
63. Amaya-Jackson L, Reynolds V, Murray M, et al. Cognitive behavioral treatment for pediatric posttraumatic stress disorder: protocol and application in school and community settings. Cognit Behav Pract 2003;10:204–13.
64. March J, Amaya-Jackson L, Murray M, et al. Cognitive behavioral psychotherapy for children and adolescents with post-traumatic stress disorder following a single incident stressor. J Am Acad Child Adolesc Psychiatry 1998;37(6):585–93.
65. Henggeler S, Clingempeel W, Brondino M, et al. Four-year follow-up of multisystemic therapy with substance-abusing and substance-dependent juvenile offenders. J Am Acad Child Adolesc Psychiatry 2002;41(7):868–74.
66. Danielson CK, McCart MR, de Arellano MA, et al. Risk reduction for substance use and trauma-related psychopathology in adolescent sexual assault victims: findings from an open trial. Child Maltreat 2010;15:261–8.
67. Ford JD, Russo E. Trauma-focused, present-centered, emotional self-regulation approach to integrated treatment for posttraumatic stress and addiction: Trauma Adaptive Recovery Group Education and Therapy (TARGET). Am J Psychother 2006;60:335–55.
68. Ford JD, Russo E, Mallon S. Integrating post-traumatic stress disorder (PTSD) and substance use disorder treatment. J Counsel Dev 2007;85:475–89.
69. Frisman L, Ford J, Lin H, et al. Outcomes of trauma treatment using the TARGET model. J Groups Addict Recover 2008;3(3–4):285–303.
70. Ford JD. Trauma, PTSD, and ethnoracial minorities: toward diversity and cultural practices in principles and practices. Clin Psychol Sci Pract 2008;15:62–7.
71. Huey SJ, Polo AJ. Evidence-based psychosocial treatments for ethnic minority youth. J Clin Child Adolesc Psychol 2008;37:262–301.
72. Jaycox LH. Cognitive-behavioral intervention for trauma in schools. Longmont (CO): Sopris West Educational Services; 2003.
73. Miranda J, Guillermo B, Lau A, et al. State of the science on psychosocial interventions for ethnic minorities. Annu Rev Clin Psychol 2005;1:113–42.
74. Whaley AL, Davis KE. Cultural competence and evidence-based practice in mental health services: a complementary perspective. Am Psychol 2007;62:563–74.
75. Cohen JA, Deblinger E, Mannarino A, et al. The importance of culture in treating abused and neglected children: an empirical review. Child Maltreat 2001;6:148–57.

Cognitive-Behavioral Therapy for Weight Management and Eating Disorders in Children and Adolescents

Denise E. Wilfley, PhD[a],*, Rachel P. Kolko, BA[b],
Andrea E. Kass, BA[b]

KEYWORDS

- Cognitive-behavioral therapy • Eating disorders • Obesity
- Weight control

Children and adolescents who struggle with eating disorders and obesity require clinical attention. Eating- and weight-related difficulties are characterized by maladaptive daily patterns, involving distorted cognitions and problematic behavior cycles. The treatment of weight control issues requires a comprehensive approach, because disordered eating permeates individual, home, and social environments. Cognitive-behavioral therapy (CBT) emphasizes the process of changing habits and attitudes that maintain psychological disorders. Given this focus, CBT is an appropriate treatment approach for eating disorders and obesity. By restructuring the harmful patterns that infiltrate daily functioning, youth are better positioned to lead healthier lives. Understanding eating disorders and obesity, as well as their representation as a spectrum of weight control issues, is imperative to their successful treatment and prevention.

WEIGHT CONTROL ISSUES: UNDERSTANDING EATING DISORDERS AND OBESITY

The spectrum of weight control issues spans a variety of behaviors and cognitions and affects a wide range of individuals. These problems typically develop in childhood and

The authors have nothing to disclose.
[a] Department of Psychiatry, Washington University School of Medicine, 660 South Euclid, Campus Box 8134, St Louis, MO 63110, USA
[b] Department of Psychology, Washington University in St Louis, One Brookings Drive, Campus Box 1125, St Louis, MO 63130, USA
* Corresponding author.
E-mail address: wilfleyd@psychiatry.wustl.edu

Child Adolesc Psychiatric Clin N Am 20 (2011) 271–285
doi:10.1016/j.chc.2011.01.002
1056-4993/11/$ – see front matter © 2011 Elsevier Inc. All rights reserved.

adolescence. Often, unhealthy weight-related patterns are difficult to treat, especially because they are entrenched in daily life. Specifically, a heightened emphasis is placed on food, eating, body weight or shape, and control; for many, these behaviors may function as an unhealthy coping strategy. As a result, weight control issues have a significant impact on social functioning and quality of life.

The *Diagnostic and Statistical Manual of Mental Disorders*, fourth edition, text revision (*DSM-IV-TR*) includes the following eating disorder diagnoses: anorexia nervosa (AN), bulimia nervosa (BN), and eating disorder not otherwise specified (EDNOS),[1] the most commonly diagnosed of the three disorders.[2] Included within the current EDNOS category is binge eating disorder (BED); however, it has been proposed as its own formal diagnosis in the upcoming fifth edition of the *DSM (DSM-V)*.[3] Although individuals with AN are severely underweight, individuals with BN and BED often fluctuate between the normal and overweight ranges.

On the far end of the weight spectrum, childhood obesity has become a major public health concern. Over the past three decades, rates of pediatric overweight and obesity have tripled in the United States,[4] making this a national epidemic. Weight classification is used to determine overweight or obese status. For adults, body mass index (BMI) is the standard metric; for children, BMI percentile is used because it is sensitive and easy to obtain.[5] BMI is the ratio of weight (in kilograms) to height (in meters squared), and BMI percentiles refer to age- and sex-specific curves. Although this article discusses the classification, associated features and comorbidities, and treatment approaches for eating disorders and obesity, it is important to note that obesity is not considered a mental illness; it is neither an eating disorder nor an addiction.[6]

Table 1 provides an overview of the current diagnostic criteria, definitions, and prevalence rates for AN, BN, BED, and obesity.

Clinical Features

Weight control issues are associated with several medical and psychological complications. Patients with eating disorders struggle with body-related cognitive distortions (ie, body dissatisfaction over concern with weight and shape, shame, and guilt) and disordered eating behaviors (ie, body dissatisfaction, overconcern with weight and shape, shame, and guilt). In addition, these individuals often experience psychosocial problems, including social isolation, low self-esteem, secretiveness about eating, and stigmatization.[7,8] Eating disorders are also highly comorbid with other psychological disorders, such as depression, anxiety, and impulse control disorders.[9,10] Severe medical complications, such as a result of the starvation associated with AN, and the repeated binge/purge cycle characteristic of BN, are common. These include metabolic changes (eg, electrolyte imbalances); osteoporosis; dental, gastric, and renal abnormalities; dysregulated body temperature; irregular or loss of menses; appetite control dysregulation; and weight fluctuation.[11–13] Adolescent binge and loss of control eating are related to excessive weight gain, which is associated with multiple problems (discussed later).[13–15] Although the physical presentation may look similar to that of obese youth, children and adolescents with BED or those who exhibit loss of control eating, which is a defining feature of a binge, also experience distinct psychopathological symptoms related to eating, mood, and anxiety disorders that are not reported by their non–eating-disordered obese counterparts.[16]

Youth who struggle with overweight and obesity often face medical and psychological complications as well. Depression, feelings of worthlessness, low self-esteem, stigmatization, and teasing are associated psychological sequelae.[17–19] Additional difficulties include poor academic performance and behavioral problems.[20] Excessive weight is correlated with cardiovascular problems (eg, heart disease, hypertension, high blood pressure, and high lipid profiles), diabetes, stroke, joint and bone pain or disease, cancer, and obstructive sleep apnea.[20] Moreover, these children and adolescents often engage in disordered eating behaviors,[21] which exacerbate the negative medical and psychological consequences of maladaptive eating patterns.

Thus, weight control issues represent serious problems that need to be addressed. Given that children and adolescents who display maladaptive eating behaviors are likely to develop additional weight-related difficulties,[14,22-24] treating their current weight issues can both reduce the resultant medical and psychological problems and prevent future unhealthy patterns. Understanding the current risk factors and treatment approaches for weight management issues will improve the clinical responsiveness to youth who present with these problems.

Developing and Maintaining Factors

Multiple factors increase youths' risk for the development of weight control issues. Body dissatisfaction, dietary restriction, overvaluation of weight and shape, negative affect, and low self-esteem are the core cognitions that place individuals at risk.[25] Specific vulnerabilities, known as appetitive traits, have been linked to eating behavior and physical activity preferences.[26] Satiety responsiveness (eg, failure to recognize hunger cues), impulsivity (eg, inability to postpone immediate rewards), and high motivation to eat are heritable and predictive of excessive weight gain.[27] Interpersonal difficulties, including sensitivity and teasing,[28,29] can propel the use of or control over food as a negative coping strategy. In addition, history of depression and history of teasing by a teacher or coach have been linked to the onset of an eating disorder.[30] Weight control issues in childhood represent another critical risk factor. Being overweight as a child can lead to later development of eating disorder psychopathology and/or obesity.[22,23,31] Loss of control and/or binge eating at a young age places youth at risk for developing the symptoms consistent with diagnostic criteria for BED[32] and for becoming obese.[14,24]

A child's environment further complicates the risk for weight gain and disordered eating pathology. Negative parental role modeling of unhealthy eating and activity patterns can lead children to develop maladaptive habits. Furthermore, recent trends toward increased sedentary behavior, meals eaten away from home, and consumption of foods and drinks that are high in energy density (ie, high in calories, fat, or sugar) have hindered healthy lifestyle choices for youth.[33,34]

Although these factors place individuals at risk, they also serve to maintain disordered weight control patterns. For example, there is often a negative cyclic relationship between weight-related behavior and depression[35] and interpersonal difficulties.[17,25] As these patterns continue, they become more strongly entrenched in daily life and more difficult to modify. Thus, the need to intervene early is evident.

TREATMENT CONSIDERATIONS: THE NEED FOR EARLY INTERVENTION

Habits start young, and in turn, interventions should follow suit. Interventions that break maladaptive behavior patterns before they become ingrained have greater potential for success. This is noteworthy because shorter duration and reduced severity of symptoms are associated with better outcomes[5,36-39]; recovery rates for adolescents with eating disorders are higher than those for adults.[8] Thus, through early intervention, children and adolescents are more likely to respond to treatment.

When intervening with youth, it is important to include the parents and family in the treatment process. Parents can facilitate positive behavior change by creating

Table 1
Overview of the current diagnostic criteria, definitions, and prevalence rates for AN, BN, BED, and obesity

Anorexia Nervosa	Bulimia Nervosa	Binge Eating Disorder	Obesity
Refusal to maintain body weight at or above a minimally normal weight for age and height (eg, weight loss leading to maintenance of body weight <85% of that expected or failure to make expected weight gain during period of growth, leading to body weight <85% of that expected).	Recurrent episodes of binge eating, characterized by: Eating, in a discrete period of time (eg, within 2 hours), an amount of food that is definitely larger than most people would eat during a similar period of time or circumstances; A sense of lack of control overeating during the episode (eg, a feeling that one cannot stop eating or control what or how much one is eating).	Recurrent episodes of binge eating, characterized by: Eating, in a discrete period of time (eg, within 2 hours), an amount of food that is definitely larger than most people would eat during a similar period of time or circumstances; A sense of lack of control overeating during the episode (eg, a feeling that one cannot stop eating or control what or how much one is eating).	Overweight: 85th to <95th BMI [a]percentile Obesity: ≥95th BMI percentile
Intense fear of gaining weight or becoming fat, even though underweight.	Recurrent inappropriate compensatory behavior, such as self-induced vomiting; misuse of laxatives, diuretics, enemas, or other medications; fasting; or excessive exercise.	Binge eating episodes are associated with 3 (or more) of the following: Eating much more rapidly than usual; Eating until uncomfortably full; Eating large amounts of food when not feeling physically hungry; Eating alone because of being embarrassed by how much one is eating; Feeling disgusted with oneself, depressed, or very guilty after overeating.	—
Disturbance in the way one's body weight or shape is experienced, undue influence of body weight or shape on self-evaluation, or denial of the seriousness of current low body weight.	The binge eating and inappropriate compensatory behaviors both occur, on average, ≥2 times a week for 3 months. [b]	Marked distress regarding binge eating is present.	—
In postmenarcheal women, amenorrhea (absence of ≥3 consecutive menstrual cycles). [c]	Self-evaluation is unduly influenced by body shape and weight.	The binge eating occurs, on average, ≥2 days a week for 6 months. [d]	—
—	The disturbance does not occur exclusively during episodes of AN.	The binge eating is not associated with the regular use of inappropriate compensatory behaviors and does not occur exclusively during episodes of AN or BN.	—
Prevalence estimates: 0.3%–3.7%.	Prevalence estimates: 1.0%–4.2%.	Prevalence estimates: 0.7%–3.0%.	Prevalence estimates: Obesity: 16.3%; Overweight and obesity: 31.9%.

[a] BMI, weight (kilograms)/height (meters²); BMI percentile, age- and sex-specific curves.

[b] Reduction of this criterion to 1 time per week for 3 months has been proposed for DSM-V.

[c] Removal of this criterion has been proposed for DSM-V.

[d] Reduction of this criterion to 1 time per week for 3 months has been proposed for DSM-V

a healthful home environment and minimizing negative stimuli to support healthy habits. For those children and adolescents who may be resistant to treatment, parents are able to serve as enforcers of necessary modifications. Furthermore, parents can model healthy lifestyle choices and reinforce the youth's progress.

Although early intervention is effective, it is equally crucial to direct focus on prevention. Prevention efforts offer the opportunity to reduce the onset and prevalence of weight-related problems. As understanding of risk factors and predictors of treatment outcome has evolved, clinical scientists are well equipped to develop appropriate preventive strategies. Furthermore, because obesity is cyclic (ie, overweight parents are more likely to have overweight children, who are also more likely to become overweight adults),[40,41] increased initiatives for parents and children would enable a necessary decline in the increasing weight trends. Successful pioneering research in this domain demonstrates the utility of preventive work.[42-48]

EMPIRICAL SUPPORT FOR THE TREATMENT OF EATING DISORDERS AND OBESITY IN YOUTH
Eating Disorders

CBT is the most established psychological treatment for BN and BED,[49] with demonstrated efficacy over pharmacologic and other psychological therapeutic options.[50] The goal of treatment is to identify, monitor, and tackle the cognitions and behaviors that maintain the disorder while heightening the motivation for change.[49,51-53] Given that the need for treatment far outweighs the availability of practitioners,[54] current efforts are focused on increasing dissemination by modifying the traditional CBT manual into guided self-help[55-57] and computer- and Internet-based versions.[58,59]

Interpersonal psychotherapy (IPT) is the only psychological treatment for BN and BED to show comparable efficacy to CBT,[60] and for certain groups, there may be increased benefits.[57,61] IPT helps patients connect their binge and/or purge behaviors to interpersonal difficulties; the therapist highlights how a social arena can function as both a causal and maintaining factor for binge eating but can also be used as an avenue through which to build support for recovery. Given the emphasis of IPT on current relationships, it is particularly effective for youth, for whom the social network is of heightened importance.[62,63] IPT has been effective for use in individual[57,64] and group formats[65-67] and has demonstrated positive results for the prevention of excessive weight gain in overweight adolescents.[13,68] Recent studies have found that IPT, as adapted for youth, can also be effectively disseminated into community-based settings.[63] Current efforts are under way to improve IPT dissemination for the eating disorder population.

Treatment research on AN has been more scant, in part due to difficulties with participant recruitment and retention.[37,69] Results of studies have provided little support for specialized psychotherapies or pharmacotherapies, conducted with both underweight and weight-restored individuals.[70-79] Family-based therapy—one established form of which is the Maudsley approach—has been effective in treating adolescents with AN.[80,81] The treatment focuses on empowering the family to serve as agents of change in helping an ill adolescent reach recovery. A therapist works collaboratively with the family to help the patient regain weight, regulate disordered eating behaviors, and promote healthy adolescent development and independence.

Although the DSM-IV-TR uses a categorical classification system of mutually exclusive diagnoses, patients with eating disorders often develop symptoms consistent with more than one diagnosis over the course of their illness, demonstrating shifts between diagnoses, known as diagnostic crossover.[82,83] To more effectively address this, an enhanced, transdiagnostic approach to CBT has been established,[84] with the goal of treating eating disorder psychopathology across diagnoses rather than a specific diagnosis. The treatment addresses the shared, underlying core beliefs (ie, overvaluation and control of one's weight and shape) to break the maladaptive cognitive and behavior patterns that have maintained the eating disorder.[25,85,86]

There are two forms of the enhanced CBT (CBT-E): focused and broad. Focused CBT-E is considered the default version and targets the eating disorder psychopathology. The broad version addresses these same issues but includes an additional focus on external factors that maintain the disorder and make behavior change more difficult. In particular, patients with low self-esteem, poor mood-regulation strategies, high interpersonal problems, and high levels of clinical perfectionism are well suited for broad CBT-E, in which these four core features are targeted. Both forms of treatment are delivered weekly for 20 sessions in an outpatient setting. CBT-E consists of four phases that modify maladaptive behaviors and negative pathology and teach strategies for relapse prevention. For those entering treatment at low weight (BMI ≤17.5), 40 weekly sessions are recommended with an additional focus on weight regain.

Obesity

Lifestyle interventions represent the most successful treatment for childhood obesity[5,38] and have been shown more effective than psychoeducation alone.[87] Furthermore, the US Preventive Services Task Force recommends that children ages 6 to 18 years old be screened by pediatricians and offered multicomponent, moderate-to-intense treatment to address obesity[88]; this recommended treatment is directly in line with the lifestyle intervention approach. Lifestyle interventions use a multicomponent approach to modify children's daily practices into healthy habits (ie, healthier diets and increased physical activity), which promotes long-term behavior maintenance.[5,89] These interventions include behavioral components and cognitive skills training to target weight-related behavior. For the majority of programs, the behavioral aspects of weight treatment are central; however, programs that supplement the behavioral approaches with cognitive restructuring and relapse-prevention techniques may result in increased treatment effectiveness.[90–92]

Interventions with behavioral components that modify both diet and activity (ie, physical activity and/or sedentary behavior, during which few or no calories are burned, such as watching TV) have been demonstrated as the most effective for overweight youth[93–96] and are recommended by the US Preventive Services Task Force.[88] Another key component of lifestyle interventions is the involvement of the family for support. Family-based behavioral interventions, which include parents in the treatment process, have been demonstrated as effective in promoting weight control and healthy habit development over the past 30 years.[87,94,97,98]

Among treatment programs, several behavioral change components have been shown to support healthy weight control. Specifically, intervention strategies focus on stimulus control (eg, restructuring the home to encourage healthy behaviors and limit unhealthy behaviors associated with eating and activity) and self-monitoring of weight, eating, and physical activity.[89,90,95,99,100] In family-based interventions, parents take an active role in treatment. They are instructed to serve as models for their children by monitoring and modifying their own behaviors, because parent success with weight control is predictive of child success.[101] Parents are also encouraged to use a behavioral reward system, in which successful goal completion (eg, weight loss, reduced caloric intake, and increased physical activity) is reinforced with rewards that are interpersonal and/or promote healthy behavior (eg, family outings, bike riding, or ice skating).[102] Family praise is also encouraged to reinforce positive behaviors. In addition, parents are educated about key parenting behaviors, including modeling, providing consistent reinforcement, and using stimulus control techniques to restructure the home environment. All of these skills help families to develop healthy behaviors.

FROM A CLINICAL PERSPECTIVE: EXTENDING BEYOND THE INDIVIDUAL TREATMENT MILIEU

Although successful treatments programs have been established, relapse and nonrecovery remain significant problems.[8,38] Within the eating disorder field, many recovered patients subsequently resume their binge and/or purge behaviors and individuals with AN often do not complete treatment, dropping out prematurely.[37,75,103] Family-based behavioral treatment for obesity has been shown to be successful in the short term,[87] but the targeted healthy behaviors are difficult to sustain over time. Many people who lose weight during the intervention experience weight regain.[99,104,105]

Although relapse prevention is addressed in each of these treatments, more effective strategies are necessary that extend beyond the individual treatment milieu. The persistence of weight-related problems may occur because environmental stimuli, which had fostered the previously learned maladaptive behaviors, have not been modified.[106] Given that individual behaviors related to eating and activity are influenced by complex interactions between socioenvironmental factors and biologic phenomena, multiple drivers of behavior must be considered to encourage sustained behavior change.[107] Thus, without addressing the environmental context, children and adolescents are cued to relapse into prior behavior patterns.

The multiple behavioral drivers can be conceptualized together within a socioecologic model,[108] which can then be incorporated into a weight management treatment program. Specifically, this model posits that factors within the individual/family, peer/social, and community domains serve as foci throughout treatment.[107,108] The social and physical environments include the availability of peers and resources to support and promote healthy eating and activity patterns (Fig. 1). For individuals who do not receive treatment, harmful patterns are cued; for those who do receive treatment, healthful behaviors are reinforced.

Throughout treatment, exploring each domain for stimuli that encourage or hinder healthy behaviors is important; this provides the foundation on which to promote positive behavior change. Key areas to assess include interpersonal relationships and difficulties as well as the accessibility and use of healthy resources within the home, peer network, and community (Fig. 2).

The socioecologic model was tested in a large-scale randomized controlled trial.[91] This study was designed to target weight maintenance in children and was the first to focus on pediatric long-term weight control. The results indicate that continued contact and focus on a child's social ecology are critical treatment components.[91] Furthermore, data from computer biosimulation models suggest a socioecologic emphasis within family-based maintenance interventions produces sustained behavior changes due to the extension into multiple contexts.[106] The results also provide support for the increased duration and intensity of weight maintenance treatment to improve effectiveness over time.

DISCUSSION AND FUTURE DIRECTIONS

The socioecologic approach helps enhance an individual's likelihood of success. The treatment targets extend beyond the individual to incorporate a supportive

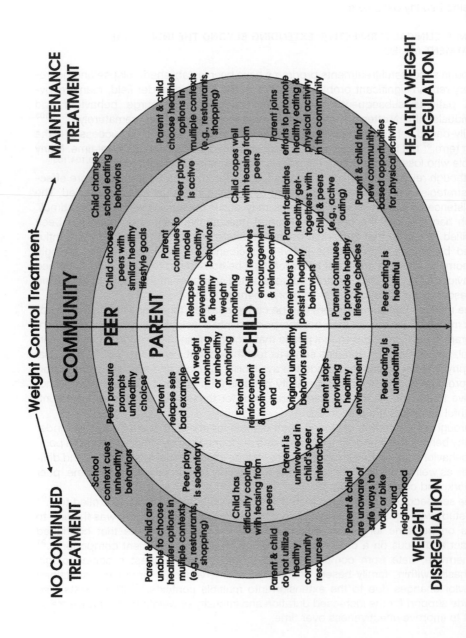

Fig. 1. Socioecologic model of cued behaviors. (*From* Wilfley DE, Van Buren DJ, Theim KR, et al. The use of biosimulation in the design of a novel multi-level weight loss maintenance program for overweight children. Obesity (Silver Spring) 2010;18(Suppl 1):S91–8; with permission.)

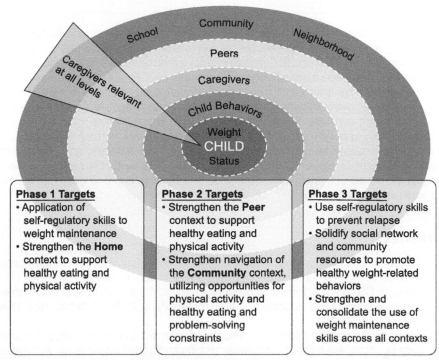

Phase 1 Targets
- Application of self-regulatory skills to weight maintenance
- Strengthen the **Home** context to support healthy eating and physical activity

Phase 2 Targets
- Strengthen the **Peer** context to support healthy eating and physical activity
- Strengthen navigation of the **Community** context, utilizing opportunities for physical activity and healthy eating and problem-solving constraints

Phase 3 Targets
- Use self-regulatory skills to prevent relapse
- Solidify social network and community resources to promote healthy weight-related behaviors
- Strengthen and consolidate the use of weight maintenance skills across all contexts

Fig. 2. The socioecologic model treatment targets.

environment, which more comprehensively addresses the multicontextual problem of weight control. Involving the network of family, peers, schools, health care providers, and community resources is crucial. For example, families should take responsibility to create a healthy home environment: eat regular meals together, avoid bringing home foods that encourage unhealthy eating or electronics that promote sedentary behavior, plan fun and active family outings, and facilitate open communication with youth about daily pressures. Leaders in schools should advocate for healthier meal and snack options as well as more physically active classes and school-wide events. Communities should offer facilities, clubs, and activities that promote healthy lifestyles, including fitness classes, healthy restaurants, and farmers' markets. Educating people and providers across the various contexts will enable effective and long-lasting change on a broader scale.

Given the establishment of effective treatments for eating disorders and weight control, the next step is to disseminate this work. Translational research promotes the extension of laboratory findings into everyday practice; this is particularly relevant for addressing the national obesity epidemic. Training community leaders and care providers to recognize disordered eating patterns and unhealthy weight status will likely make early detection and intervention more feasible and, in turn, has the potential to further prevention efforts. Moreover, instructing providers in the delivery of the established, manual-based treatments will advance treatment practices and reach. Additionally, research across populations should continue to be expanded. Studying additional ages, racial/ethnic groups, and cultural factors may offer insight into the manifestation of disordered weight control patterns and key treatment factors that need to be addressed to ensure widespread treatment success.

SUMMARY

The parallels between eating disorders and obesity allow for the discussion of these issues along a weight control continuum. Within the eating disorders field, specialized psychotherapies (eg, CBT and IPT) remain effective modalities for the individual eating disorder diagnoses, and a transdiagnostic approach (ie, CBT-E) has been developed to better address symptom fluctuation between diagnostic categories. For obesity, family-based behavioral treatment programs are the most effective, and the incorporation of targeted cognitive skills is a useful addition. These lifestyle interventions are enhanced when applied through a socioecologic framework. Across the spectrum, treatment approaches should encourage the family, peer network, and community to create supportive environments. Ultimately, early intervention is needed to have the best likelihood of helping children and adolescents to improve daily functioning and lead healthy lives.

REFERENCES

1. American Psychiatric Association. Diagnostic and statistical manual of mental disorders. text rev. 4th edition. Washington, DC: Author; 2000.
2. Fairburn CG, Bohn K. Eating disorder NOS (EDNOS): an example of the troublesome "not otherwise specified" (NOS) category in DSM-IV. Behav Res Ther 2005;43(6):691–701.
3. American Psychiatric Association. Proposed draft revisions to DSM disorders and criteria. 2010. Available at: http://www.dsm5.org/Pages/Default.aspx. Accessed February 15, 2010.
4. Ogden CL, Carroll MD, Curtin LR, et al. Prevalence of overweight and obesity in the United States, 1999–2004. JAMA 2006;295(13):1549–55.
5. Barlow SE. Expert committee recommendations regarding the prevention, assessment, and treatment of child and adolescent overweight and obesity: summary report. Pediatrics 2007;120(Suppl 4):S164–92.
6. Wilson GT. Eating disorders, obesity and addiction. Eur Eat Disord Rev 2010; 18(5):341–51.
7. Goldschmidt AB, Hilbert A, Manwaring JL, et al. The significance of overvaluation of shape and weight in binge eating disorder. Behav Res Ther 2010;48(3): 187–93.
8. American Psychiatric Association. Treatment of patients with eating disorders, third edition. American Psychiatric Association. Am J Psychiatry 2006;163(Suppl 7): 4–54.
9. Beumont PJ. Clinical presentation of anorexia nervosa and bulimia nervosa. In: Fairburn CG, Brownell KD, editors. Eating disorders and obesity: a comprehensive handbook. 2nd edition. New York: Guilford Press; 2002. p. 162–70.
10. Bulik CM. Anxiety, depression, and eating disorders. In: Fairburn CG, Brownell KD, editors. Eating disorders and obesity: a comprehensive handbook. 2nd edition. New York: Guilford Press; 2002. p. 193–8.
11. Pomeroy C, Mitchell JE. Medical complications of anorexia nervosa and bulimia nervosa. In: Fairburn CG, Brownell KD, editors. Eating disorders and obesity: a comprehensive handbook. 2nd edition. New York: Guilford Press; 2002. p. 278–85.
12. Goldstein MA, Herzog DB, Misra M, et al. Case records of the Massachusetts General Hospital. Case 29-2008. A 19-year-old man with weight loss and abdominal pain. N Engl J Med 2008;359(12):1272–83.

13. Tanofsky-Kraff M, Wilfley DE, Young JF, et al. Preventing excessive weight gain in adolescents: interpersonal psychotherapy for binge eating. Obesity (Silver Spring) 2007;15(6):1345–55.

14. Tanofsky-Kraff M, Cohen ML, Yanovski SZ, et al. A prospective study of psychological predictors of body fat gain among children at high risk for adult obesity. Pediatrics 2006;117(4):1203–9.

15. Tanofsky-Kraff M. Binge eating among children and adolescents. In: Jelalian E, Steele R, editors. Handbook of child and adolescent obesity. New York: Springer; 2008. p. 42–57.

16. Glasofer DR, Tanofsky-Kraff M, Eddy KT, et al. Binge eating in overweight treatment-seeking adolescents. J Pediatr Psychol 2007;32(1):95–105.

17. Goldschmidt AB, Sinton MM, Aspen VP, et al. Psychosocial and familial impairment among overweight youth with social problems. Int J Pediatr Obes 2010; 5(5):428–35.

18. BeLue R, Francis LA, Colaco B. Mental health problems and overweight in a nationally representative sample of adolescents: effects of race and ethnicity. Pediatrics 2009;123(2):697–702.

19. Hayden-Wade HA, Stein RI, Ghaderi A, et al. Prevalence, characteristics, and correlates of teasing experiences among overweight children vs. non-overweight peers. Obes Res 2005;13(8):1381–92.

20. August GP, Caprio S, Fennoy I, et al. Prevention and treatment of pediatric obesity: an endocrine society clinical practice guideline based on expert opinion. J Clin Endocrinol Metab 2008;93(12):4576–99.

21. Goldschmidt AB, Aspen VP, Sinton MM, et al. Disordered eating attitudes and behaviors in overweight youth. Obesity (Silver Spring) 2008;16(2):257–64.

22. Fairburn CG, Welch SL, Doll HA, et al. Risk factors for bulimia nervosa. A community-based case-control study. Arch Gen Psychiatry 1997;54(6): 509–17.

23. Stice E, Whitenton K. Risk factors for body dissatisfaction in adolescent girls: a longitudinal investigation. Dev Psychol 2002;38(5):669–78.

24. Stice E, Presnell K, Spangler D. Risk factors for binge eating onset in adolescent girls: a 2-year prospective investigation. Health Psychol 2002;21(2):131–8.

25. Fairburn CG, Cooper Z, Shafran R. Cognitive behaviour therapy for eating disorders: a "transdiagnostic" theory and treatment. Behav Res Ther 2003;41(5): 509–28.

26. Carnell S, Wardle J. Appetitive traits and child obesity: measurement, origins and implications for intervention. Proc Nutr Soc 2008;67(4):343–55.

27. Carnell S, Wardle J. Appetitive traits in children. New evidence for associations with weight and a common, obesity-associated genetic variant. Appetite 2009; 53(2):260–3.

28. Taylor CB, Bryson S, Celio Doyle AA, et al. The adverse effect of negative comments about weight and shape from family and siblings on women at high risk for eating disorders. Pediatrics 2006;118(2):731–8.

29. Warschburger P. The unhappy obese child. Int J Obes (Lond) 2005;29(Suppl 2): S127–9.

30. Jacobi C, Fittig E, Bryson SW, et al. Who is really at risk: identifying risk factors for subthreshold and full eating disorders in a high-risksample. Psychol Med 2011;31:1–11.

31. Striegel-Moore RH, Fairburn CG, Wilfley DE, et al. Toward an understanding of risk factors for binge-eating disorder in black and white women: a community-based case-control study. Psychol Med 2005;35(6):907–17.

32. Tanofsky-Kraff M, Shomaker LB, Roza CA, et al. A prospective study of pediatric loss of control eating and psychological outcomes. J Abnorm Psychol 2011; 20(1):108–18.

33. Ayala GX, Rogers M, Arredondo EM, et al. Away-from-home food intake and risk for obesity: examining the influence of context. Obesity (Silver Spring) 2008; 16(5):1002–8.

34. Gordon-Larsen P, Nelson MC, Popkin BM. Longitudinal physical activity and sedentary behavior trends: adolescence to adulthood. Am J Prev Med 2004; 27(4):277–83.

35. Luppino FS, de Wit LM, Bouvy PF, et al. Overweight, obesity, and depression: a systematic review and meta-analysis of longitudinal studies. Arch Gen Psychiatry 2010;67(3):220–9.

36. Epstein LH, Valoski AM, Kalarchian MA, et al. Do children lose and maintain weight easier than adults: a comparison of child and parent weight changes from six months to ten years. Obes Res 1995;3(5):411–7.

37. Agras WS, Brandt HA, Bulik CM, et al. Report of the National Institutes of Health workshop on overcoming barriers to treatment research in anorexia nervosa. Int J Eat Disord 2004;35(4):509–21.

38. Spear BA, Barlow SE, Ervin C, et al. Recommendations for treatment of child and adolescent overweight and obesity. Pediatrics 2007;120(Suppl 4):S254–88.

39. Berkman ND, Lohr KN, Bulik CM. Outcomes of eating disorders: a systematic review of the literature. Int J Eat Disord 2007;40(4):293–309.

40. Whitaker RC, Wright JA, Pepe MS, et al. Predicting obesity in young adulthood from childhood and parental obesity. N Engl J Med 1997;337(13):869–73.

41. Serdula MK, Ivery D, Coates RJ, et al. Do obese children become obese adults? A review of the literature. Prev Med 1993;22(2):167–77.

42. Neumark-Sztainer D, Flattum CF, Story M, et al. Dietary approaches to healthy weight management for adolescents: the New Moves model. Adolesc Med State Art Rev 2008;19(3):421–30, viii.

43. Taylor CB, Bryson S, Luce KH, et al. Prevention of eating disorders in at-risk college-age women. Arch Gen Psychiatry 2006;63(8):881–8.

44. Kohn M, Rees JM, Brill S, et al. Preventing and treating adolescent obesity: a position paper of the Society for Adolescent Medicine. J Adolesc Health 2006;38(6):784–7.

45. Shaw H, Stice E, Becker CB. Preventing eating disorders. Child Adolesc Psychiatr Clin N Am 2009;18(1):199–207.

46. Franko DL, Mintz LB, Villapiano M, et al. Food, mood, and attitude: reducing risk for eating disorders in college women. Health Psychol 2005;24(6):567–78.

47. Austin SB, Kim J, Wiecha J, et al. School-based overweight preventive intervention lowers incidence of disordered weight-control behaviors in early adolescent girls. Arch Pediatr Adolesc Med 2007;161(9):865–9.

48. Jones M, Luce KH, Osborne MI, et al. Randomized, controlled trial of an internet-facilitated intervention for reducing binge eating and overweight in adolescents. Pediatrics 2008;121(3):453–62.

49. Wilson GT, Grilo CM, Vitousek KM. Psychological treatment of eating disorders. Am Psychol 2007;62(3):199–216.

50. Wilson GT. Psychological treatment of eating disorders. Annu Rev Clin Psychol 2005;1:439–65.

51. Wilson GT, Fairburn CG, Agras WS. Cognitive-behavioral therapy for bulimia nervosa. In: Garner DM, Garfinkel PE, editors. Handbook of treatment for eating disorders. 2nd edition. New York: Guilford Press; 1997. p. 67–93.

52. Wilfley DE. Psychological treatment of binge eating disorder. In: Fairburn CG, Brownell KD, editors. Eating disorders and obesity: a comprehensive handbook. 2nd edition. New York: The Guilford Press; 2002. p. 350–3.
53. Fairburn CG. Overcoming binge eating. New York: Guilford Press; 1995.
54. Insel TR. Translating scientific opportunity into public health impact: a strategic plan for research on mental illness. Arch Gen Psychiatry 2009;66(2):128–33.
55. Schmidt U, Lee S, Beecham J, et al. A randomized controlled trial of family therapy and cognitive behavior therapy guided self-care for adolescents with bulimia nervosa and related disorders. Am J Psychiatry 2007;164(4):591–8.
56. Striegel-Moore RH, Wilson GT, DeBar L, et al. Cognitive behavioral guided self-help for the treatment of recurrent binge eating. J Consult Clin Psychol 2010; 78(3):312–21.
57. Wilson GT, Wilfley DE, Agras WS, et al. Psychological treatments of binge eating disorder. Arch Gen Psychiatry 2010;67(1):94–101.
58. Sanchez-Ortiz VC, Munro C, Stahl D, et al. A randomized controlled trial of internet-based cognitive-behavioural therapy for bulimia nervosa or related disorders in a student population. Psychol Med 2011;41(2):407–17.
59. Schmidt U, Andiappan M, Grover M, et al. Randomised controlled trial of CD-ROM-based cognitive-behavioural self-care for bulimia nervosa. Br J Psychiatry 2008;193(6):493–500.
60. Wilson GT, Shafran R. Eating disorders guidelines from NICE. Lancet 2005; 365(9453):79–81.
61. Chui W, Safer DL, Bryson SW, et al. A comparison of ethnic groups in the treatment of bulimia nervosa. Eat Behav 2007;8(4):485 91.
62. Young JF, Mufson L. Manual for interpersonal psychotherapy-adolescent skills training (IPT-AST). New York: Columbia University; 2003.
63. Mufson L. Interpersonal psychotherapy for depressed adolescents (IPT-A): extending the reach from academic to community settings. Child Adolesc Ment Health 2010;15(2):66–72.
64. Marcus MD, Wing RR, Fairburn CG. Cognitive behavioral treatment of binge eating vs. behavioral weight control on the treatment of binge eating disorder. Ann Behav Med 1995;17:S090.
65. Telch CF, Agras WS, Rossiter EM, et al. Group cognitive-behavioral treatment for the nonpurging bulimic: an initial evaluation. J Consult Clin Psychol 1990;58(5): 629–35.
66. Wilfley DE, Agras WS, Telch CF, et al. Group cognitive-behavioral therapy and group interpersonal psychotherapy for the nonpurging bulimic individual: a controlled comparison. J Consult Clin Psychol 1993;61(2):296–305.
67. Wilfley DE, Welch RR, Stein RI, et al. A randomized comparison of group cognitive-behavioral therapy and group interpersonal psychotherapy for the treatment of overweight individuals with binge-eating disorder. Arch Gen Psychiatry 2002;59(8):713–21.
68. Tanofsky-Kraff M, Wilfley DE, Young JF, et al. A pilot study of interpersonal psychotherapy for preventing excess weight gain in adolescent girls at-risk for obesity. Int J Eat Disord 2010;43(8):701–6.
69. Halmi KA. The perplexities of conducting randomized, double-blind, placebo-controlled treatment trials in anorexia nervosa patients. Am J Psychiatry 2008; 165(10):1227–8.
70. Channon S, de Silva P, Hemsley D, et al. A controlled trial of cognitive-behavioural and behavioural treatment of anorexia nervosa. Behav Res Ther 1989;27(5):529–35.

71. Pike KM, Walsh BT, Vitousek K, et al. Cognitive behavior therapy in the posthospitalization treatment of anorexia nervosa. Am J Psychiatry 2003;160(11): 2046–9.

72. McIntosh VV, Jordan J, Carter FA, et al. Three psychotherapies for anorexia nervosa: a randomized, controlled trial. Am J Psychiatry 2005;162(4):741–7.

73. Serfaty MA, Turkington D, Heap M, et al. Cognitive therapy versus dietary counseling in the outpatient treatment of anorexia nervosa: effects of the treatment phase. Eur Eat Disord Rev 1999;7:334–50.

74. Halmi KA. A multi-site study of AN treatment involving CBT and fluoxetine treatment in prevention of relapse: a 6-month treatment analysis. Paper presented at: Annual meeting of the Eating Disorders Research Society. San Diego (CA), November, 1999.

75. Halmi KA, Agras WS, Crow S, et al. Predictors of treatment acceptance and completion in anorexia nervosa: implications for future study designs. Arch Gen Psychiatry 2005;62(7):776–81.

76. Ball J, Mitchell P. A randomized controlled study of cognitive behavior therapy and behavioral family therapy for anorexia nervosa patients. Eat Disord 2004; 12(4):303–14.

77. Walsh BT, Kaplan AS, Attia E, et al. Fluoxetine after weight restoration in anorexia nervosa: a randomized controlled trial. JAMA 2006;295(22):2605–12.

78. Attia E, Haiman C, Walsh BT, et al. Does fluoxetine augment the inpatient treatment of anorexia nervosa? Am J Psychiatry 1998;155(4):548–51.

79. Kaye WH, Nagata T, Weltzin TE, et al. Double-blind placebo-controlled administration of fluoxetine in restricting- and restricting-purging-type anorexia nervosa. Biol Psychiatry 2001;49(7):644–52.

80. Lock J, le Grange D. Family-based treatment of eating disorders. Int J Eat Disord 2005;37(Suppl):S64–7 [discussion: S87–9].

81. Lock J. Treating adolescents with eating disorders in the family context. Empirical and theoretical considerations. Child Adolesc Psychiatr Clin N Am 2002; 11(2):331–42.

82. Eddy KT, Dorer DJ, Franko DL, et al. Diagnostic crossover in anorexia nervosa and bulimia nervosa: implications for DSM-V. Am J Psychiatry 2008;165(2):245–50.

83. Fairburn CG, Harrison PJ. Eating disorders. Lancet 2003;361(9355):407–16.

84. Fairburn CG, Cooper Z, Doll HA, et al. Transdiagnostic cognitive-behavioral therapy for patients with eating disorders: a two-site trial with 60-week follow-up. Am J Psychiatry 2009;166(3):311–9.

85. Murphy R, Straebler S, Cooper Z, et al. Cognitive behavioral therapy for eating disorders. Psychiatr Clin North Am 2010;33(3):611–27.

86. Fairburn CG. Cognitive behavior therapy and eating disorders. New York: Guilford Press; 2008.

87. Wilfley DE, Tibbs TL, Van Buren DJ, et al. Lifestyle interventions in the treatment of childhood overweight: a meta-analytic review of randomized controlled trials. Health Psychol 2007;26(5):521–32.

88. U.S. Preventive Services Task Force. Screening for obesity in children and adolescents: US Preventive Services Task Force recommendation statement. Pediatrics 2010;125(2):361–7.

89. Faith MS, Saelens BE, Wilfley DE, et al. Behavioral treatment of childhood and adolescent obesity: Current status, challenges, and future directions. In: Thompson JK, Smolak L, editors. Body Image, eating disorders, and obesity in youth: assessment, prevention, and treatment. Washington, DC: American Psychological Association; 2001. p. 313–9.

90. Graves T, Meyers AW, Clark L. An evaluation of parental problem-solving training in the behavioral treatment of childhood obesity. J Consult Clin Psychol 1988;56(2):246–50.
91. Wilfley DE, Stein RI, Saelens BE, et al. Efficacy of maintenance treatment approaches for childhood overweight: a randomized controlled trial. JAMA 2007;298(14):1661–73.
92. Herrera EA, Johnston CA, Steele RG. A comparison of cognitive and behavioral treatments for pediatric obesity. Child Health Care 2004;33:151–67.
93. Jelalian E, Saelens BE. Empirically supported treatments in pediatric psychology: pediatric obesity. J Pediatr Psychol 1999;24(3):223–48.
94. Tsiros MD, Sinn N, Coates AM, et al. Treatment of adolescent overweight and obesity. Eur J Pediatr 2008;167(1):9–16.
95. Young KM, Northern JJ, Lister KM, et al. A meta-analysis of family-behavioral weight-loss treatments for children. Clin Psychol Rev 2007;27(2):240–9.
96. Epstein LH, Paluch RA, Gordy CC, et al. Decreasing sedentary behaviors in treating pediatric obesity. Arch Pediatr Adolesc Med 2000;154(3):220–6.
97. Epstein LH, Wing RR, Woodall K, et al. Effects of family-based behavioral treatment on obese 5- to 8-year-old children. Behav Ther 1985;16:205–12.
98. Epstein LH, Paluch RA, Roemmich JN, et al. Family-based obesity treatment, then and now: twenty-five years of pediatric obesity treatment. Health Psychol 2007;26(4):381–91.
99. Epstein LH, Myers MD, Raynor HA, et al. Treatment of pediatric obesity. Pediatrics 1998;101(3 Pt 2):554–70.
100. Wilfley DE, Saelens BE. Epidemiology and causes of obesity in children. In: Fairburn CG, Brownell KD, editors. Eating disorders and obesity: a comprehensive handbook. 2nd edition. New York: Guilford Press; 2002. p. 429–32.
101. Wrotniak BH, Epstein LH, Paluch RA, et al. Parent weight change as a predictor of child weight change in family-based behavioral obesity treatment. Arch Pediatr Adolesc Med 2004;158(4):342–7.
102. Dietz WH, Robinson TN. Clinical practice. Overweight children and adolescents. N Engl J Med 2005;352(20):2100–9.
103. Stein RI, Saelens BE, Dounchis JZ, et al. Treatment of eating disorders in women. Couns Psychol 2001;29:695–732.
104. Jeffery RW, Drewnowski A, Epstein LH, et al. Long-term maintenance of weight loss: current status. Health Psychol 2000;19(Suppl 1):5–16.
105. Wadden TA, Butryn ML, Byrne KJ. Efficacy of lifestyle modification for long-term weight control. Obes Res 2004;12(Suppl):151S–62S.
106. Wilfley DE, Van Buren DJ, Theim KR, et al. The use of biosimulation in the design of a novel multilevel weight loss maintenance program for overweight children. Obesity (Silver Spring) 2010;18(Suppl 1):S91–8.
107. Huang TT, Drewnosksi A, Kumanyika S, et al. A systems-oriented multilevel framework for addressing obesity in the 21st century. Prev Chronic Dis 2009; 6(3):A82.
108. Glass TA, McAtee MJ. Behavioral science at the crossroads in public health: extending horizons, envisioning the future. Soc Sci Med 2006;62(7):1650–71.

Cognitive-Behavioral Therapy for Youth with Body Dysmorphic Disorder: Current Status and Future Directions

Katharine A. Phillips, MD[a,b,*], Jamison Rogers, MD[a,c]

KEYWORDS

- Body dysmorphic disorder • Treatment
- Cognitive-behavioral therapy • Children • Adolescents

Body dysmorphic disorder (BDD) is an often severe disorder that usually begins during early adolescence and appears to be common in youth. BDD consists of preoccupation with a nonexistent or slight defect in physical appearance that causes clinically significant distress or impairment in functioning; the symptoms are not better accounted for by an other mental disorder (eg, anorexia nervosa).[1] BDD is characterized by substantial impairment in psychosocial functioning and markedly high rates of

---

This work was supported by Grant No. K24 MH063975 from the National Institute of Mental Health to Dr Phillips.

Disclosure for Dr Phillips (current): Rhode Island Hospital (salary support), Warren Alpert Medical School of Brown University (salary support), National Institute of Mental Health (salary support and research funding), Food and Drug Administration (research funding), Forest Laboratories (medication only for a study sponsored and funded by the National Institute of Mental Health), Oxford University Press (royalties), Guilford Press (potential future royalties), The Free Press (potential future royalties). Disclosure for Dr Rogers (current): Bradley Hospital (salary support).

The authors thank Martha Niemiec, AB, for assistance with the references.

[a] Department of Psychiatry and Human Behavior, Warren Alpert Medical School of Brown University, Rhode Island Hospital, Coro Center West, Suite 2.030, 1 Hoppin Street, Providence, RI 02903, USA

[b] Department of Psychiatry and Human Behavior, Rhode Island Hospital, Coro Center West, 1 Hoppin Street, Providence, RI 02903, USA

[c] Adolescent Inpatient Unit, Bradley Hospital, 1011 Veterans Memorial Parkway, East Providence, RI 02915, USA

* Corresponding author. Rhode Island Hospital, Coro Center West, 1 Hoppin Street, Providence, RI 02903.

E-mail address: Katharine_Phillips@Brown.edu

Child Adolesc Psychiatric Clin N Am 20 (2011) 287–304

doi:10.1016/j.chc.2011.01.004

1056-4993/11/$ – see front matter © 2011 Elsevier Inc. All rights reserved.

childpsych.theclinics.com

suicidality.[2–6] However, despite its severity and description for more than a century, BDD remains underrecognized in both youth and adults.[4,5,7–12]

Because BDD usually begins during early adolescence,[13,14] is often chronic,[15] and causes substantial morbidity in youth,[16,17] early intervention is critical. Cognitive-behavioral therapy (CBT) is the best tested and most promising psychosocial treatment for adults with BDD.[4,5,18–20] However, CBT has not been developed for or tested in youth. In fact, no evidence-based psychosocial treatment of any type is available for youth with this common and severe illness. Thus, there is a pressing need for an efficacious psychosocial treatment for this age group. A BDD treatment practice guideline from the United Kingdom's National Institute for Health and Clinical Excellence[21] underscores the paucity of treatment research on BDD and calls for more treatment research, especially in youth.

AN ADOLESCENT WITH BDD

J, a normal-appearing 12-year-old boy, was preoccupied with the belief that his head was "too big," his arms looked like "toothpicks," and his hair looked "ugly and weird." He was convinced that he looked abnormal, and he thought about these "defects" for 5 to 6 hours a day. J's preoccupations caused severe distress and depressed mood. He spent 4 to 5 hours a day checking his appearance in mirrors, asking his parents if he looked okay, and combing his hair to try to make it "look right." He sometimes stayed in the bathroom for hours at a time, scrutinizing himself in the mirror, frantically combing his hair, and crying because he was so distressed over how he looked. These time-consuming repetitive behaviors and preoccupations interfered with his concentration, causing his grades to plummet. J went to school only because his parents insisted, and he missed school at least once a week because he felt so ugly. He stopped all athletic activities because they "messed up" his hair. J avoided classmates, friends, and most social events because he was convinced that others thought he was ugly. He often felt angry because he erroneously believed that other people mocked his appearance.

BDD IS A COMMON DISORDER

In a study of 566 high school students, BDD's prevalence, based on a self-report questionnaire, was 2.2%.[22] A study of psychiatric inpatients found that 14% of 21 adolescents had BDD.[10] In a larger study of adolescent psychiatric inpatients, 6.7% of 208 consecutively admitted adolescents met *Diagnostic and Statistical Manual of Mental Disorders* (DSM)-IV criteria for definite or probable BDD.[23] And in a subsequent study of 327 consecutive psychiatric inpatients ages 12 to 17, 7.1% met DSM-IV criteria for BDD (Dyl and colleagues, unpublished data, 2010).

In adults, three nationwide studies in the United States and Germany found a point prevalence of 1.7%, 1.8%, and 2.4%,[24–26] making BDD more common than many other mental disorders.[1] BDD is even more common in adults in inpatient and outpatient psychiatric settings as well as dermatology, cosmetic surgery, cosmetic dental, and orthodontia settings.[3,5,27,28] BDD is underrecognized, however, in both adults and youth. Studies that systematically assessed patients for BDD found that those with BDD rarely or never had the diagnosis recorded in their medical record.[9–12,23,29] BDD patients typically do not disclose their appearance concerns to clinicians unless asked about them, most often because they are too embarrassed to do so.[10,29]

BDD USUALLY BEGINS DURING EARLY ADOLESCENCE

In a study of 293 individuals with BDD, the mean age at BDD onset was 16.0 ± 6.9 (range, 4–43).[30] In a more broadly ascertained sample of 200 individuals with BDD, the mean age at BDD onset was 16.4 ± 7.0 years (range, 5–49).[14] The mode was 13 in both samples, and 70% of cases had onset of BDD before age 18. In the latter sample, subclinical BDD began at a mean age of 12.9 ± 5.8 years.[14] Among adults ascertained for major depressive disorder who had BDD, the mean age at BDD onset was 17.5 ± 10.0 years.[31]

CLINICAL FEATURES OF BDD

Available data, although limited, indicate that BDD's clinical features are very similar in youth and adults.[16,17] Preoccupations may focus on any body area, most often the skin (eg, scarring, acne) and hair (eg, balding, excessive facial or body hair).[11,13,14,16,17,32–34] Concern with multiple body areas is common.[13,14] Appearance preoccupations occur, on average, for 3 to 8 hours a day.[35] The preoccupations are usually difficult to control and are distressing.[35] In 33 youth with BDD, the appearance concerns caused severe or extreme, disabling distress in 72% of the sample.[16]

Insight is usually poor or absent; many patients have delusional appearance beliefs[36–39] (ie, complete conviction that they look disfigured). Some describe themselves as looking like a monster or a burn victim.[4] In a study that compared adults (n = 164) and adolescents (n = 36) with BDD on the Brown Assessment of Beliefs Scale,[40] adolescents had poorer insight regarding their appearance "defects" than adults did (P<.001), and a higher proportion of youth had delusional BDD beliefs (59% vs 33%, P = .006).[17] This finding may reflect youth's poorer metacognitive skills, which may continue developing into adolescence[41] and are hypothesized to mediate poor insight in some mental disorders.[42] Two-thirds of patients have ideas or delusions of reference, believing others take special notice of the "defect" (eg, mock the patient).[36,37]

Self-esteem is often poor[33,43–45]; in youth, body image may be the most important contributor to adolescents' global self-esteem.[46,47] Mean levels of depressive symptoms, anxiety, and social anxiety are high.[23,29,48–51] In two of the above-noted inpatient studies in youth, those with BDD had significantly greater depression and anxiety than youth without significant body image concerns; in one of these studies, youth with BDD also had higher levels of posttraumatic stress disorder symptoms and dissociation (Dyl and colleagues, unpublished data, 2010).[23]

Nearly all persons with BDD perform time-consuming repetitive behaviors in response to their appearance concerns. These include: frequently checking their appearance in mirrors and other reflecting surfaces, comparing their appearance with that of other people, excessively grooming, and seeking reassurance about how they look.[11,13,14] Compulsive skin picking intended to improve the skin's appearance can cause significant lesions and scarring, bodily injury, and even life-threatening injuries.[52–54] In one study, lifetime skin picking was more common in adolescents than in adults at a trend level (58% vs 41%, P = .06) (Phillips KA, unpublished data, 2010). Comorbidity is common in both youth and adults, with major depressive disorder, substance use disorders, social phobia, and obsessive-compulsive disorder (OCD) most commonly comorbid.[14,16,17,30]

INDIVIDUALS WITH BDD HAVE SUBSTANTIAL FUNCTIONAL IMPAIRMENT

The literature describes both youth and adults with BDD as severely distressed and impaired, often to a debilitating degree.[34,55–59] Case descriptions indicate that they may avoid activities, stop working, or drop out of school because they think they look ugly or deformed.[60–65] They often avoid dating and other social interactions.[4,32,59] Some become extremely isolated, even housebound for years.[60,66]

On standardized measures, studies have found that youth with BDD have very poor psychosocial functioning and quality of life.[16,17] Mean scores on the Global Assessment of Functioning (44.9–45.7) indicate serious symptoms or serious impairment, and mean scores on the Social Adjustment Scale (SAS) and Quality of Life Enjoyment and Satisfaction Scale (Q-LES-Q) are markedly poor.[16,17] In a study of 33 youth with BDD, 18% had dropped out of elementary school or high school primarily because of BDD symptoms,[16] and in a more broadly ascertained sample of 36 youth with BDD, 22% had dropped out of school primarily because of BDD symptoms.[17] Twenty six percent of the 36 youth wanted to work but were unable to because of psychopathology (BDD was the primary diagnosis for most).[17] Adults with BDD, too, have markedly poor functioning and quality of life on standardized measures.[2,67] For example, among 176 broadly ascertained individuals with BDD, SAS and Q-LES-Q scores were approximately 2 SD units poorer than normative data.[2] In two samples, SF-36 mental health scores were 1.7–2.2 SD units poorer than United States population norms, 0.4–0.7 SD units poorer than norms for depression, and poorer than norms for medical illnesses.[2,67]

SUICIDALITY AND AGGRESSION APPEAR COMMON IN BDD

In two studies, 67% of 33 youth and 81% of 36 youth with BDD had lifetime suicidal ideation,[16,17] which is far higher than rates reported in the community (15%–27%).[68,69] In these studies, 21% and 44% of youth, respectively, had attempted suicide.[16,17] In the latter study, suicide attempts were more common in youth than adults (44% vs 24%, $P = .01$).[17] In two studies of psychiatric inpatients[23] (Dyl and colleagues, unpublished data, 2010), youth with BDD had higher scores than youth without significant body image concerns on the Suicide Probability Scale ($P<.001–P<.0001$), which reflects suicide risk.[70] In adolescents, greater body image dissatisfaction more generally is associated with higher suicidality risk.[71]

Lifetime suicidal ideation (78%–81%) and suicide attempts (24%–28%) are also common in adults with BDD.[6,13,32,33,72,73] In a recent nationwide epidemiologic study, 31% of adults with BDD reported thoughts about committing suicide due to appearance concerns, and 22% had attempted suicide due to appearance concerns.[24] Data on completed suicide are very preliminary; however, the standardized mortality ratio appears markedly elevated[73–75] (Phillips KA, unpublished data, 2010). Indeed, persons with BDD have many suicide risk factors.[6,76–80]

BDD-related aggressive and violent behavior may also occur,[81] with 22% to 38% of youth with BDD reporting lifetime physical aggression or violence due primarily to BDD.[16,82] In a survey of 265 cosmetic surgeons,[83] 12% reported being physically threatened by a BDD patient due to dissatisfaction with surgery, which appears to usually be ineffective for BDD.[33,84–86] High mean levels of anger-hostility have been reported.[50] Clinical observations suggest that aggression or violence may be fueled by: (1) anger about looking "deformed," (2) inability to fix the "defect," (3) delusions of reference, and (4) feeling rejected because of the "defect."[5] Persons with BDD appear particularly sensitive to social rejection,[31] which is associated with aggressive and hostile behavior.[87] They also tend to misinterpret other people's facial expressions as contemptuous and angry,[88] which may have the potential to fuel aggressive behavior.

DIAGNOSING BDD IN YOUTH

The clinical features described above indicate that BDD is not simply normal adolescent concern with appearance; rather, it is a severe and even life-threatening disorder.[89] Thus, all youth should be asked about appearance concerns, and BDD should be diagnosed when present.[89] **Box 1** contains questions clinicians can ask to diagnose BDD in youth, which follow DSM-IV criteria.[5] The Body Dysmorphic Disorder Questionnaire, a self-report screening questionnaire for BDD, has an adolescent version with good psychometric properties.[4,10] Clues to BDD's presence include the clinical features described above (eg, excessive mirror checking). Although some clues (eg, being housebound) are not specific to BDD, youth who display any of these behaviors should be asked about BDD and whether the behaviors are related to appearance concerns.

TREATMENT OF BDD

A Cochrane Review on BDD and a treatment practice guideline on OCD and BDD from the United Kingdom's National Institute for Health and Clinical Excellence (National Health Service) recommend CBT and serotonin reuptake inhibitors (SRIs) as first-line treatments for BDD.[21,90] Although virtually no treatment research has been done in children and adolescents with BDD, these treatments are considered the first-line treatments for this age group.[5,21,90] Other types of psychosocial interventions for BDD are virtually unstudied; thus, they are not recommended as monotherapy for BDD.

CBT

CBT for adults with BDD
CBT that specifically targets BDD symptoms is currently recommended as the psychosocial treatment of choice for BDD.[4,5,18–21,90] Because BDD is a unique disorder, CBT for other disorders is not suitable for BDD. While BDD may be related to major depressive disorder, social phobia, or OCD, it differs from them in important ways and does not appear to be identical to any of them.[4,35,43,51,91–102] For example, BDD patients have more delusional beliefs, greater suicidality, and a higher

---

Box 1
Questions to diagnose BDD in children and adolescents[a]

1. Are you very worried about how you look?
   If yes, What don't you like?
   Do you think (body part) looks really bad?
2. Is there anything else you don't like about how you look? What about your face, skin, hair, nose, or the shape, size or other things about any other part of your body?
3. Do you think about (body part) a lot? Do you wish you could worry about it less?
4. Do other people say you worry about it too much?
5. How does this problem with how you look affect your life?
6. Does it upset you a lot?
7. Has your worry affected your family or friends?

[a] These questions will help determine whether DSM-IV criteria for BDD are met.

prevalence of major depressive disorder than patients with OCD.[35,98–101] Patients with BDD are concerned with more body areas (typically not weight) than eating disorder patients are, and they have more negative self-evaluation and self-worth, more avoidance of activities, and poorer functioning and quality of life due to appearance concerns.[43,97] Unlike patients with social phobia, those with BDD have prominent repetitive behaviors and perceptual distortions involving body image.[4,102] In a prospective longitudinal study, BDD symptoms persisted in a sizable proportion of subjects who remitted from comorbid OCD, major depressive disorder, or social phobia, suggesting that BDD is not simply a symptom of these disorders.[93]

Most published studies of CBT for BDD have included cognitive restructuring, exposure (eg, to avoided social situations), and response (ritual) prevention (eg, not seeking reassurance) that is tailored specifically to BDD symptoms.[18,20,103] Additional strategies (used in combination with the above approaches) include perceptual retraining with mirrors, habit reversal for BDD-related skin picking or hair plucking, cognitive approaches that target core beliefs, incorporation of behavioral experiments into exposure exercises, motivational interviewing tailored to BDD, and other approaches.[103]

BDD patients typically need more intensive engagement and ongoing motivational interventions than patients with other disorders such as OCD, because many BDD patients have poor or absent insight[36–39,101,104] and are thus reluctant to initiate or remain in psychiatric care. Cognitive interventions are more complex and intensive for BDD than for OCD or social phobia because of the delusional nature of BDD beliefs and delusions of reference. Exposure exercises and behavioral experiments are needed for prominent social avoidance, unlike treatment for OCD, depression, or eating disorders.[102] And intensive ritual prevention is a core component of treatment for BDD, which is not needed for depression or social phobia.[102] Treatment must also target other problematic symptoms unique to BDD, such as surgery seeking and skin picking or hair pulling done in an attempt to improve one's appearance.

Several investigators have developed cognitive behavioral models of BDD's development and maintenance, which provide a foundation for CBT treatment for BDD.[19,103,105–107] BDD likely results from a combination of biologic, psychological, and sociocultural factors.[4,5,108] CBT models additionally and more specifically propose that persons with BDD selectively attend to specific aspects of appearance or minor appearance flaws. This hypothesis is supported by clinical observations and neurocognitive (eg, functional MRI) research findings that indicate that persons with BDD excessively focus on detail rather than on larger configural elements of visual stimuli.[109–112] BDD patients consider their perceived flaws to be important and to reflect personal defectiveness and lack of self-worth[33] (eg, "If I don't get chin surgery, I will always be alone. I am completely worthless."). The CBT model further proposes that patients react to perceived imperfections and related maladaptive interpretations with negative emotions (eg, shame, depression, anxiety) that further increase selective attention to perceived flaws. To try to neutralize their distressing feelings, patients avoid social situations and other triggers,[49,51] and they perform repetitive ritualistic behaviors (eg, excessive grooming, mirror checking). Patients' misperception of situations and faces as threatening or angry[88,113,114] may further contribute to neutralizing behaviors such as social avoidance and rituals. Rituals and avoidance are negatively reinforced because they sometimes temporarily diminish painful emotions. Thus, these behaviors are posited to maintain maladaptive BDD beliefs.[103]

CBT for BDD that is based on this or similar models, and that incorporates strategies described above, appears to often be efficacious for adults. In a randomized trial of 54 adults who received 8 weekly 2-hour group sessions of CBT for BDD or were assigned to a waitlist condition, CBT was more efficacious than no treatment.[115] Improvement was sustained at follow-up 4.5 months later.[115] A study that randomized 19 adults to individual CBT or a waitlist found that CBT led to greater improvement than no treatment.[107] In single cases and case series of adults (n = 10–17), symptoms improved significantly at posttest.[18,116–118] For example, a study of group CBT for BDD (n = 13) found that BDD symptoms and depressive symptoms significantly improved.[117] One small study suggested that delusional BDD beliefs predict a poorer outcome,[119] although this finding requires replication. Session number and frequency have varied greatly across studies, from 12 weekly hour-long sessions to 12 weeks of daily 90-minute sessions. To more adequately establish CBT's efficacy for BDD, CBT must be directly compared with other psychosocial interventions that control for therapist time, attention, and other nonspecific treatment elements.

CBT for youth with BDD

Reports are limited to a small number of case studies. The reports below used approaches similar to those for adults. Greenberg and colleagues[120] described individual CBT with family involvement for a 17-year-old female who was horrified by her "flabby" stomach, "bushy" eyebrows, "frizzy" hair, and the size and symmetry of her ears, which made her feel "totally ugly." The patient thought about these perceived flaws for more than 8 hours a day, which caused intense anxiety, shame, disgust, and depression. To try to reduce her distress and "fix" her appearance, she spent 3 to 8 hours a day performing BDD rituals, such as excessive mirror checking, reassurance seeking, clothes changing, hair styling (to cover her ears), and excessive makeup application. Her preoccupations and behaviors made it difficult to get to school on time, sit through class, or focus on her schoolwork. As a result of these concerns, she avoided gym class and stopped socializing with friends. She argued with family members about their involvement in her BDD rituals.

Treatment consisted of 12 50-minute sessions (twice weekly for 4 weeks followed by 4 weekly sessions). Initial sessions focused on assessment, obtaining information from the family to better understand their involvement in the illness, and psychoeducation. The therapist and patient developed a CBT model of the patient's BDD. The patient listed pros and cons of changing versus not changing her BDD behaviors, and treatment goals were established. Cognitive strategies consisted of recognizing self-defeating thoughts and developing more accurate and helpful beliefs. The patient then developed a hierarchy of BDD-related rituals and avoidance behaviors and did in-session and out-of-session exposure exercises while not ritualizing (ritual prevention), starting with less anxiety-provoking situations on her hierarchy. Perceptual retraining using mirrors helped the patient learn to see her entire body (without excessive checking) rather than focusing on disliked details, and to describe herself in neutral and nonjudgmental ways. Treatment increasingly focused on re-establishing friendships and activities. Throughout treatment, the parents assisted with behavioral assignments, reduced their accommodation of BDD symptoms (eg, did not provide reassurance), positively rewarded their daughter for participating in non-BDD activities, and helped maintain her motivation for treatment. Finally, strategies for relapse prevention were discussed. CBT homework was assigned throughout treatment. The patient's score on the Yale-Brown Obsessive-Compulsive Scale Modified for BDD (BDD-YBOCS)[121] decreased from 36 (severe) to 8 (subclinical). Self-esteem, mood, and quality of life improved on standardized measures. At 3-month follow-up, the patient's intrusive thoughts and related distress remained low, and she reported no deliberate avoidance, although her compulsive behaviors had returned to baseline, suggesting that she may have benefitted from longer treatment or booster sessions.

Aldea and colleagues[122] used intensive CBT to treat a 16-year-old girl with BDD who had previously been misdiagnosed with social phobia because of her prominent social avoidance. The patient was convinced that her face, freckles, ears, and hair color and texture were ugly. To diminish anxiety over her "ugliness," she spent 4 to 6 hours a day changing her clothes, applying make-up, blow-drying and straightening her hair, seeking reassurance, and checking her appearance in windows and mirrors. Because she thought other people noticed her "flaws" and were disgusted by her, she did not leave her house during the day, did not attend school, and rarely saw friends.

The patient received 14 90-minute sessions of CBT on consecutive weekdays, with three additional follow-up sessions during the next 3 months that included bolstering relapse prevention skills. The first three sessions focused on building rapport, providing psychoeducation about BDD and its treatment, and developing a hierarchy of situations that caused BDD-related distress. In these initial sessions, rather than trying to convince the patient that she needed treatment, or challenging her irrational beliefs, the therapist focused on her BDD-related distress. Subsequent sessions focused on exposure and response prevention, plus cognitive restructuring that included challenging the patient's perfectionism, self-criticism, and need for approval. In-session exposures were done; for example, walking outside in bright sunlight without hiding her face. The patient completed CBT homework assignments (eg, exposure and ritual prevention), which were reviewed at each session. The parents were asked to not respond to their daughter's requests for reassurance about her appearance and to refrain from buying her an excessive amount of beauty products. The patient's score on the BDD-YBOCS decreased from 27 (moderate) to 10 (subclinical). Gains were maintained at 3-month follow-up.

Horowitz and colleagues[123] used CBT in addition to other treatment modalities for a 16-year-old girl who had a series of referrals to a plastic surgeon for a breast surgery consultation. The patient then presented to an outpatient psychiatric treatment center with a chief complaint of "I want to have surgery soon to remove my breasts, because they don't look like breasts; they look like flaps of skin hanging." The patient thought her breasts were too large; she also worried about the appearance of her face, and she applied creams and bleaches to her face, hair, eyelashes, and eyebrows, and at times picked her skin. These rituals kept her in the bathroom or looking at the mirror during class and before school, causing her academic performance to suffer. Because the patient thought her peers laughed at her appearance in school, she sometimes hid in the bathroom or walked down the hallway pressed up against the walls so she could hide her face and breasts. At home, she sometimes kept the shades drawn or hid under the bed or in the closet because she believed other people were looking at her face and breasts. As a result of her appearance concerns, she became increasingly socially isolated.

Initially, treatment focused on establishing an alliance with the patient and her parents, as the patient believed she was going to therapy to convince her psychiatrist that she needed a bilateral mastectomy. Subsequently, treatment included multiple treatment modalities: elements of CBT, psychodynamic psychotherapy, medication (fluvoxamine 400 mg/day), and consultations with other physicians. CBT focused on cognitive restructuring and exposure and response prevention, which the patient was initially reluctant to engage in. Over time, she made some progress; for example, she developed a hierarchy of activities for exposure therapy, did exposure exercises, and used some therapy time to walk outside. Ritual prevention focused on decreasing mirror checking and other repetitive behaviors. Family sessions focused on psychoeducation about BDD, parenting skills, and improving communication. With this multimodal approach, the patient improved although she had some remaining symptoms.

Sobanski and Schmidt[124] used primarily behavioral approaches (exposure and response prevention) for a 16-year-old girl who was convinced that her pubic bone was becoming increasingly dislocated and prominent, and that everyone stared at it and talked about it. She was convinced that she could be helped only by surgery. In an attempt to achieve a smaller hip girth and change her pubic bone, she reduced her weight to a body mass index of 15.8 kg/m^2, which caused amenorrhea. As a result of her constant preoccupation with her hipbone and shame over her appearance, she become completely housebound, spending most of the day in her bedroom. She frequently measured her pubic bone and camouflaged her pelvis with large clothes.

The patient was treated with exposure, response prevention, and 125 mg/day of doxepin. An anxiety hierarchy of avoided situations was established, with increasing degrees of difficulty: (1) wearing jeans in her own room; (2) wearing jeans in the hospital ward and meeting others; (3) wearing jeans, going to town and visiting a pub; and (4) visiting her school and meeting classmates. She received thirty 60- to 90-minute sessions. The patient was gradually able to face avoided situations. Her BDD symptoms improved; she felt less distressed and had no impairment in functioning. These gains were maintained at 6-month follow-up.

Needed research on CBT for youth with BDD and possible adaptations for youth

Currently, no evidence-based psychosocial treatment of any type is available for children or adolescents with BDD, and CBT has not been studied in this age group. Using CBT for youth has face validity, because BDD's clinical features appear largely similar in youth and adults,[17] CBT for adults with BDD is very promising (see previous discussion), and CBT is efficacious for youth with other disorders that have similarities to BDD.[125–128] However, CBT must be developed for and tested specifically in youth to ensure that it is feasible to implement and efficacious.

The authors recommend that CBT for youth with BDD incorporate both cognitive and behavioral approaches, as in the cases described above. However, CBT must be adapted for youth. For example, while establishing a therapeutic alliance is important for all patients, regardless of their age, building rapport and engaging the patient is especially important before beginning CBT with youth. Often, parents bring youth with BDD to treatment, and many youth do not want to be in treatment. Furthermore, youth are likely to have less insight into their illness than adults.[17] Thus, it may be helpful for therapists to use a motivational interviewing style and not directly challenge a youth's defenses and resistance at the beginning of treatment. Spending initial sessions learning about the youth's interests, what is important in his or her world, and how he or she views BDD can go a long way toward establishing rapport. Using humor may help facilitate rapport, although this should be done with care, as patients with BDD tend to be rejection sensitive, and humor about BDD or the patient's appearance is not advised. Another helpful technique to aid rapport building is respecting the youth's need for autonomy. Although parental involvement is necessary for successful treatment of youth with BDD, paying close attention to topics the youth wants to be kept confidential builds trust. Clarifying at the beginning of treatment with the youth which topics cannot be kept confidential (those involving safety) helps foster a good therapeutic relationship. Once rapport is well-established, CBT for BDD can proceed.

CBT for youth must be modified so it is age appropriate. For example, treatment forms should use modified language and graphics, and the therapist's communication style must be age appropriate (eg, when providing psychoeducation about BDD or using metaphors). Types of external reinforcement and rewards for treatment attendance and adherence should also be appropriate for the patient's age.

CBT for BDD in youth must also address developmental transitions and tasks. Body image more broadly is an important aspect of psychological and interpersonal development in youth[46,47]; it is particularly salient during adolescence because substantial physical development occurs. In addition, at puberty, across species, the brain appears to increasingly attend to indicators of social status, including appearance, as well as cues of social rejection.[5] Body image may influence normative developmental transitions and tasks, such as affiliation transitions (greater autonomy from the family and peer affiliations, development of romantic affiliations), achievement transitions (eg, school and work), and identity transitions (eg, changes in self-definition).[129] Thus, treatment should address issues such as relationships with family and peers, dating, and school-related difficulties. Because severe psychopathology, including BDD, may adversely affect key developmental transitions,[130] some patients may benefit from an additional focus on skills training to address developmental deficits such as a lack of peer relationships or not completing school.[120]

Parents or guardians need to be involved in psychoeducation and treatment. Younger patients will likely require more parental involvement than older adolescents. Parents can learn to decrease their participation in BDD rituals, encourage and help their child with CBT homework assignments, enhance motivation for treatment, reinforce positive behaviors and activities, and develop realistic expectations for their child's progress.[5] Teachers may need to be informed about treatment and advised about recommended approaches for students who are struggling in school because of their symptoms. In some cases, alternative education plans or home tutoring may be needed for youth who cannot attend school because they are too ill.

CBT may need to be modified for more severely depressed youth to ensure that depressive symptoms that may interfere with treatment are addressed (for example, via activity scheduling). Treatment modification will also be needed for youth who are more highly suicidal or appear at risk for violent behavior, so the safety of the patient and others is adequately addressed. In the authors' opinion (based on their clinical experience), patients with very severe BDD or depressive symptoms, and those who are suicidal, should receive an SRI in addition to CBT.[4,5]

Pharmacotherapy

SRIs are considered the medication of choice for BDD.[5,21,90,131,132] Randomized, double-blind, controlled studies in adults demonstrated that fluoxetine was more efficacious than placebo and that the SRI clomipramine was more efficacious than the non-SRI antidepressant desipramine.[133,134] Methodologically rigorous open-label studies[131,135–138] and large clinical series[37,139] also support SRI efficacy in adults. Response rates (intention-to-treat analyses) are 53% to 77%.[131,132] Patients with delusional BDD beliefs are as likely to respond to SRI monotherapy as patients with nondelusional beliefs.[37,133–136,140] In adults, relatively high SRI doses are often needed, and a 12 to 16 week trial is recommended to determine efficacy.[5,131,132]

In children and adolescents, SRI efficacy has been reported in case reports[65,141–144] and a series of 33 patients, in which a majority of patients had clinically significant improvement in BDD with SRIs but no improvement with non-SRI medications.[16] Given concerns about suicidality and SRI use in youth,[145] caution should be used when prescribing these medications in this age group. In patients with BDD age 18 and older, SRIs have been shown to decrease suicidality[135] and to exert a protective effect against worsening of suicidality.[146]

Cosmetic Treatment

Studies have found that 41% to 63% of youth with BDD seek dermatologic, surgical, dental, or other cosmetic treatment for BDD concerns; most requested treatments are received.[16,84,85] Such treatment appears to virtually never improve overall BDD symptoms in youth or adults, and some patients develop new appearance concerns.[16,28,33,84,85,147] Thus, cosmetic treatment is not recommended for youth or adults with BDD.

SUMMARY

Because BDD is common, usually begins in early adolescence, and is associated with substantial impairment in psychosocial functioning and markedly elevated suicidality rates, there is a pressing need for the development of evidence-based treatments for youth. CBT that is tailored to BDD's unique symptoms is the best-tested and most promising psychosocial treatment for adults with BDD. Because no evidence-based psychosocial treatment of any type is available for youth, there is a critical need to develop and test CBT and other interventions in this age group.

REFERENCES

1. American Psychiatric Association. Diagnostic and statistical manual of mental disorders: DSM-IV-TR. Washington, DC: American Psychiatric Association; 2000.
2. Phillips KA, Menard W, Fay C, et al. Psychosocial functioning and quality of life in body dysmorphic disorder. Compr Psychiatry 2005;46:254–60.
3. Didie ER, Kelly MM, Phillips KA. Clinical features of body dysmorphic disorder. Psychiatr Ann 2010;40:310–6.
4. Phillips KA. The broken mirror: understanding and treating body dysmorphic disorder. Revised and expanded edition. New York: Oxford University Press; 2005.
5. Phillips KA. Understanding body dysmorphic disorder: an essential guide. New York: Oxford University Press; 2009.
6. Phillips KA, Coles ME, Menard W, et al. Suicidal ideation and suicide attempts in body dysmorphic disorder. J Clin Psychiatry 2005;66:717–25.
7. Morselli E. Sulla dismorfofobia e sulla tafefobia. Bolletinno della R Accademia di Genova 1891;6:110–9 [in Italian].
8. Thompson CM, Durrani AJ. An increasing need for early detection of body dysmorphic disorder by all specialties. J R Soc Med 2007;100:61–2.
9. Phillips KA, Nierenberg AA, Brendel G, et al. Prevalence and clinical features of body dysmorphic disorder in atypical major depression. J Nerv Ment Dis 1996; 184:125–9.
10. Grant JE, Kim SW, Crow SJ. Prevalence and clinical features of body dysmorphic disorder in adolescent and adult psychiatric inpatients. J Clin Psychiatry 2001;62:517–22.
11. Phillips KA, McElroy SL, Keck PE Jr, et al. Body dysmorphic disorder: 30 cases of imagined ugliness. Am J Psychiatry 1993;150:302–8.
12. Zimmerman M, Mattia JI. Body dysmorphic disorder in psychiatric outpatients: recognition, prevalence, comorbidity, demographic, and clinical correlates. Compr Psychiatry 1998;39:265–70.
13. Phillips KA, Diaz SF. Gender differences in body dysmorphic disorder. J Nerv Ment Dis 1997;185:570–7.

14. Phillips KA, Menard W, Fay C, et al. Demographic characteristics, phenomenology, comorbidity, and family history in 200 individuals with body dysmorphic disorder. Psychosomatics 2005;46:317–25.

15. Phillips KA, Pagano ME, Menard W, et al. A 12-month follow-up study of the course of body dysmorphic disorder. Am J Psychiatry 2006;163:907–12.

16. Albertini RS, Phillips KA. Thirty-three cases of body dysmorphic disorder in children and adolescents. J Am Acad Child Adolesc Psychiatry 1999;38:453–9.

17. Phillips KA, Didie ER, Menard W, et al. Clinical features of body dysmorphic disorder in adolescents and adults. Psychiatry Res 2006;141:305–14.

18. Neziroglu F, Khemlani-Patel S. A review of cognitive and behavioral treatment for body dysmorphic disorder. CNS Spectr 2002;7:464–71.

19. Veale D. Cognitive behavioral therapy for body dysmorphic disorder. Psychiatr Ann 2010;40:333–40.

20. Buhlmann U, Reese HE, Renaud S, et al. Clinical considerations for the treatment of body dysmorphic disorder with cognitive-behavioral therapy. Body Image 2008;5:39–49.

21. National Collaborating Centre for Mental Health. Core interventions in the treatment of obsessive compulsive disorder and body dysmorphic disorder (a guideline from the National Institute for Health and Clinical Excellence, National Health Service). 2006. Available at: www.nice.org.uk/page.aspx?o=289817. Accessed January 6, 2011.

22. Mayville S, Katz RC, Gipson MT, et al. Assessing the prevalence of body dysmorphic disorder in an ethnically diverse group of adolescents. J Child Fam Stud 1999;8:357–62.

23. Dyl J, Kittler J, Phillips KA, et al. Body dysmorphic disorder and other clinically significant body image concerns in adolescent psychiatric inpatients: prevalence and clinical characteristics. Child Psychiatry Hum Dev 2006;36: 369–82.

24. Buhlmann U, Glaesmer H, Mewes R, et al. Updates on the prevalence of body dysmorphic disorder: a population-based survey. Psychiatry Res 2010;178: 171–5.

25. Koran LM, Abujaoude E, Large MD, et al. The prevalence of body dysmorphic disorder in the United States adult population. CNS Spectr 2008;13:316–22.

26. Rief W, Buhlmann U, Wilhelm S, et al. The prevalence of body dysmorphic disorder: a population-based survey. Psychol Med 2006;36:877–85.

27. Phillips KA, Feusner J. Assessment and differential diagnosis of body dysmorphic disorder. Psychiatr Ann 2010;40:317–24.

28. Crerand CE, Sarwer DB. Cosmetic treatments and body dysmorphic disorder. Psychiatr Ann 2010;40:344–8.

29. Conroy M, Menard W, Fleming-Ives K, et al. Prevalence and clinical characteristics of body dysmorphic disorder in an adult inpatient setting. Gen Hosp Psychiatry 2008;30:67–72.

30. Gunstad J, Phillips KA. Axis I comorbidity in body dysmorphic disorder. Compr Psychiatry 2003;44:270–6.

31. Nierenberg AA, Phillips KA, Petersen TJ, et al. Body dysmorphic disorder in outpatients with major depression. J Affect Disord 2002;69:141–8.

32. Perugi G, Giannotti D, Frare F, et al. Prevalence, phenomenology and comorbidity of body dysmorphic disorder (dysmorphophobia) in a clinical population. Int J Psychiatry Clin Pract 1997;1:77–82.

33. Veale D, Boocock A, Gournay K, et al. Body dysmorphic disorder. A survey of fifty cases. Br J Psychiatry 1996;169:196–201.

34. Yamada M, Kobashi K, Shigemoto T, et al. On dysmorphophobia. Bull Yamaguchi Med Sch 1978;25:47–54.
35. Phillips KA, Gunderson CG, Mallya G, et al. A comparison study of body dysmorphic disorder and obsessive-compulsive disorder. J Clin Psychiatry 1998; 59:568–75.
36. Phillips KA. Psychosis in body dysmorphic disorder. J Psychiatr Res 2004;38: 63–72.
37. Phillips KA, McElroy SL, Keck PE Jr, et al. A comparison of delusional and non-delusional body dysmorphic disorder in 100 cases. Psychopharmacol Bull 1994;30:179–86.
38. Mancuso SG, Knoesen NP, Castle DJ. Delusional versus nondelusional body dysmorphic disorder. Compr Psychiatry 2010;51:177–82.
39. Phillips KA, Menard W, Pagano ME, et al. Delusional versus nondelusional body dysmorphic disorder: clinical features and course of illness. J Psychiatr Res 2006;40:95–104.
40. Eisen JL, Phillips KA, Baer L, et al. The Brown Assessment of Beliefs Scale: reliability and validity. Am J Psychiatry 1998;155:102–8.
41. Ormond C, Luszcz MA, Mann L, et al. A metacognitive analysis of decision making in adolescence. J Adolesc 1991;14:275–91.
42. Koren D, Seidman LJ, Poyurovsky M, et al. The neuropsychological basis of insight in first-episode schizophrenia: a pilot metacognitive study. Schizophr Res 2004;70:195–202.
43. Rosen JC, Ramirez E. A comparison of eating disorders and body dysmorphic disorder on body image and psychological adjustment. J Psychosom Res 1998; 44:441–9.
44. Phillips KA, Pinto A, Jain S. Self-esteem in body dysmorphic disorder. Body Image 2004;1:385–90.
45. Bohne A, Wilhelm S, Keuthen NJ, et al. Prevalence of body dysmorphic disorder in a German college student sample. Psychiatry Res 2002;109:101–4.
46. Levine M, Smolak M, Cash T, et al. Body image development in adolescence. In: Cash T, Pruzinsky T, editors. Body image: a handbook of theory, research, and clinical practice. New York: Guilford Press; 2002. p. 74–82.
47. Harter S, Marold D, Whitesell N. Model of psychosocial risk factors leading to suicidal ideation in young adolescents. Dev Psychopathol 1992;4:167–88.
48. Phillips KA, Didie ER, Menard W. Clinical features and correlates of major depressive disorder in individuals with body dysmorphic disorder. J Affect Disord 2007;97:129–35.
49. Pinto A, Phillips KA. Social anxiety in body dysmorphic disorder. Body Image 2005;2:401–5.
50. Phillips KA, Siniscalchi JM, McElroy SL. Depression, anxiety, anger, and somatic symptoms in patients with body dysmorphic disorder. Psychiatr Q 2004;75: 309–20.
51. Kelly MM, Walters C, Phillips KA. Social anxiety and its relationship to functional impairment in body dysmorphic disorder. Behav Ther 2010;41:143–53.
52. Grant JE, Menard W, Phillips KA. Pathological skin picking in individuals with body dysmorphic disorder. Gen Hosp Psychiatry 2006;28:487–93.
53. O'Sullivan RL, Phillips KA, Keuthen NJ, et al. Near-fatal skin picking from delusional body dysmorphic disorder responsive to fluvoxamine. Psychosomatics 1999;40:79–81.
54. Phillips KA, Taub SL. Skin picking as a symptom of body dysmorphic disorder. Psychopharmacol Bull 1995;31:279–88.

55. Cotterill JA. Dermatological non-disease: a common and potentially fatal disturbance of cutaneous body image. Br J Dermatol 1981;104:611–9.
56. Hollander E, Cohen LJ, Simeon D. Body dysmorphic disorder. Psychiatr Ann 1993;23:359–64.
57. Koblenzer CS. The dysmorphic syndrome. Arch Dermatol 1985;121:780–4.
58. Munro A, Chmara J. Monosymptomatic hypochondriacal psychosis: a diagnostic checklist based on 50 cases of the disorder. Can J Psychiatry 1982;27:374–6.
59. Phillips KA. Body dysmorphic disorder: the distress of imagined ugliness. Am J Psychiatry 1991;148:1138–49.
60. Braddock LE. Dysmorphophobia in adolescence: a case report. Br J Psychiatry 1982;140:199–201.
61. Olley PC. Aspects of plastic surgery. Psychiatric aspects of referral. Br Med J 1974;3:248–9.
62. Philippopoulos GS. The analysis of a case of dysmorfophobia. Can J Psychiatry 1979;24:397–401.
63. Zaidens SH. Dermatologic hypochondriasis; a form of schizophrenia. Psychosom Med 1950;12:250–3.
64. Bezoari M, Falcinelli D. Immagine del corpo e relazioni oggetuali: note sulla dismorfofobia. Rass Studi Psichiatr 1977;66:489–510 [in Italian].
65. Phillips KA, Atala KD, Albertiini RS. Body dysmorphic disorder in adolescents. J Am Acad Child Adolesc Psychiatry 1995;34:1216–20.
66. Neziroglu FA, Yaryura-Tobias JA. Exposure, response prevention, and cognitive therapy in the treatment of body dysmorphic disorder. Behav Ther 1993;24:431–8.
67. Phillips KA. Quality of life for patients with body dysmorphic disorder. J Nerv Ment Dis 2000;188:170–5.
68. Ackerman GL. A congressional view of youth suicide. Am Psychol 1993;48:183–4.
69. Sells W, Blum R. Current trends in adolescent health. In: DiClemente R, Hansen W, Ponton L, editors. Handbook of adolescent health risk behavior. New York: Plenum Press; 1996. p. 5–33.
70. Cull JG, Gill WS. Suicide Probability Scale (SPS) manual. Los Angeles (CA): Western Psychological Services; 1982.
71. Crow S, Eisenberg ME, Story M, et al. Suicidal behavior in adolescents: relationship to weight status, weight control behaviors, and body dissatisfaction. Int J Eat Disord 2008;41:82–7.
72. Phillips KA. Suicidality in body dysmorphic disorder. Prim Psychiatry 2007;14:58–66.
73. Phillips KA, Menard W. Suicidality in body dysmorphic disorder: a prospective study. Am J Psychiatry 2006;163:1280–2.
74. Harris EC, Barraclough B. Suicide as an outcome for mental disorders: a meta-analysis. Br J Psychiatry 1997;170:205–28.
75. American Psychiatric Association. Practice guideline for the assessment and treatment of patients with suicidal behaviors. Am J Psychiatry 2003;160:1–60.
76. Moscicki EK. Identification of suicide risk factors using epidemiologic studies. Psychiatr Clin North Am 1997;20:499–517.
77. Brown GK, Beck AT, Steer RA, et al. Risk factors for suicide in psychiatric outpatients: a 20-year prospective study. J Consult Clin Psychol 2000;68:371–7.
78. Cohen Y, Spirito A, Brown L. Suicide and suicidal behavior. In: DiClemente R, Hansen W, Ponton L, editors. Handbook of adolescent health risk behavior. New York: Plenum Press; 1996. p. 193–224.

79. Henricksson M, Aro H, Marttunen M, et al. Mental disorders and comorbidity in suicide. Am J Psychiatry 1993;150:939–40.
80. Qin P, Agerbo E, Mortensen P. Suicide risk in relation to socioeconomic, demographic, psychiatric, and familial factors: a national register-based study of all suicides in Denmark. Am J Psychiatry 2003;160:765–72.
81. Lucas P. Violence may be serious in men with body dysmorphic disorder. BMJ 2002;324:678.
82. Christopher P, Menard W, Stuart G, et al. Aggressive and violent behavior in individuals with body dysmorphic disorder. In: 13th Annual Research Symposium on Mental Health Sciences. Providence (RI); 2009. p. 14.
83. Sarwer DB. Awareness and identification of body dysmorphic disorder by aesthetic surgeons: results of a survey of American Society for Aesthetic Plastic Surgery Members. Aesthet Surg J 2002;22:531–5.
84. Phillips KA, Grant J, Siniscalchi J, et al. Surgical and nonpsychiatric medical treatment of patients with body dysmorphic disorder. Psychosomatics 2001; 42:504–10.
85. Crerand CE, Phillips KA, Menard W, et al. Nonpsychiatric medical treatment of body dysmorphic disorder. Psychosomatics 2005;46:549–55.
86. Crerand CE, Menard W, Phillips KA. Surgical and minimally invasive cosmetic procedures among persons with body dysmorphic disorder. Ann Plast Surg 2010;65:11–6.
87. Leary MR, Twenge JM, Quinlivan E. Interpersonal rejection as a determinant of anger and aggression. Pers Soc Psychol Rev 2006;10:111–32.
88. Buhlmann U, Etcoff NL, Wilhelm S. Emotion recognition bias for contempt and anger in body dysmorphic disorder. J Psychiatr Res 2006;40:105–11.
89. Hadley SJ, Greenberg J, Hollander E. Diagnosis and treatment of body dysmorphic disorder in adolescents. Curr Psychiatry Rep 2002;4:108–13.
90. Ipser J, Sander C, Stein D. Pharmacotherapy and psychotherapy for body dysmorphic disorder. Cochrane Database Syst Rev 2009;1:CD005332.
91. Jaisoorya TS, Reddy YC, Srinath S. The relationship of obsessive-compulsive disorder to putative spectrum disorders: results from an Indian study. Compr Psychiatry 2003;44:317–23.
92. Phillips KA. Body dysmorphic disorder and depression: theoretical considerations and treatment strategies. Psychiatr Q 1999;70:313–31.
93. Phillips KA, Stout RL. Associations in the longitudinal course of body dysmorphic disorder with major depression, obsessive-compulsive disorder, and social phobia. J Psychiatr Res 2006;40:360–9.
94. Phillips KA. The obsessive-compulsive spectrums. Psychiatr Clin North Am 2002;25:791–809.
95. Phillips KA, McElroy SL, Hudson JI, et al. Body dysmorphic disorder: an obsessive-compulsive spectrum disorder, a form of affective spectrum disorder, or both? J Clin Psychiatry 1995;56:41–51.
96. Cohen LJ, Simeon D, Hollander E, et al. Obsessive-compulsive spectrum disorders. In: Hollander E, Stein DJ, editors. Obsessive-compulsive disorders: diagnosis, etiology, treatment. New York: Marcel Dekker Inc; 1997. p. 47–74.
97. Hrabosky JI, Cash TF, Veale D, et al. Multidimensional body image comparisons among patients with eating disorders, body dysmorphic disorder, and clinical controls: a multisite study. Body Image 2009;6:155–63.
98. Phillips KA, Pinto A, Menard W, et al. Obsessive-compulsive disorder versus body dysmorphic disorder: a comparison study of two possibly related disorders. Depress Anxiety 2007;24:399–409.

99. Frare F, Perugi G, Ruffolo G, et al. Obsessive-compulsive disorder and body dysmorphic disorder: a comparison of clinical features. Eur Psychiatry 2004; 19:292–8.

100. McKay D, Neziroglu F, Yaryura-Tobias JA. Comparison of clinical characteristics in obsessive-compulsive disorder and body dysmorphic disorder. J Anxiety Disord 1997;11:447–54.

101. Eisen JL, Phillips KA, Coles ME, et al. Insight in obsessive compulsive disorder and body dysmorphic disorder. Compr Psychiatry 2004;45:10–5.

102. Phillips KA, Stein DJ, Rauch SL, et al. Should an obsessive-compulsive spectrum grouping of disorders be included in DSM-V? Depress Anxiety 2010;27:528–55.

103. Wilhelm S, Phillips KA, Steketee G. Cognitive-behavioral therapy for body dysmorphic disorder: a modular treatment manual. Guilford Press, in press.

104. Phillips KA, Wilhelm S, Koran LM, et al. Body dysmorphic disorder: some key issues for DSM-V. Depress Anxiety 2010;27:573–91.

105. Wilhelm S, Buhlmann U, Cook L, et al. Cognitive-behavioral treatment approach for body dysmorphic disorder. Cogn Behav Pract 2010;17:241–7.

106. Wilhelm S, Neziroglu F. Cognitive theory of body dysmorphic disorder. In: Frost R, Steketee G, editors. Cognitive approaches to obsessions and compulsions: theory, assessment, and treatment. Amsterdam (Netherlands): Pergamon/Elsevier Science Inc; 2002. p. 203–14.

107. Veale D, Gournay K, Dryden W, et al. Body dysmorphic disorder: a cognitive behavioural model and pilot randomised controlled trial. Behav Res Ther 1996;34: 717–29.

108. Feusner JD, Neziroglu F, Wilhelm S, et al. What causes BDD: research findings and a proposed model. Psychiatr Ann 2010;40:349–55.

109. Deckersbach T, Savage CR, Phillips KA, et al. Characteristics of memory dysfunction in body dysmorphic disorder. J Int Neuropsychol Soc 2000;6:673–81.

110. Feusner JD, Townsend J, Bystritsky A, et al. Visual information processing of faces in body dysmorphic disorder. Arch Gen Psychiatry 2007;64:1417–25.

111. Feusner JD, Moller H, Altstein L, et al. Inverted face processing in body dysmorphic disorder. J Psychiatr Res 2010;44:1088–94.

112. Feusner JD, Moody T, Hembacher E, et al. Abnormalities of visual processing and frontostriatal systems in body dysmorphic disorder. Arch Gen Psychiatry 2010;67:197–205.

113. Buhlmann U, Wilhelm S, McNally RJ, et al. Interpretive biases for ambiguous information in body dysmorphic disorder. CNS Spectr 2002;7:435–6, 41–3.

114. Buhlmann U, McNally RJ, Etcoff NL, et al. Emotion recognition deficits in body dysmorphic disorder. J Psychiatr Res 2004;38:201–6.

115. Rosen JC, Reiter J, Orosan P. Cognitive-behavioral body image therapy for body dysmorphic disorder. J Consult Clin Psychol 1995;63:263–9.

116. Neziroglu F, McKay D, Todaro J, et al. Effect of cognitive behavior therapy on persons with body dysmorphic disorder and comorbid Axis II diagnosis. Behav Ther 1996;27:67–77.

117. Wilhelm S, Otto MW, Lohr B, et al. Cognitive behavior group therapy for body dysmorphic disorder: a case series. Behav Res Ther 1999;37:71–5.

118. McKay D, Todaro J, Neziroglu F, et al. Body dysmorphic disorder: a preliminary evaluation of treatment and maintenance using exposure with response prevention. Behav Res Ther 1997;35:67–70.

119. Neziroglu F, Stevens KP, McKay D, et al. Predictive validity of the overvalued ideas scale: outcome in obsessive-compulsive and body dysmorphic disorders. Behav Res Ther 2001;39:745–56.

120. Greenberg JL, Markowitz S, Petronko MR, et al. Cognitive-behavioral therapy for adolescent body dysmorphic disorder. Cogn Behav Pract 2010;17:248–58.

121. Phillips KA, Hollander E, Rasmussen SA, et al. A severity rating scale for body dysmorphic disorder: development, reliability, and validity of a modified version of the Yale-Brown Obsessive Compulsive Scale. Psychopharmacol Bull 1997; 33:17–22.

122. Aldea MA, Storch EA, Geffken GR, et al. Intensive cognitive-behavioral therapy for adolescents with body dysmorphic disorder. Clin Case Stud 2009;8:113–21.

123. Horowitz K, Gorfinkle K, Lewis O, et al. Body dysmorphic disorder in an adolescent girl. J Am Acad Child Adolesc Psychiatry 2002;41:1503–9.

124. Sobanski E, Schmidt MH. 'Everybody looks at my pubic bone'–a case report of an adolescent patient with body dysmorphic disorder. Acta Psychiatr Scand 2000;101:80–2.

125. Albano AM, Barlow DH. Breaking the vicious cycle: cognitive-behavioral group treatment for socially anxious youth. In: Hibbs ED, Jensen PS, editors. Psychosocial treatments for child and adolescent disorders: empirically based strategies for clinical practice. Washington, DC: American Psychological Association; 1996. p. 43–62.

126. Franklin ME, Kozak MJ, Cashman LA, et al. Cognitive-behavioral treatment of pediatric obsessive-compulsive disorder: an open clinical trial. J Am Acad Child Adolesc Psychiatry 1998;37:412–9.

127. Piacentini J, Langley A, Roblek T. Cognitive-behavioral treatment of childhood OCD: it's only a false alarm, therapist guide. New York: Oxford University Press; 2007.

128. March JS, Franklin M, Nelson A, et al. Cognitive-behavioral psychotherapy for pediatric obsessive-compulsive disorder. J Clin Child Psychol 2001;30:8–18.

129. Schulenberg J, Maggs J, Hurrelmann K. Negotiating developmental transitions during adolescence and young adulthood: health risks and opportunities. In: Schulenberg J, Maggs J, Hurrelmann K, editors. Health risks and developmental transitions during adolescence. Cambridge (UK): Cambridge University Press; 1997. p. 1–22.

130. Brown BB, Dolcini MM, Leventhal A. Transformations in peer relationships at adolescence: implications for health-related behavior. In: Schulenberg J, Maggs J, Hurrelmann K, editors. Health risks and developmental transitions during adolescence. Cambridge (UK): Cambridge University Press; 1997. p. 161–89.

131. Phillips KA, Hollander E. Treating body dysmorphic disorder with medication: evidence, misconceptions, and a suggested approach. Body Image 2008;5: 13–27.

132. Phillips KA. Pharmacotherapy for body dysmorphic disorder. Psychiatr Ann 2010;40:325–32.

133. Hollander E, Allen A, Kwon J, et al. Clomipramine vs desipramine crossover trial in body dysmorphic disorder: selective efficacy of a serotonin reuptake inhibitor in imagined ugliness. Arch Gen Psychiatry 1999;56:1033–9.

134. Phillips KA, Albertini RS, Rasmussen SA. A randomized placebo-controlled trial of fluoxetine in body dysmorphic disorder. Arch Gen Psychiatry 2002;59:381–8.

135. Phillips KA. An open-label study of escitalopram in body dysmorphic disorder. Int Clin Psychopharmacol 2006;21:177–9.

136. Phillips KA, Najjar F. An open-label study of citalopram in body dysmorphic disorder. J Clin Psychiatry 2003;64:715–20.

137. Phillips KA, Dwight MM, McElroy SL. Efficacy and safety of fluvoxamine in body dysmorphic disorder. J Clin Psychiatry 1998;59:165–71.

138. Perugi G, Giannotti D, Di Vaio S, et al. Fluvoxamine in the treatment of body dysmorphic disorder (dysmorphophobia). Int Clin Psychopharmacol 1996;11: 247–54.

139. Phillips KA. Pharmacologic treatment of body dysmorphic disorder. Psychopharmacol Bull 1996;32:597–605.

140. Phillips KA, McElroy SL, Dwight MM, et al. Delusionality and response to open-label fluvoxamine in body dysmorphic disorder. J Clin Psychiatry 2001;62: 87–91.

141. Albertini RS, Phillips KA, Guevremont D. Body dysmorphic disorder in a young child [letter]. J Am Acad Child Adolesc Psychiatry 1996;35:1425–6.

142. el-Khatib HE, Dickey TO. Sertraline for body dysmorphic disorder. J Am Acad Child Adolesc Psychiatry 1995;34:1404–5.

143. Heimann SW. SSRI for body dysmorphic disorder. J Am Acad Child Adolesc Psychiatry 1997;36:868.

144. Sondheimer A. Clomipramine treatment of delusional disorder-somatic type. J Am Acad Child Adolesc Psychiatry 1988;27:188–92.

145. US Food and Drug Administration: antidepressant use in children, adolescents, and adults. 2010. Available at: http://www.fda.gov/Drugs/DrugSafety/InformationbyDrugClass/ucm096273.htm. Accessed January 6, 2011.

146. Phillips KA, Kelly MM. Suicidality in a placebo-controlled fluoxetine study of body dysmorphic disorder. Int Clin Psychopharmacol 2009;24:26–8.

147. Tignol J, Biraben-Gotzamanis L, Martin-Guehl C, et al. Body dysmorphic disorder and cosmetic surgery: evolution of 24 subjects with a minimal defect in appearance 5 years after their request for cosmetic surgery. Eur Psychiatry 2007;22:520–4.

Cognitive-Behavioral Therapy for Externalizing Disorders in Children and Adolescents

John E. Lochman, PhD, ABPP*, Nicole P. Powell, PhD, MPH,
Caroline L. Boxmeyer, PhD, Luis Jimenez-Camargo, MA

KEYWORDS

- Cognitive-behavioral therapy • Oppositional defiant disorder
- Conduct disorder

This article describes the use of cognitive and behavioral therapy (CBT) strategies with children and adolescents with externalizing disorders. The externalizing disorders that are the focus of this article include conduct disorder (CD) and oppositional defiant disorder (ODD). CD is a repetitive and persistent pattern of behavior that violates societal norms or the basic rights of others,[1] covering 4 symptom areas: (1) aggressive behavior that threatens or causes physical harm to other people or animals (eg, bullies, threatens or intimidates others; this symptom area typically coincides with most forms of CD); (2) nonaggressive conduct that causes property loss or damage (eg, fire-setting); (3) deceitfulness or theft (eg, breaking into someone's house or car); and (4) serious violation of rules (eg, truancy). To be diagnosed, at least 3 of 15 possible symptoms must have been displayed during the previous 12 months. Childhood-onset CD is differentiated from adolescent-onset when at least one of the behavioral characteristics is evident before age 10. However, if criteria are met for CD and no symptoms are present before age 10, the child is classified adolescent-onset type.

ODD is defined as a recurrent pattern of negativistic, defiant, disobedient, and hostile behavior toward authority figures that persists for at least 6 months and is characterized by the frequent occurrence of at least 4 of the following behaviors: losing temper, arguing with adults, actively defying or refusing to comply with requests or rules of adults, deliberately doing things that will annoy other people, blaming others

Department of Psychology, Center for the Prevention of Youth Behavior Problems, The University of Alabama, 200 Hackberry Lane, 101 McMillan Building, PO Box 870348, Tuscaloosa, AL 35487-0348, USA
* Corresponding author.
E-mail address: jlochman@ua.edu

Child Adolesc Psychiatric Clin N Am 20 (2011) 305–318
doi:10.1016/j.chc.2011.01.005
1056-4993/11/$ – see front matter
childpsych.theclinics.com

for his or her own mistakes or misbehavior, being touchy or easily annoyed by others, being angry and resentful, or being spiteful or vindictive.

CONTEXTUAL SOCIAL-COGNITIVE MODEL

The contextual social-cognitive model that serves as the basis of our Anger Coping[2] and Coping Power[3] programs has been based on empirically identified risk factors that predict children's antisocial behavior.[4] As children develop, they can begin to display a progressively larger set of risk factors, increasing the probability that they will eventually display severe antisocial behavior. These risk factors can be conceptualized as falling within 5 categories: biologic and temperamental child factors, family context, neighborhood context, peer context, and later-emerging child factors involving their social cognitive processes and related emotional regulation abilities.

Biologic and Temperament Factors

Aggression is often the result of interactions between child risk factors and environmental factors, in a diathesis-stress framework. Thus, risk factors such as birth complications, genetic loading, cortisol reactivity, testosterone, abnormal serotonin levels, and temperament all contribute to children's conduct problems, but often only when environmental factors such as harsh parenting, interparental violence, or low socioeconomic status are present. For example, some male children have been found to have a gene that expresses only low levels of MAOA (monoamine oxidase A) enzyme. MAOA metabolizes and gets rid of excess neurotransmitters, including serotonin, norepinephrine, epinephrine, and melatonin. Low MAOA leads to violent behavior, but only if children were maltreated—an indicator of diathesis-stress.[5]

Community and Neighborhood Contextual Factors

Neighborhood environments have also been found to be risk factors for aggression and delinquency, over and above the variance accounted for by family characteristics. High neighborhood crime rates, low social cohesion, and neighborhood disadvantage have been found to predict children's beliefs about aggression and their disruptive and aggressive behavior (eg, see Guerra and colleagues[6]), especially proactive aggressive behavior.[7] Neighborhood effects can begin to create heightened risk during middle childhood,[8] as children become more independent in moving around their community and become more directly exposed to community risks. Early onset of aggression and violence has been associated with neighborhood disorganization and poverty, partly because children who live in poor and disorganized neighborhoods are likely to have less supervision and engage in more risk-taking behaviors.

Family Contextual Factors

There are a wide array of factors in the family that can affect child aggression, ranging from poverty to more general stress and discord within the family. Children's aggression has been linked to family background factors such as parent criminality, substance use, depression, poverty, marital conflict, stressful life events, and single and teenage parenthood.[9,10] All of these family risk factors intercorrelate, especially with socioeconomic status,[9] and can influence child behavior through their effect on parenting processes. For example, aggressive marital conflict influences maternal harsh punishment, which in turn predicts children's aggressive-disruptive behavior.[11] Parenting processes linked to children's aggression[12] include nonresponsive parenting, coercive, escalating cycles of harsh parental nattering and child noncompliance, unclear directions and commands, lack of warmth and involvement, and lack of effective parental supervision and monitoring. The relation between parenting factors and childhood aggression is often bidirectional, as child temperament and behavior can affect parenting behaviors, and visa versa.[13]

Peer Contextual Factors

Children with disruptive behaviors are often rejected by their peers[14] and can often have inflated and inaccurate perceptions of their levels of peer acceptance.[15] Aggressive children who are also socially rejected exhibit more severe antisocial behavior than children who are either aggressive or rejected only.[16] As children with conduct problems enter adolescence, they tend to associate with deviant peers. Adolescents who are reactively aggressive and who have been rejected from more prosocial peer groups sometimes turn to antisocial cliques for social support. Other aggressive children who are more likely to display proactive (rather than reactive) aggressive behaviors also are at risk to enter into deviant peer groups, but not because they were rejected by the larger peer group. Aggressive children's movement into deviant peer groups increases the probability that they will begin to display increasingly severe antisocial behavior.[17]

Social Cognition

As children develop, they begin to form stable patterns of processing social information and regulating their emotions. The patterns of social information processing and emotional regulation that children develop are influenced by children's temperament and biologic dispositions as well as children's contextual experiences with their family, peers, and community. Aggressive children have cognitive distortions at the appraisal phases of social-cognitive processing because of difficulties in encoding incoming social information, partially because of neurocognitive difficulties in their executive functions,[18] and in accurately interpreting social events and others' intentions. In the appraisal phases of social information processing, aggressive children have been found to recall fewer relevant nonhostile cues about events.[19] Aggressive children also have cognitive deficiencies at the problem solution phases of social-cognitive processing. They have dominance and revenge-oriented social goals,[20] which guides the maladaptive action-oriented and nonverbal solutions they generate for perceived problems.[19] In addition, aggressive children evaluate aggressive behavior in a positive way and they expect that aggressive behavior will lead to positive outcomes for them.[19]

CBT STRATEGIES FOR CHILDREN AND ADOLESCENTS WITH EXTERNALIZING DISORDERS

Externalizing behavior problems are among the most commonly cited reasons for youth referrals to mental health clinics.[21] This is likely because of the substantial toll that youth conduct problems exact on those around them. Thus, it is important to intervene with children with externalizing disorders as early as possible, before their maladaptive behaviors become increasingly stable and impairing.[22] The ways in which children typically present conduct problems can vary from relatively minor oppositional behaviors, such as yelling or temper tantrums, to more serious antisocial behaviors such as aggression, physical destructiveness, and stealing.[23] Several programs using CBT techniques have been shown to be efficacious in reducing externalizing behavior problems in at-risk and clinic-referred youth, including the Coping Power Program,[3,24,25] The Life Skills Training Program,[26] and The Art of Self-Control[27] program. Youth-focused treatment components most common to these types of CBT-based programs include the following: Emotion Awareness, Perspective Taking, Anger Management, Social Problem Solving, and Goal Setting. For the purpose of this article, each of these components is described using the Coping Power Program as a model.[28]

Emotion Awareness

Before addressing problem behaviors, it is necessary for children to understand from where their behaviors stem. Emotion awareness strategies typically allow children to learn to recognize the emotions that lead them to engage in externalizing behaviors. Recognition of negative emotions, and the degree to which they are experienced, enables children to determine the conditions under which they are most prone to act out. CBT-oriented clinicians use a range of techniques to teach emotion awareness in children. In Coping Power, child clients first learn to describe their emotions in terms of physiologic sensations (eg, heart racing, tight muscles, face becomes flushed), behaviors (eg, raising your voice, making a threatening gesture, pushing or shoving), and cognitions (eg, I hate my mom; my teacher always picks on me; I am going to show that kid he can't mess with him). Using a thermometer analogy, children are taught to identify varying intensities of particular emotions. Situational triggers and thought patterns associated with varying levels of such emotions are then identified (eg, an extra homework assignment might make you a little bit upset, whereas someone making fun of a family member might make you enraged). Through in-session activities and self-monitoring homework assignments, children are taught to identify common situational triggers for their own anger arousal.

Perspective Taking

This component is designed to teach children the difficulty involved in accurately determining others' intentions. Children who exhibit externalizing behaviors tend to overly interpret others' intentions as hostile; thus, it is necessary to teach children about other more benign alternate explanations for others' behaviors.[19,29,30] To implement this component, the clinician can have children role-play different characters in an ambiguous situation. On completion of the role-play, children are encouraged to discuss the different viewpoints of each of the characters portrayed. Children are also asked to recall real-life incidents in which they later realized they had misinterpreted the reason for another person's actions in an overly hostile light. In school settings, clinicians may also wish to have children interview their teachers to allow children the opportunity to obtain a firsthand account of common student misconceptions regarding disciplinary procedures and classroom management.

Anger Management

Emotion regulation, specifically anger control, is key to the successful decrease of conduct problems. As previously noted, deficits in emotion regulation are thought to contribute to externalizing behaviors; thus, it is essential to incorporate anger management in any CBT-based intervention. Additionally, with a working knowledge of personal emotion awareness and perspective-taking skills, children are more likely to successfully implement anger management techniques before becoming inundated by an unmanageable level of anger. A number of strategies can be taught to children to help them manage their anger arousal, including distraction, relaxation, and coping self-statements. With regard to relaxation, guided imagery and progressive muscle relaxation techniques may be taught to prevent escalation of low levels of anger. In terms of distraction, exercises through which the child is taught to divert his or her attention away from the anger-provoking stimulus can be conducted. For example, in a group setting, a child may be given a set of letters or numbers to memorize while the rest of the group is instructed to taunt and disturb the child as much as possible. By focusing on the task at hand, the child learns that he or she can prevent his or her anger from escalating by ignoring, or focusing attention away from the anger-evoking stimulus.

The use of coping self-statements can be taught through a series of graded exposure role-plays. Initially, children can be provided with a list of coping self-statements that they may find helpful to lower their anger (eg, "It's not worth it to get angry"; "He is trying to make me mad, but I am not going to let him get to me"). Children are also encouraged to generate their own coping statements, which may have a greater impact on their anger management. Children are given time to become familiar with the coping statements and choose the ones that they find the most helpful. Upon selection of coping statements, children are first exposed to a situation in which they practice using coping statements in a relatively benign and impersonal anger-arousing scenario. For example, in a group setting, children can use puppets to tease a specific child's puppet. The child controlling the puppet being teased can state aloud the coping statements his puppet is using to avoid anger escalation. With increasing proficiency in the use of coping statements, children can be progressively challenged with more personal anger arousal scenarios until they get to the point at which they can role-play and declare the coping statements used in a scenario in which they are taunted verbally. With this type of technique, it is important to monitor children closely to avoid situations in which the teasing gets out of hand.

Social Problem Solving

Children are encouraged to practice the anger-reducing techniques described in the previous section to allow them time to generate more adaptive solutions to anger-evoking problem situations. Variations on the Antecedents-Behavior-Consequences (ABC) model, in which children identify the antecedents to a particular problem and how different behaviors in response to those antecedents can result in different outcomes, can be used to demonstrate problem-solving techniques. The PICC (Problem Identification, Choices, Consequences) model used in Coping Power, for example, teaches children how to first identify a problem by defining it in objective and behavioral terms. The children are then encouraged to generate a variety of choices in response to the problem that lead to both positive and negative outcomes. The children are then asked to discuss the consequences of each choice, evaluate all choices in terms of their benefits and disadvantages, and choose the outcome with the most positive consequences. This model can be applied to a variety of child problems, including peer or sibling conflict, teacher-student relations, parental conflict, and neighborhood problems. Children can practice and consolidate their problem-solving skills using several methods, such as role-plays, creation of a video illustrating problem solving in action, and story writing. While learning these skills, children should be encouraged to apply them to their own daily problems and to share with the group successful applications of the PICC model.

Goal Setting

Throughout the implementation of the previously mentioned CBT components, clinicians can also help children learn to set personal goals. As a first step, clinicians can introduce the concept of personal goal setting and have each child identify 1 to 2 long-term goals that he or she would like to accomplish in the next 6 to 12 months. The clinician can then work with the child to help him or her break the long-term goals into short-term goals that can be accomplished within a day or week. Before initiating the goal-setting process, it is beneficial for clinicians to consult with parents and teachers to elicit their input on goals that may improve the child's functioning in the school or home setting. The clinician's role is to synthesize the ideas for goals generated by the child, parent, and teacher, as well as the goals on the treatment plan, and to work collaboratively with the child to generate a list and hierarchy of goals that the child is motivated to work to reach. This process can be executed using a weekly goal sheet. For example, a child wishing to raise his or her grades to be eligible to play on the basketball team may work on short-term goals of completing homework every day, bringing books home, and paying attention in class. Each of these goals can be assigned on a weekly sheet and assessed by the child's parent or teacher. Upon mastering a goal, the child can move toward a more difficult goal. Throughout the goal-setting process, clinicians seek to incorporate goals that allow children opportunities to practice the skills they are learning in the program. For example, children who are consistently disrespectful toward their parents may be given the goal to follow parental directions every day. Parents are instructed to assess this goal daily, and upon the child's return (assuming successful completion), the clinician can inquire about the coping skills used to achieve the goal. If unsuccessful, the clinician can work with the child to remind him or her of skills that could improve goal achievement in the future. Goal setting works well when used in combination with a point-rewards system to motivate children to attain their goals.

The components described are central to many CBT-based interventions for children with externalizing behavior problems. The Coping Power program has additional treatment components for coexisting problems and developmental concerns. For example, given the high rate of attention problems in children with ODD and CD and the important role of academic achievement, additional sessions focus on teaching children organization and study skills. Other sessions focus on peer relationships and seek to teach children how to identify and establish friendships with prosocial peers rather than deviant peers. Children are also taught specific skills to resist peer pressure and to handle problems faced in the family and neighborhood contexts. See Lochman and colleagues[28] for greater detail about how each of these intervention components is implemented in the Coping Power Program.

CBT STRATEGIES FOR PARENTS OF CHILDREN WITH EXTERNALIZING DISORDERS

The Coping Power parent program[31] will also be described to illustrate the use of CBT strategies with parents of children with externalizing disorders. Many elements of the Coping Power parent sessions derive from well-established behavioral parent training programs[32,33] and focus on improving the parent-child bond and helping parents use positive parenting skills. Additional sessions that are more specific to Coping Power focus on stress management, building family cohesion and communication, and family problem solving. The Coping Power parent component includes content for 16 intervention sessions for the primary caregivers of children simultaneously participating in the child component. An important objective of each parent session is to inform parents about what their children are learning in the child group and to discuss ways that the parents can reinforce their children's use of these skills at home. A small group format has been used most often in outcome studies of the Coping Power parent component; however, the intervention materials have also been adapted for use with individual parents and families.[34]

Parent group sessions follow a consistent sequence. Time is reserved at the beginning and end of each session to allow parents to visit with each other, which helps to develop group cohesion and supportive relationships among the group members. The session then opens with a review of prior content, including discussion of parents' use of new parenting strategies at home and the observed impact on their relationships with their child and on the child's behavior. New discussion topics are then introduced and group activities are used to facilitate skill acquisition (eg, interactive worksheets, role-plays). Homework assignments are given at the end of each session to facilitate generalization of parenting skills outside of the intervention setting. Clinicians deliver the intervention content in a flexible manner, with a goal of adapting session activities to best address the specific problems and issues of the group members.

The following Coping Power parent component sections are reflective of the skills taught in a number of well-established parent training programs for child disruptive behavior problems.

Basic Social Learning Theory, Praise, and Improving the Parent-Child Relationship

In the beginning of the program, the clinician seeks to present the basic social learning model using the concepts of antecedents (A), behavior (B), and consequences (C). The clinician teaches parents how they can modify their own patterns of responding to their child's behavior to increase desirable behaviors (eg, following directions, sharing, compromising) and decrease undesirable behaviors (eg, noncompliance, aggression). The clinician introduces a monitoring system to help parents become more aware of their child's positive and negative behaviors. The clinician also helps parents identify positive consequences (eg, increased parental attention, a favorite dessert, labeled praise) that they can provide to increase their child's desirable behavior. To reestablish positive parent-child bonds, the clinician also emphasizes the importance of "special time" between parents and children, helps parents set goals for having regular "special time" with their child, and provides tips for how to minimize conflict during special time.

Ignoring Minor Disruptive Behavior

Parents are then taught to manage and reduce children's minor disruptive behaviors through ignoring. Minor disruptive behaviors that might be appropriate to ignore are first identified (eg, changing the television channel repeatedly, fussing after the child does not get his or her way) and distinguished from more serious behaviors that cannot be ignored (eg, beating up a sibling, overt defiance). Interactive role-plays are then used to model effective ignoring, which includes removing eye contact and verbal interaction with the child until the minor disruptive behavior ceases. Common challenges in the use of ignoring (eg, how to handle it when the child escalates his or her disruptive behavior to try to get the parent's attention) are also discussed and acted out.

Antecedent Control: Giving Effective Instructions and Establishing Rules and Expectations

Next, clinicians seek to teach parents how their own actions can serve as helpful/ unhelpful antecedents to children's compliant or noncompliant behaviors. In particular, parents' use of clear instructions is illustrated as an important aspect of antecedent control. Ineffective instructions often precede child noncompliance, whereas clear instructions often precede child compliance. Through discussion and role play, the clinician seeks to identify and model the qualities of "good" and "bad" instructions (eg, obtain child's eye contact first, state request clearly, give one instruction at a time, avoid lengthy or overly complicated instructions, only make a request if you plan to follow-up and ensure the child complies). After practicing giving effective instructions in session, parents are encouraged to make an effort to give more clear instructions at home and to monitor the differential impact on child compliance.

Parents' use of household rules and expectations is described as another important aspect of antecedent control. Behavior rules establish the behaviors that children should decrease (eg, hitting, noncompliance), whereas behavior expectations establish the behaviors that children should increase (eg, making the bed, talking nicely to family members). In discussing rules and expectations with parents, clinicians emphasize the importance of labeling rule violations (eg, "Lamar, you just hit your sister and that is against the rules we set for our family") so that children are made more aware of the rules. Clinicians also emphasize the importance of keeping expectations age-appropriate. Parents are coached in how to establish behavior rules and expectations at home and are encouraged to track their child's compliance, their own positive reinforcement of compliance, and their labeling of noncompliance.

Discipline and Punishment

Next, clinicians introduce the concept of punishment and define punishment as any response to problem behavior that results in a decrease in the behavior. Clinicians elicit parents' current punishment strategies and their perceived effectiveness. The clinician seeks to expand parents' "tool box" in terms of the range of punishment strategies they use. Parents are also taught a specific sequence of steps for responding systematically to punish noncompliance and other forms of misbehavior.

The specific punishment techniques taught include "time out" (using a specific series of steps), the removal of privileges, and the assignment of additional work chores. The parents are taught to follow a sequence in which they (1) give their child a clear instruction, (2) assess for compliance, (3) praise compliance or provide a warning describing the punishment that will be instituted if the child does not comply, and (4) institute the punishment if the instruction is not followed. This sequence is continued, adding additional punishments as needed, until the child complies with the initial instruction. The parents and clinician role-play this sequence in a variety of parent-child scenarios to practice adhering to the above steps, even in the face of significant child escalation. The clinician also engages parents in a discussion about appropriate punishment for major misbehavior, with an aim of helping parents find alternatives to physical punishment and lengthy, unspecified grounding.

The following Coping Power parent component sections describe additional topics and skills covered with parents.

Family Cohesion Building, Family Problem Solving, and Family Communication

During these sessions, the clinician seeks to elicit and discuss parents' hopes and concerns for their children as they mature. The clinician emphasizes that having a positive, healthy parent-child relationship will become increasingly important as the child grows older and more independent. The group brainstorms strategies for how families can build their cohesion both in the home (eg, family game nights) and outside of the home (eg, going to a park). Parents are encouraged to follow-through with family cohesion-building activities on a consistent basis.

Parents are also taught the PICC problem-solving model that the children are learning and discuss ways they can use this model to resolve family conflicts at home. For example, if the family members get into arguments nearly every morning as they rush to get ready for school and work, they can work together to brainstorm choices for solving this problem (eg, wake up 15 minutes earlier, create a schedule for sharing the bathroom, eat breakfast in the car instead of at the table, lay out your clothes the night before) and the likely consequences of each choice. The family can then decide together which choice(s) they are going to implement.

The clinician also leads parents in a discussion about their ongoing family communication patterns. Questions the clinician might ask include the following: Does your family have a way of talking with each other about their concerns? How do they set family rules, or negotiate desired changes to family rules? Are all of the family members satisfied with the way they communicate? The clinician then introduces the notion of holding regular family meetings as one way to preserve positive parent involvement in children's lives and tackle potential problems before they arise. The clinician guides parents in a discussion about how they might establish family meetings at home and how to make them desirable to all family members. Another important topic the clinician addresses with parents is the importance of continuing to monitor children's involvement with peers and in the community as they become more independent. A specific communication system is described for helping parents monitor who their child spends time with, what activities they engage in, and what types of supervision and rules are in place.

Academic Support in the Home

Parents are also given strategies for supporting their child's academic work at home. Parents are taught to use a "homework completion system" (eg, a school-to-home assignment notebook) that allows for increased parent-teacher communication about homework assignments and parental monitoring of homework completion. Parents are also encouraged to proactively schedule a parent-teacher conference, rather than waiting until problems arise. Parents are provided with potential questions and topics for the parent-teacher conference, and role-play this interaction in the therapeutic setting.

Stress Management

One of the intervention topics rated most favorably by parents is stress management. In this portion of the intervention, the fact that parenting can be very stressful is normalized and discussed. The clinician seeks to describe how stress can undermine positive parenting behaviors and negatively impact the parent-child relationship. Role-plays are used to illustrate how parents' own stress can lead to overreaction to their children's behavior. Parents are encouraged to find ways to take part in enjoyable, stress-reducing activities and to schedule this time for themselves regularly. The clinician also leads parents in specific relaxation techniques, including guided imagery, deep breathing, and progressive muscle relaxation. Parents are also taught to monitor how their own thoughts ("my child is driving me crazy" vs "he is irritable today because he did not sleep well last night") and feelings affect their parenting behaviors. Parents who have marked difficulty modulating their own emotions are advised to seek adjunctive individual therapy for themselves.

EFFECTIVENESS OF CBT STRATEGIES FOR EXTERNALIZING DISORDERS

This section summarizes the evidence for the effectiveness of CBT strategies for externalizing disorders and presents specific outcome research on several programs that include CBT techniques, including the Coping Power Program. Results of several meta-analyses have provided support for CBT interventions in the prevention and remediation of aggressive and disruptive behaviors. Sukhodolsky and colleagues[35] conducted a meta-analytical study of 40 treatment outcome evaluations of CBT programs targeting anger and aggression in youth. Studies included youth ages 7.0

to 17.2 years (with a mean of 12.5 years) and included a total of 1953 children, most of whom received a group form of therapy. Most treatments were considered short-term, with a treatment length of 8 to 18 hours. Across all studies, the mean effect size was 0.67, in the medium range, with larger effect size values for youth in the moderate range of problem severity (0.80) as compared with children with severe (0.59) or mild (0.57) levels. Differences in effectiveness were also found for 4 categories of CBT, including skills development (0.79), multimodal treatment (0.74), problem solving (0.67), and affective education (0.36), suggesting that a focus on actual behavioral change is important in the reduction of aggressive behavior.

Robinson and colleagues[36] found similar results in their meta-analysis of 23 studies investigating CBT effects on externalizing behavior symptoms. Across studies specifically targeting aggression, the mean effect size was 0.64, with 88% of studies reporting positive results. McCart and colleagues[37] found an effect size in the small range (0.35), and noted that CBT had a stronger effect for adolescents than for younger children, possibly as a result of adolescents' more advanced cognitive development.

As demonstrated by meta-analytic results, treatment outcome studies indicate that CBT can produce significant reductions in children's and adolescents' externalizing behavior problems. For both intervention research and clinical application, manualized interventions have been developed to apply CBT to disruptive behaviors in youth. Several such programs can be considered empirically supported or evidence-based treatments (EBTs) based on positive effects of well-conducted outcome research. Eyberg and colleagues[38] provide a review of EBTs for youth with externalizing behavior problems, identifying programs at several levels of efficacy. Examples of several EBTs incorporating CBT principles and techniques for externalizing problems in youth are provided as follows.

In Kazdin's Problem-Solving Skills Training (PSST),[39] children attend 12 weekly core sessions in which they learn a sequence of problem-solving steps to apply when faced with interpersonal conflicts. Homework assignments, called "supersolvers," help children generalize the application of PSST to everyday life. Several treatment outcome studies support the effectiveness of PSST, both as a stand-alone intervention and in combination with Parent Management Training (PMT), a manualized behavioral program delivered to parents. Alone and with PMT, PSST has been shown to reduce externalizing behavior problems in the home and school settings and to increase prosocial behaviors; however, the combined PSST and PMT treatment results in greater improvements. Gains have been found immediately following intervention and up to 1 year later. See Kazdin[39] for a review of outcome research results.

Another EBT incorporating CBT elements is the Incredible Years (IY),[40] a multimodal program that includes parent training and teacher training curricula in addition to the cognitive-behavioral intervention for 3- to 8-year-olds (IY-CT). Delivery of IY-CT takes place over 22 weeks and is based on a series of DVDs that illustrate problem-solving and social skills. Although the child and parent programs are typically delivered together, IY-CT alone has been shown to effectively reduce children's aggression, to increase positive social skills, and to improve children's problem-solving and conflict management skills. Stronger effects are found when the parent and child components are delivered together. A review of outcome research results is available in Webster-Stratton and Reid.[40]

The Anger Coping Program,[41] an 18-session intervention targeting children in the fourth through sixth grades, uses CBT to help children develop skills in emotion recognition and awareness, anger coping through self-talk and distraction, perspective taking, goal setting, and social problem solving. In outcome research studies,[42,43] Anger Coping has produced reductions in parent-reported aggression and observers' ratings of disruptive classroom behavior, reductions in teacher-rated aggression, and improvements in self-esteem and perceived social competence. Follow-up research indicates maintenance of improvements in classroom behavior after 7 months and lower levels of substance use after 3 years.[42]

The Coping Power Program was developed to extend and expand on Anger Coping, with the goal of strengthening outcome effects, particularly in the area of delinquency prevention. Coping Power's extended length allows for more in-depth coverage of core topic areas, as well as additional sessions on study skills, social skills, and peer pressure resistance. As described previously, Coping Power also includes a companion parenting component.

Several randomized controlled trials have supported Coping Power's efficacy and effectiveness. In the first study,[25] boys whose teachers rated them as aggressive were randomly assigned to 1 of 3 groups: Coping Power child component only, Coping Power child and parent components, or an untreated control condition. Results indicated that, compared with the control group, both Coping Power conditions demonstrated lower rates of delinquency and parent-rated substance use, and greater teacher-rated behavioral improvements at a 1-year follow-up. The first 2 intervention effects were enhanced for the combined treatment condition. Additional analyses indicated that outcomes were mediated by changes in the targets of the intervention, including children's social cognitive processes, schemas, and parenting processes.[3] Another study evaluated the addition of a universal intervention to the full Coping Power Program.[24] The universal intervention consisted of 5 in-service training sessions for teachers, which focused on strategies for improving children's academic, social, and emotional skills and increasing parents' school involvement. The universal intervention also included 4 large-scale parent meetings for all parents of children in universal intervention classrooms and included discussion of strategies for improving children's academic, social, and emotional skills, and preparing children for the middle-school transition. Compared with an untreated control group, children who received both Coping Power and the universal intervention had lower rates of self-reported substance use and teacher-rated aggression, higher perceived social competence, and greater teacher-reported improvement in classroom behavior. At a 1-year follow-up, children who received Coping Power, the universal program, or both programs all demonstrated lower rates of delinquency and substance use than controls.

Coping Power has also yielded positive outcomes effects in evaluations involving clinic populations. Dutch children diagnosed with disruptive behavior disorders were randomly assigned to receive an abbreviated version of Coping Power or to clinic treatment as usual. Although both groups demonstrated improvements in disruptive behaviors at posttreatment, the Coping Power group's reductions in overt aggression were significantly greater.[44] Reductions in disruptive behaviors were maintained for both groups at a 6-month follow-up. At a 4-year follow-up, the Coping Power children had significantly lower rates of tobacco and marijuana use than the treatment as usual condition, although rates of alcohol use were similar for both groups.[45]

SUMMARY AND IMPLICATIONS

This article has sought to describe the contextual, social, and cognitive risk factors for children's development of externalizing disorders, the types of cognitive and behavioral treatment strategies that can be used to address these risk factors, and the evidence base for CBT-based interventions for externalizing behavior disorders. Based on the existing research, it is clear that cognitive and behavioral intervention strategies can produce significant reductions in children's externalizing behavior problems, particularly when interventions are multimodal (ie, incorporate parents, children, and other key stakeholders in treatment) and focus on development of specific skills, such as those described in this article.

REFERENCES

1. American Psychiatric Association. Diagnostic and statistical manual of mental disorders. 4th edition. Washington, DC: American Psychiatric Association; 1994. DSM-IV.
2. Lochman JE, Nelson WM III, Sims JP. A cognitive behavioral program for use with aggressive children. J Clin Child Psychol 1981;10:146–8.
3. Lochman JE, Wells KC. Contextual social-cognitive mediators and child outcome: a test of the theoretical model in the coping power program. Dev Psychopathol 2002;14:971–93.
4. Matthys W, Lochman JE. Oppositional defiant disorder and conduct disorder in childhood. Oxford (England): Wiley-Blackwell; 2010.
5. Caspi A, McClay J, Moffitt T, et al. Role of genotype in the cycle of violence in maltreated children. Science 2002;297:851–4.
6. Guerra NG, Huesmann LR, Spindler A. Community violence exposure, social cognition, and aggression among urban elementary school children. Child Dev 2003;74:1561–76.
7. Fite PJ, Wynn P, Lochman JE, et al. The effect of neighborhood disadvantage on proactive and reactive aggression. J Community Psychol 2009;37:542–6.
8. Ingoldsby EM, Shaw DS. Neighborhood contextual factors and early starting antisocial pathways. Clin Child Fam Psychol Rev 2002;5:21–55.
9. Luthar SS. Children in poverty: risk and protective factors in adjustment. Thousand Oaks (CA): Sage; 1999.
10. Odgers CL, Milne BJ, Caspi A, et al. Predicting prognosis for the conduct-problem boy: can family history help? J Am Acad Child Adolesc Psychiatry 2007;46:1240–9.
11. Erath SA, Bierman KL, the Conduct Problems Prevention Research Group. Aggressive marital conflict, maternal harsh punishment, and child aggressive-disruptive behavior: evidence for direct and indirect relations. J Fam Psychol 2006;20:217–26.
12. Jaffee SR, Caspi A, Moffitt TE, et al. Physical maltreatment victim to antisocial child: evidence of an environmentally mediated process. J Abnorm Psychol 2004;113:44–55.
13. Fite PJ, Colder CR, Lochman JE, et al. The mutual influence of parenting and boys' externalizing behavior problems. J Appl Dev Psychol 2006;27:151–64.
14. Cillessen AH, Van Ijzendoorn HW, Van Lieshout CF, et al. Heterogeneity among peer-rejected boys: subtypes and stabilities. Child Dev 1992;63:893–905.
15. Pardini DA, Barry TD, Barth JM, et al. Self-perceived social acceptance and peer social standing in children with aggressive-disruptive behaviors. Soc Dev 2006; 15:46–64.
16. Lochman JE, Wayland KK. Aggression, social acceptance and race as predictors of negative adolescent outcomes. J Am Acad Child Adolesc Psychiatry 1994;33:1026–35.
17. Fite PJ, Colder CR, Lochman JE, et al. Pathways from proactive and reactive aggression to substance use. Psychol Addict Behav 2007;21:355–64.

18. Ellis ML, Weiss B, Lochman JE. Executive functions in children: associations with aggressive behavior and social appraisal processing. J Abnorm Child Psychol 2009;37:945–56.
19. Lochman JE, Dodge KA. Social-cognitive processes of severely violent, moderately aggressive and nonaggressive boys. J Consult Clin Psychol 1994;62: 366–74.
20. Lochman JE, Wayland KK, White KJ. Social goals: relationship to adolescent adjustment and to social problem solving. J Abnorm Child Psychol 1993;21: 135–51.
21. Steiner H, Remsing L. Practice parameter for the assessment and treatment of children and adolescents with oppositional defiant disorder. J Am Acad Child Adolesc Psychiatry 2007;46(1):126–41.
22. Frick PJ, Silverthorn P. Psychopathology in children. In: Sutker PB, Adams HE, editors. Comprehensive handbook of psychopathology. 3rd edition. New York (NY): Kluwer Academic; 2001. p. 881–920.
23. McMahon R, Frick P. Conduct and oppositional disorders. Assessment of childhood disorders. 4th edition. New York: Guilford Press; 2007. p. 132–83.
24. Lochman JE, Wells KC. Effectiveness study of coping power and classroom intention with aggressive children: outcomes at a one-year follow-up. Behav Ther 2003;34:493–515.
25. Lochman JE, Wells KC. The coping power program for preadolescent aggressive boys and their parents: outcome effects at the 1-year follow-up. J Consult Clin Psychol 2004;72:571–8.
26. Botvin GJ, Griffin KW. Life skills training: empirical findings and future directions. J Prim Prev 2004;25:211–32.
27. Feindler EL, Ecton RB. Adolescent anger control: cognitive-behavior techniques. New York: Pergamon Books; 1986.
28. Lochman JE, Wells KC, Lenhart LA. Coping Power child group program: facilitator guide. New York: Oxford; 2008.
29. Lansford J, Malone P, Dodge K, et al. A 12-year prospective study of patterns of social information processing problems and externalizing behaviors. J Abnorm Child Psychol 2006;34:715–24.
30. Dodge KA, Lochman JE, Harnish JD, et al. Reactive and proactive aggression in school children and psychiatrically impaired chronically assaultive youth. J Abnorm Psychol 1997;106:37–51.
31. Wells KC, Lochman JE, Lenhart LA. Coping Power parent group program: facilitator guide. New York: Oxford; 2008.
32. Forehand R, Sturgis ET, McMahon RJ, et al. Parent behavioral training to modify child noncompliance: treatment generalization across time and from home to school. Behav Modif 1979;3:3–25.
33. Patterson GR, Reid JB, Jones RR, et al. A social learning approach: families with aggressive children. vol. I. Eugene (OR): Castalia; 1975.
34. Wells K, Lochman J, Goldman E. The integrated psychotherapy consortium. In: Project liberty enhanced services program: disruptive behavior symptoms intervention manual. New York (NY): Columbia University; 2007.
35. Sukhodolsky DG, Kassinove H, Gorman BS. Cognitive-behavioral therapy for anger in children and adolescents: a meta-analysis. Aggress Violent Behav 2004;9:247–69.
36. Robinson TR, Smith SW, Miller MD, et al. Cognitive behavior modification of hyperactivity-impulsivity and aggression: a meta-analysis of school-based studies. J Educ Psychol 1999;91:195–203.

37. McCart MR, Priester PE, Davies WH, et al. Differential effectiveness of behavioral parent training and cognitive-behavioral therapy for antisocial youth: a meta-analysis. J Abnorm Child Psychol 2006;34(4):527–43.

38. Eyberg SM, Nelson MM, Boggs SR. Evidence-based psychosocial treatments for children and adolescents with disruptive behavior. J Clin Child Adolesc Psychol 2008;37(1):215–37.

39. Kazdin AE. Problem-solving skills training and parent management training for oppositional defiant disorder and conduct disorder. In: Weisz JR, Kazdin AE, editors. Evidence-based psychotherapies for children and adolescents. 2nd edition. New York: Guilford; 2010. p. 211–26.

40. Webster-Stratton C, Reid JM. The Incredible Years parents, teachers, and children training series. In: Weisz JR, Kazdin AE, editors. Evidence-based psychotherapies for children and adolescents. 2nd edition. New York: Guilford; 2010. p. 194–210.

41. Larson J, Lochman JE. Helping schoolchildren cope with anger: a cognitive-behavioral intervention. New York: Guilford; 2002.

42. Lochman JE. Cognitive-behavioral interventions with aggressive boys: three-year follow-up and preventive effects. J Consult Clin Psychol 1992;60:426–32.

43. Lochman JE, Burch PP, Curry JF, et al. Treatment and generalization effects of cognitive-behavioral and goal setting interventions with aggressive boys. J Consult Clin Psychol 1984;52:915–6.

44. van de Weil NMH, Matthys W, Cohen-Kettenis PT, et al. The effectiveness of an experimental treatment when compared with care as usual depends on the type of care as usual. Behav Modif 2007;31:298–312.

45. Zonnevylle-Bender MJS, Matthys W, van de Wiel NMH, et al. Preventive effects of treatment of disruptive behavior disorder in middle childhood on substance use and delinquent behavior. J Am Acad Child Adolesc Psychiatry 2007;46:33–9.

Cognitive-Behavioral Therapy for Childhood Repetitive Behavior Disorders: Tic Disorders and Trichotillomania

Christopher A. Flessner, PhD[a,b,*]

KEYWORDS

- Children • CBT • Tic disorders
- Trichotillomania • Habit reversal

This brief review provides an overview of cognitive-behavioral therapy (CBT) for repetitive behavior disorders. The term repetitive behavior disorder encompasses a variety of conditions, including tic disorders (ie, Tourette syndrome [TS], chronic tic disorders, transient tic disorder), trichotillomania (TTM), skin picking, nail-biting, and bruxism (teeth grinding). In an effort to avoid repetition, no pun intended, the focus of this discussion is centered on the most often studied and most debilitating of these conditions: tic disorders and TTM. After an introduction to each disorder, an overview of CBT for children presenting with these concerns is provided. In particular, the article focuses on a therapeutic technique called habit reversal training (HRT) that is at the core of most CBT-based interventions. Two recent empirical studies on the immense potential of CBT for the treatment of childhood repetitive behavior disorders and some future areas of research are also discussed. First, a disclaimer is necessary.

Tic disorders and TTM are the focus of this review. However, CBT (broadly defined) and the unique therapeutic techniques described herein demonstrate similar benefit across most repetitive behavior disorders. The author hopes that with this brief review, readers will get a better understanding of these child-onset disorders, the

This work was supported by grant No. R01 DA023134 01A2 from the National Institutes of Health.

[a] Division of Child and Family Psychiatry, Rhode Island Hospital, Warren Alpert School of Medicine at Brown University, Providence, RI 02903, USA
[b] Bradley Hasbro Children's Research Center, 1 Hoppin Street, Suite 204, Coro West, Providence, RI 02903, USA
* Bradley Hasbro Children's Research Center, 1 Hoppin Street, Suite 204, Coro West, Providence, RI 02903.
E-mail address: cflessner@lifespan.org

cognitive-behavioral interventions available to children (and their families) afflicted with these conditions, and the important areas for further investigation.

AN INTRODUCTION TO TIC DISORDERS AND TTM
Tic Disorders

The *Diagnostic and Statistical Manual of Mental Disorders, Fourth Edition, Text Revision (DSM-IV-TR)*[1] describes tic disorders as involving the presence of 1 or more motor and/or vocal tics (ie, sudden, rapid, recurrent, nonrhythmic motor movements or sounds). The most studied tic disorder, and most often referenced in the popular media, is the TS. TS is characterized by multiple motor tics and 1 or more vocal tics present for at least 1 year. Other tic disorder diagnoses include chronic tic disorder (ie, presence of motor or vocal tics [but not both] for >1 year), transient tic disorder (ie, presence of motor or vocal tics for <1 year), and tic disorder, not otherwise specified.[1] Tics can vary in location and/or topography, wax and wane over time, and can be simple or complex. Simple tics may include facial grimacing, head and shoulder jerking, leg kicking, stomach tensing, grunting, coughing, and throat clearing. Complex tics include touching objects or other people, hopping, tapping or straightening objects, obscene gestures, echolalia, and shouting insults or obscenities (coprolalia). Although coprolalia is frequently depicted in the media, it actually occurs relatively infrequently among those with a tic disorder diagnosis.

Tic disorders (ie, TS, chronic tic disorder, transient tic disorder) occur in as many as 6.6% of children and adolescents.[2] More specifically, TS demonstrates a prevalence of approximately 1% in the general population, although estimates vary considerably from about 0.04% to 3.00%.[1–4] TS is more common in men than in women,[1,5] with an average age of onset at 5 to 7 years.[1,6] Children with TS often report experiencing a premonitory urge. This urge is often described as an aversive itching, tickling, or tensing sensation in the area of the body where a tic is about to occur.[7–10] Tics usually result in a temporary reduction or amelioration of the premonitory urge. As many as 93% of persons diagnosed with tic disorders experience some form of urge, feeling, or need to engage in a tic.[9] Most typically, premonitory urges are experienced by older children (ie, older than 10 years), yet children as young as 7 years may also report such urges. There is some evidence to suggest that in younger children, the urge is present but not well formed.[10] Woods and colleagues[10] developed a measure, the Premonitory Urge for Tics Scale (PUTS), designed to assess the presence of these urges in children. From a therapeutic perspective, identification of a child's premonitory urge may be especially useful for enhancing the implementation and efficacy of certain behavioral interventions (eg, HRT).

Perhaps, the greatest concern for individuals diagnosed with a tic disorder is the presence of comorbid psychiatric diagnoses.[11,12] Research suggests that as many as 95% of individuals diagnosed with a tic disorder meet the diagnostic criteria for another psychiatric condition,[13] with attention-deficit/hyperactivity disorder (ADHD) and obsessive-compulsive disorder (OCD) among the most common comorbid concerns.[12,14] Research also suggests elevated rates of mood and anxiety disorders among those with tic disorders.[4,15–17] The affected children also demonstrate increased rates of disruptive behavior problems (eg, conduct and oppositional defiant disorder).[4,5,13]

TTM

TTM is classified as an impulse control disorder in the *DSM-IV-TR*.[1] Hairpulling is the trademark symptom of the disorder, yet according to the *DSM-IV-TR*, hairpulling must also be accompanied by an increasing sense of tension before or while attempting to resist pulling (criterion B) and by gratification, relief, or pleasure after pulling (criterion C). However, most clinical researchers confer a diagnosis of TTM in the absence of criterion B and/or criterion C.[18–20] Proposed changes to the *Diagnostic and Statistical Manual of Mental Disorders* (Fifth Edition) indicate that the inclusion of criteria B and C will likely no longer be a prerequisite for diagnosis of the disorder. This change may be particularly beneficial for younger children because they may lack the cognitive ability to adequately describe the experience that these criteria are meant to assess. Children with TTM pull their hair from anywhere it grows, including (but not limited to) the scalp; eyebrows; eyelashes; and, among older children and adolescents, pubic regions.[21] As is the case with most psychiatric conditions (although tic disorders are an exception), the child also experiences clinically significant impairment in 1 or more areas of daily functioning (eg, interpersonal relationships, academics) as a result of hairpulling.

Recent estimates suggest that the prevalence of TTM is approximately 1.2% in the general population (when omitting criteria B and C).[22] However, some believe that the disorder is more prevalent in children than in adults[23] and that the female to male ratio may be lower in children.[24] Unlike OCD, TTM does not demonstrate a bimodal age of onset. The average age of onset is approximately 9 to 10 years,[25] although evidence suggests that hairpulling can begin as young as 18 months.[20,26] Importantly, children (and adults) with TTM report experiencing 2 disparate styles of pulling referred to as automatic and focused. Automatic pulling is characterized as pulling without one's awareness (ie, while watching television or reading a book). Focused pulling is characterized by pulling in response to an urge (ie, reduce tension), an impulse (ie, experience pleasure or gratification), or a negative emotional state (ie, anxiety, depression, or stress). The vast majority (approximately 96%) of children report experiencing both styles of pulling.[27] Flessner and colleagues[28] developed an assessment tool, the Milwaukee Inventory for Styles of Trichotillomania–Child Version (MIST-C), to more adequately measure these disparate pulling styles. Akin to the PUTS, the MIST-C is validated only for children aged 10 years and older and may be useful for informing the selection of appropriate treatments.

Empirical evidence suggests that about 70% of children with TTM may also meet the diagnostic criteria for other psychiatric diagnoses.[29] Recent data from a treatment-seeking sample demonstrated that 39.1% of children with TTM presented with a comorbid psychiatric diagnosis. Of these children, 30.4% and 10.9% presented with anxiety and externalizing disorders, respectively.[25] Generalized anxiety (13.0%), social phobia (8.7%), OCD (6.5%), ADHD (8.7%), and oppositional defiant disorder (6.5%) were among the most common diagnoses. A larger Internet-based study found that 38.3% of children had been previously diagnosed with at least 1 other mental health disorder. Among these diagnoses, anxiety disorders (24.1%), mood disorders (18.8%), and ADHD (16.5%) were the most common.[30] Very young children with TTM also present with marked comorbidity. One study found that 50% of toddlers who pulled their hair met the requirements for a comorbid anxiety disorder, 40% displayed developmental problems, and 100% of the sample had family stressors (ie, parental separation, homelessness, or parent mental illness).[26] These data suggest that early childhood TTM is not just a benign habit.

CBT FOR CHILDHOOD REPETITIVE BEHAVIOR DISORDERS

The term CBT implies the use of cognitive- or acceptance-based strategies. In contrast to many other childhood psychiatric conditions (ie, anxiety and mood disorders), CBT for repetitive behavior disorders does not always use such strategies. More typically, if anything, such strategies (eg, cognitive restructuring) are used as only 1 small part of a larger treatment protocol. As a result, CBT for TTM, tic disorders, and other repetitive behavior disorders can be thought of as a comprehensive approach to treatment that includes a variety of therapeutic techniques: (1) awareness training, (2) function-based interventions, (3) self-monitoring, (4) HRT, (5) aversion, (6) massed practice, (7) relaxation training, (8) social support, and (9) stimulus control.[31,32] Not all of these treatment techniques are used regularly. For example, massed practice involves asking the patient to engage in their targeted behavior (ie, motor/vocal tics) as quickly, accurately, and putting forth as much effort as possible for a predetermined amount of time with brief periods of rest interspersed (ie, engage in the tic for 3 minutes, rest for 1 minute, and so on).[33] In general, however, the use of massed practice does not hold much empirical support. In addition, these therapeutic techniques are rarely used in isolation. That is, most CBT protocols incorporate several of these techniques. Although this incorporation provides for a more comprehensive approach to the treatment, it also makes identifying the critical components of therapeutic success or comparing results across studies difficult. One treatment technique, however, is generally considered the gold standard or the core component of CBT protocols for repetitive behaviors, namely, the HRT.

HRT

HRT was first developed nearly 40 years ago by Azrin and Nunn[34] for the treatment of nervous habits and tics. Originally, HRT was a comprehensive procedure consisting of several steps. However, the technique has changed somewhat in the past several decades. A recent study by Flessner and colleagues[31] surveyed 67 experts and found that self-monitoring (eg, asking patients to track their hairpulling and motor/vocal tics), awareness training, competing response training, and stimulus control procedures (ie, modifying the environment to reduce cues for hairpulling) were the most frequently endorsed elements of HRT used for the treatment of TTM. Stimulus control procedures, as defined earlier, are generally not used often for the treatment of tic disorders. An abbreviated version of HRT has been demonstrated to be equally effective as and easier to administer than the original procedure developed by Azrin and Nunn.[35] Germane to the aims of this review, the abbreviated (simplified) version of HRT is applicable across all childhood repetitive behavior disorders and consists of 3 primary components: awareness training, competing response training, and social support.[36–38]

Awareness training consists of several key elements. First, the therapist asks the child to describe in great detail and reenact the repetitive behavior (such as hairpulling, motor or vocal tics) that is the target of the treatment. Subsequently, the child-therapist dyad play a game in which the child must accurately detect instances of his/her target behavior as well as instances in which the therapist mimics the behavior. If the child's behavior does not occur naturally (as is likely to be the case for children with TTM), he/she is instructed to simulate the behavior. This exercise continues until the child has correctly identified 4 of 5 instances of his/her and the therapist's behaviors. The child-therapist dyad then proceed to identify the warning signs for the behavior in question. For example, a child may report a tickling sensation before clearing the throat (ie, a premonitory urge) or moving the head down and to the left, accompanied by an upward movement of the left arm, before pulling hair from the scalp. Again, the child must correctly identify 4 of 5 warning signs for the targeted behavior before proceeding to the second component of simplified HRT, that is, competing response training.

In *competing response training*, children are taught a behavior that is incompatible with the target behavior. For example, children who pull their hair might clench their fists or place their hands underneath their legs on identifying a warning sign for hair-pulling. Alternatively, children who exhibit a throat-clearing tic might practice regulated or relaxed breathing (ie, breathing in through their nose and out through the mouth) on becoming aware of a tickling sensation in their throat. The same children might bring their hands to their sides or cross their arms in response to an arm-jerking tic. However, 3 rules are common to all competing responses: (1) the chosen response must be opposite to the targeted behavior, (2) the chosen response must be maintained for 1 minute or until the urge to pull hair or the tic subsides (whichever is longer), and (3) the chosen response should be socially inconspicuous. Children are taught to initiate their competing response on identifying either a warning sign for the targeted behavior (ideally) or the targeted behavior itself (eg, hairpulling, throat clearing). In case of identifying the targeted behavior, the third component of simplified HRT social support may be critical.

The *social support* component of simplified HRT consists of identifying a family member (most typical) or friend to provide encouragement and support in the children's use of their competing response. Specifically, the social support person (or the entire family, if deemed more appropriate) is instructed to praise the children when they practice competing responses. The social support person is also asked to remind the children, in a nonpejorative manner, to use the competing response when they fail to detect an occurrence of the targeted behavior (ie, "Don't forget to use the exercises that Dr Smith showed you"). Although research suggests that the social support component of HRT may not be essential for adults,[39] it is generally considered an important component in the treatment of children.

EMPIRICAL EVIDENCE SUPPORTING HRT FOR THE TREATMENT OF REPETITIVE BEHAVIOR DISORDERS

A substantial body of research using single-subject research designs and a growing body of randomized controlled trials support the efficacy of HRT for the treatment of both tic disorders and TTM (see later discussion). The components of HRT, however, do not differ significantly whether the treatment is administered to children or adults, although use of the social support component may be less important for adults. As a result, the studies described later include empirical evidence from studies including both the children and adult populations. These studies generally recruit participants with tic disorders or TTM (not both); hence, the following section is partitioned accordingly.

Tic Disorders

Carr and Chong[40] reviewed 20 studies that collectively treated more than 100 individuals with tic disorders using HRT and found the procedure to be generally effective. Although methodological shortcomings limited conclusions from this examination, the investigators acknowledged HRT as probably efficacious according to the guidelines outlined by the Task Force on Promotion and Dissemination of Psychological Procedures.[41]

Azrin and Nunn[34] conducted the first examination of HRT for the treatment of patients engaged in hairpulling, nail-biting, and thumb-sucking as well as individuals with tic disorders. Although important methodological limitations are noteworthy (eg, self-reporting as the sole dependent measure, lack of a comparison group), results demonstrated that HRT was effective in completely eliminating these repetitive behaviors in 83.3% (10 of 12) of patients. In a subsequent study, Azrin and Peterson[42] randomly assigned 14 participants with TS to HRT or waiting-list condition. Tic frequency was measured via videotaped observation (rather than patient self-report). At 12-month follow-up, the investigators noted 89% and 92% reductions in tics in the clinic and home, respectively. Patients in the waiting-list condition demonstrated no treatment benefit at 3-month follow-up; they were offered HRT, and by the end of the treatment, they demonstrated similar reductions in tic frequency to those in the experimental condition. A larger study involving 47 participants with chronic tic disorders compared HRT with waiting-list control.[43] At 4-month follow-up, participants who underwent HRT reported significant (75%–100%) control over their tics. More recently, Wilhelm and colleagues[44] compared HRT with supportive psychotherapy for individuals with TS and found that HRT produced significantly greater improvement than supportive psychotherapy. After treatment, those who underwent HRT demonstrated a 35% reduction in tic severity when compared with a 1% increase in tic severity among those in the supportive condition. These results suggest that treatment-specific factors implemented in HRT are likely responsible for the change. Discrepancies in treatment effects across studies are likely because of variations in methodology (such as stringency of research design, outcome measures).

TTM

Although treatment outcome research for TTM is generally considered to lag far behind that of other psychiatric disorders (even tic disorders), recent adult research suggests that CBT is superior to waiting-list condition,[45,46] pharmacotherapy,[46,47] pill placebo,[47] and supportive therapy.[48] As described earlier, HRT represents a core component of these tested CBT packages. In addition, a meta-analysis by Bloch and colleagues[49] found that HRT was superior to pharmacotherapy with clomipramine for the treatment of adults with the disorders. In contrast, there is some limited evidence from single-subject experimental designs[37] and 1 open-label CBT trial as to the efficacy of HRT in pediatric TTM.[25] Because (1) the basic components of CBT are thought to be analogous when comparing the treatment of children with that of adults and (2) there are no published well-controlled studies of CBT for children with TTM, a brief overview of CBT for adults is provided. Later in this article, the lone open trial of CBT among this population is discussed (see the section "CBT Solidifies its Case as a Viable Treatment Option for repetitive behavior disorders").

van Minnen and colleagues[46] compared CBT with fluoxetine therapy and a waiting-list control for individuals diagnosed with TTM and found significantly greater reductions in hairpulling for those treated with HRT than fluoxetine therapy or waiting-list control. In another study, Mouton and Stanley[50] examined the effectiveness of group-delivered CBT with 5 adult hair pullers. The investigators found that CBT was effective in reducing the severity of hairpulling posttreatment and that treatment gains were maintained at 1 month for 3 participants and at 6 months for 2 participants. More recently, however, group-based CBT for TTM has not demonstrated similar positive results.[47] In a review of available treatments of TTM, Elliott and Fuqua[32] concluded that HRT was the most effective behavioral treatment of the disorder, although they acknowledged the need for further well-controlled outcome studies. In a unique look at the social validity of HRT as a treatment of TTM, Elliot and Fuqua[51] distributed several vignettes to college students and found HRT to be a more acceptable form of treatment than hypnosis, medication, or punishment. Although the study was an analogue study using college students, the results nonetheless support that HRT may be a socially valid treatment option for TTM.

Collectively, these findings highlight the potential efficacy of CBT, with HRT often used as a core component in the treatment of TTM, tic disorders, and repetitive behavior disorders. This summary also highlights the limitations to existing research. For example, to date, only 1 moderate-sized open trial of CBT for childhood TTM exists.[25] For CBT to gain widespread use and recognition as a viable alternative to pharmacologic interventions, large-scale randomized controlled trials are necessary to confirm the results of the preliminary studies described earlier. Recently, researchers have begun to address these limitations. Described later are 2 recent studies and impending lines of research that, to varying degrees, may help to dramatically affect how CBT (as an alternative or adjunct to psychotropic medication) is viewed by child psychologists, psychiatrists, and pediatricians.

CBT SOLIDIFIES ITS CASE AS A VIABLE TREATMENT OPTION FOR REPETITIVE BEHAVIOR DISORDERS

A recent article published in the *Journal of the American Medical Association* demonstrates the potency of CBT in the treatment of tic disorders. Piacentini and colleagues[52] compared the efficacy of an 8-session comprehensive behavioral intervention for tic disorders that included a function-based intervention, HRT, psychoeducation, relaxation training, and a behavioral reward program with that of psychoeducation supportive therapy. In this study, 126 children diagnosed with either TS or a chronic tic disorder were randomized to either the behavioral intervention or the supportive therapy across 3 treatment sites (namely, University of Wisconsin-Milwaukee; University of California, Los Angeles; and Johns Hopkins University). Results demonstrated that the behavioral intervention led to a significantly greater decrease in tic severity from baseline to follow-up. Significantly, more children receiving the behavioral intervention were rated by an independent evaluator as being very much improved or much improved. Most importantly, few families (9.5%) withdrew from the study or reported worsening of symptoms (4%). In total, 87% of available treatment responders continued to exhibit benefit from the behavioral intervention at 6-month follow-up. These results provide the strongest support to date regarding the efficacy of behavior therapy for the treatment of tic disorders.

Only 1 study has sought to examine the efficacy of CBT for childhood TTM using anything more than single-subject research design methodology. Tolin and colleagues[25] conducted an open-label CBT trial (including HRT, self-monitoring, stimulus control, and cognitive restructuring) with 22 child hair pullers. Children participated in 12 sessions of CBT (8 weekly sessions + 4 biweekly relapse prevention sessions). Although limited by the lack of a comparison group, results from this study were encouraging, and an independent evaluator classified 77% and 66% of children as treatment responders at posttreatment and 6-month follow-up, respectively. Clearly, these findings are preliminary and require replication. However, this study is the first comprehensive CBT protocol ever developed for children with TTM. The first 2 investigators (David F. Tolin, PhD, and Martin E. Franklin, PhD) of this study have subsequently published a treatment manual based on the CBT protocol used in this study. After this study's completion, the second investigator (Martin E. Franklin, PhD) procured funding for a treatment development grant from the National Institute of Mental Health (NIMH, R21) to pilot test this CBT protocol using a randomized controlled design. Results will soon be published and are quite promising. Based on the results of this treatment-development grant, Dr Franklin has received funding from the NIMH (R01) for a large-scale randomized controlled trial that compares CBT with psychoeducation supportive therapy for childhood TTM. A growing body of evidence suggests that CBT is a viable treatment option for children with TTM. Of note, there is no empirical evidence supporting the efficacy of any pharmacologic intervention for the treatment of children with this disorder.

FUTURE RESEARCH DIRECTIONS AND SUMMARY

A substantial body of literature has accumulated pointing to the efficacy of CBT for childhood repetitive behavior disorders. In particular, HRT seems to be at the core of most of these interventions. However, much research is still needed. For example, the study by Piacentini and colleagues[52] must be extended to provide a more direct comparison of behavior therapy with pharmacologic interventions for the treatment of tic disorders. Research on the potential predictors or moderators of treatment is also needed. The findings by Tolin and colleagues[25] are encouraging but require replication and extension. Although this work is currently underway, independent recruitment sites and researchers must also take part in this level of examination. Akin to work in childhood OCD, empirical investigations should compare CBT alone, medication alone, and combination therapy (ie, CBT + medication) with placebo (or a stronger control condition) for the treatment of hairpulling in children. Unfortunately, CBT, in particular HRT, is not well known or used in the general community. As a result, researchers must better disseminate efficacious cognitive-behavioral interventions to better serve those children and their families afflicted with these sometimes debilitating disorders.

REFERENCES

1. American Psychiatric Association. Diagnostic and statistical manual of mental disorders. Text Revision (DSM-IV-TR). 4th edition. Washington, DC: American Psychiatric Association; 2000.
2. Khalifa N, Knorring A. Prevalence of tic disorders and Tourette syndrome in a Swedish population. Dev Med Child Neurol 2003;45:315–9.
3. Hornsey H, Banerjee S, Zeitlin H, et al. The prevalence of Tourette syndrome in 13–14-year-olds in mainstream schools. J Child Psychol Psychiatry 2001;42(8): 1035–9.
4. Mason A, Banerjee S, Eapen V, et al. The prevalence of Tourette syndrome in a mainstream school population. Dev Med Child Neurol 1998;40(5):292–6.
5. Kadesjo B, Gillberg C. Tourette's disorder: epidemiology and comorbidity in primary school children. J Am Acad Child Adolesc Psychiatry 2000;39(5): 548–55.
6. Freeman RD, Fast DK, Burd L, et al. An international perspective on Tourette syndrome: selected findings from 3,500 individuals in 22 countries. Dev Med Child Neurol 2000;42(7):436–47.
7. Leckman JF, Peterson BS, Anderson GM, et al. Pathogenesis of Tourette's syndrome. J Child Psychol Psychiatry 1997;38(1):119–42.
8. Leckman JF, Peterson BS, Pauls DL, et al. Tic disorders. Psychiatr Clin North Am 1997;20(4):839–61.
9. Leckman JF, Walker DE, Cohen DJ. Premonitory urges in Tourette's syndrome. Am J Psychiatry 1993;150(1):98–102.
10. Woods DW, Piacentini J, Himle MB, et al. Premonitory Urge for Tics Scale (PUTS): initial psychometric results and examination of the premonitory urge phenomenon in youths with tic disorders. J Dev Behav Pediatr 2005;26(6):397–403.
11. Gadow KD, Nolan EE, Sprafkin J, et al. Tics and psychiatric comorbidity in children and adolescents. Dev Med Child Neurol 2002;44(5):330–8.

12. Cohen DJ, Friedhoff AJ, Leckman JF, et al. Tourette syndrome. Extending basic research to clinical care. Adv Neurol 1992;58:341–62.
13. Coffey BJ, Biederman J, Geller DA, et al. Distinguishing illness severity from tic severity in children and adolescents with Tourette's disorder. J Am Acad Child Adolesc Psychiatry 2000;39(5):556–61.
14. Comings DE, Comings BG. Tourette syndrome: clinical and psychological aspects of 250 cases. Am J Hum Genet 1985;37(3):435–50.
15. Carter AS, Pauls DL, Leckman JF, et al. A prospective longitudinal study of Gilles de la Tourette's syndrome. J Am Acad Child Adolesc Psychiatry 1994;33(3): 377–85.
16. Coffey BJ, Biederman J, Smoller JW, et al. Anxiety disorders and tic severity in juveniles with Tourette's disorder. J Am Acad Child Adolesc Psychiatry 2000; 39(5):562–8.
17. Spencer T, Biederman J, Harding M, et al. The relationship between tic disorders and Tourette's syndrome revisited. J Am Acad Child Adolesc Psychiatry 1995; 34(9):1133–9.
18. Diefenbach GJ, Tolin DF, Hannan S, et al. Trichotillomania: impact on psychosocial functioning and quality of life. Behav Res Ther 2005;43(7):869–84.
19. Watson TS, Allen KD. Elimination of thumb-sucking as a treatment for severe trichotillomania. J Am Acad Child Adolesc Psychiatry 1993;32:830–4.
20. Watson TS, Dittmer KI, Ray KP. Treating trichotillomania in a toddler: variation on effective treatments. Child Fam Behav Ther 2000;22(4):29–40.
21. Christenson GA, Mackenzie TB, Mitchell JE. Characteristics of 60 adult chronic hair pullers. Am J Psychiatry 1991;148(3):365–70.
22. Duke DC, Keeley ML, Geffken GR, et al. Trichotillomania: a current review. Clin Psychol Rev 2010;30(2):181–93.
23. Mehregan AH. Trichotillomania. Arch Dermatol 1970;102:129–33.
24. Cohen LJ, Stein DJ, Simeon D, et al. Clinical profile, comorbidity, and treatment history in 123 hair pullers: a survey study. J Clin Psychiatry 1995;56(7):319–26.
25. Tolin DF, Franklin ME, Diefenbach GJ, et al. Pediatric trichotillomania: descriptive psychopathology and an open trial of cognitive behavioral therapy. Cognit Behav Ther 2007;36(3):129–44.
26. Wright HH, Holmes GR. Trichotillomania (hair pulling) in toddlers. Psychol Rep 2003;92(1):228–30.
27. Flessner CA, Woods DW, Franklin ME, et al. Styles of pulling in youths with trichotillomania: exploring differences in symptom severity, phenomenology, and comorbid psychiatric symptoms. Behav Res Ther 2008;46(9):1055–61.
28. Flessner CA, Woods DW, Franklin ME, et al. The Milwaukee Inventory for Styles of Trichotillomania-Child Version (MIST-C): initial development and psychometric properties. Behav Modif 2007;31(6):896–918.
29. Reeve EA, Bernstein GA, Christenson GA. Clinical characteristics and psychiatric comorbidity in children with trichotillomania. J Am Acad Child Adolesc Psychiatry 1992;31(1):132–8.
30. Franklin M, Flessner CA, Woods DW, et al. The Child and Adolescent Trichotillomania Impact Project (CA-TIP): exploring phenomenology, functional impact, and comorbid symptoms. J Dev Behav Pediatr 2007;29:493–500.
31. Flessner CA, Penzel FA, Keuthen NJ, TLC-SAB. Current treatment practices for children and adults with trichotillomania: consensus among experts. Cognit Behav Pract 2010;17:290–300.
32. Elliott AJ, Fuqua RW. Trichotillomania: conceptualization, measurement, and treatment. Behav Ther 2000;31:529–45.

33. Storms L. Massed negative practice as a behavioral treatment for Gilles de la Tourette's syndrome. Am J Psychother 1985;39(2):277–81.
34. Azrin NH, Nunn RG. Habit-reversal: a method of eliminating nervous habits and tics. Behav Res Ther 1973;11(4):619–28.
35. Miltenberger RG, Fuqua RW, McKinley T. Habit reversal with muscle tics: replication and component analysis. Behav Ther 1985;16:39–50.
36. Woods DW, Miltenberger RG. Habit reversal: a review of applications and variations. J Behav Ther Exp Psychiatry 1995;26(2):123–31.
37. Rapp JT, Miltenberger RG, Long ES, et al. Simplified habit reversal treatment for chronic hair pulling in three adolescents: a clinical replication with direct observation. J Appl Behav Anal 1998;31(2):299–302.
38. Woods DW, Twohig MP, Flessner CA, et al. Treatment of vocal tics in children with Tourette syndrome: investigating the efficacy of habit reversal. J Appl Behav Anal 2003;36(1):109–12.
39. Flessner CA, Miltenberger RG, Egemo K, et al. An evaluation of the social support component of simplified habit reversal for the treatment of nail biting. Behav Ther 2005;36:35–42.
40. Carr JE, Chong IM. Habit reversal treatment of tic disorders: a methodological critique of the literature. Behav Modif 2005;29(6):858–75.
41. Task Force on Promotion and Dissemination of Psychological Procedures. Training in and dissemination of emperically-validated psychological treatments. Clin Psychol 1995;48(1):3–23.
42. Azrin NH, Peterson AL. Treatment of Tourette's syndrome by habit reversal: a waiting-list control group comparison. Behav Ther 1990;21:305–18.
43. O'Connor KP, Brault M, Robillard S, et al. Evaluation of a cognitive-behavioural program for the management of chronic tic and habit disorders. Behav Res Ther 2001;39(6):667–81.
44. Wilhelm S, Deckersbach T, Coffey BJ, et al. Habit reversal versus supportive psychotherapy for Tourette's disorder: a randomized controlled trial. Am J Psychiatry 2003;160(6):1175–7.
45. Woods DW, Wetterneck CT, Flessner CA. A controlled evaluation of acceptance and commitment therapy plus habit reversal for trichotillomania. Behav Res Ther 2006;44(5):639–56.
46. van Minnen A, Hoogduin KA, Keijsers GP, et al. Treatment of trichotillomania with behavioral therapy or fluoxetine: a randomized, waiting-list controlled study. Arch Gen Psychiatry 2003;60(5):517–22.
47. Ninan PT, Rothbaum BO, Marsteller FA, et al. A placebo-controlled trial of cognitive-behavioral therapy and clomipramine in trichotillomania. J Clin Psychiatry 2000;61(1):47–50.
48. Diefenbach GJ, Tolin DF, Hannan S, et al. Group treatment for trichotillomania: behavior therapy versus supportive therapy. Behav Ther 2006;37(4):353–63.
49. Bloch MH, Landeros-Weisenberger A, Dombrowski P, et al. Systematic review: pharmacological and behavioral treatment for trichotillomania. Biol Psychiatry 2007;62(8):839–46.
50. Mouton SG, Stanley MA. Habit reversal training for trichotillomania: a group approach. Cognit Behav Pract 1996;3:159–82.
51. Elliott AJ, Fuqua RW. Acceptability of treatments for trichotillomania. Behav Modif 2002;26:378–99.
52. Piacentini J, Woods DW, Scahill L, et al. Behavior therapy for children with Tourette disorder: a randomized controlled trial. JAMA 2010;303(19):1929–37.

Cognitive-Behavioral Therapy for Children with Comorbid Physical Illness

Rachel D. Thompson, MA[a,b,c], Patty Delaney, LCSW[b,c], Inti Flores, BA[c,d], Eva Szigethy, MD, PhD[c,e,f],*

KEYWORDS

- Adolescent • Chronic • Stress • Adjustment • Coping
- Treatment • Physical illness

OVERVIEW

There is growing literature to support a reciprocal relationship between physical and mental illnesses: chronic medical conditions can have an adverse effect on psychological well-being, and psychopathology and stress can have a negative effect on physical health.[1–3] Although the mechanisms responsible for the brain-body interactions are still to be determined and are not yet fully understood, a wide array of pathophysiologic mechanisms seem to converge in different illnesses, resulting in common symptoms such as anxiety, depression, and pain. Promising psychosocial treatments for psychopathology can be tailored to target physical symptom relief, medical adherence, and quality of life (QoL) among individuals vulnerable to psychological and medical stress caused by their experience of chronic medical illness. One of the most promising and empirically researched therapies for medical comorbidity is cognitive-behavioral therapy (CBT), which uses an active, directive, time-limited, and structured approach

This work was supported by grant nos. R01MH077770 and 1DP2OD001210 from the National Institutes of Health.

The authors have nothing to disclose.

[a] Psychology Department, University of Cincinnati, 4150 Edwards One, Cincinnati, OH 45221-0376, USA

[b] Western Psychiatric Institute and Clinic, 3811 O'Hara Street, Pittsburgh, PA 15213, USA

[c] Medical Coping Clinic, Division of Gastroenterology, Children's Hospital of UPMC, 4401 Penn Avenue, 5-FP-Gastro, Pittsburgh, PA 15224, USA

[d] School of Medicine, University of Pittsburgh, 3550 Terrace Street, Pittsburgh, PA 15261, USA

[e] Department of Psychiatry, University of Pittsburgh, 3811 O'Hara Street, Pittsburgh, PA 15213, USA

[f] Department of Pediatrics, University of Pittsburgh, 4401 Penn Avenue, Pittsburgh, PA 15224, USA

* Corresponding author. Medical Coping Clinic, Division of Gastroenterology, Children's Hospital of UPMC, 4401 Penn Avenue, 5-FP-Gastro, Pittsburgh, PA 15224.

E-mail address: szigethye@upmc.edu

to the treatment of many psychiatric symptoms and behavioral health issues.[4–7] This review discusses the empirical evidence for using CBT to treat psychopathology and illness-related problems in youth with physical illness in 2 parts: (1) a focus on general considerations for using CBT for chronic medical illnesses; (2) emphasis on several model diseases affecting youth and their families to illustrate key points about the usefulness of CBT. These pediatric diseases of focus are diabetes, inflammatory bowel disease (IBD), cancer, and sickle cell disease (SCD). These physical illnesses were selected because they affect a large cross section of the pediatric population and also highlight prominent medical and psychological issues of concern, including treatment adherence, pain management, stigma, and psychosocial adjustment. Both similarities and differences between the problems faced in these disorders and CBT-generated solutions are addressed throughout the review.

Theoretic Applications of CBT

CBT is based on the premise that an individual's behavior and affect stems from his or her immediate cognitive experience. This immediate experience, also referred to as automatic thought, is largely determined by overarching cognitive schemas, which develop over time through life experiences.[4,8,9] In the case of individuals with chronic medical illness, these cognitive schemas develop within the context of unpleasant physical symptoms and related functional impairment, altered developmental trajectories, numerous outpatient medical visits, and inpatient hospitalizations. This is coupled with the additional stressors of invasive medical procedures and highly uncertain medical outcomes. Through collaborative exploration and discovery with a skilled CBT therapist, patients are able to become aware of their maladaptive cognitions and begin concentrating on actual events and the meanings they attribute to them. The goal of therapy is to help children and adolescents attribute realistic meanings to life events and challenge dysfunctional thought and behavioral patterns, such as emotional and situational avoidance strategies, medical nonadherence, and behavioral nonactivation.[8] Left untreated, such maladaptive coping strategies can contribute to decreased QoL and increased medical morbidity and related medical costs. For consistency, children and adolescents are referred to as youth throughout the remainder of this article.

Although CBT has consistently demonstrated efficacy for the treatment of anxiety and depressive disorders in both adults and youth, it seems particularly relevant to the treatment of behavioral health and medical coping issues in the medical comorbidity literature.[5,6,10,11] However, the efficacy of CBT has not been well studied in terms of adjustment to and coping with pediatric physical illness. Randomized controlled trials (RCTs) testing the effectiveness of CBT compared with alternative forms of treatment or support are challenging studies to conduct; thus, data are limited. Moreover, the extant literature is difficult to integrate given the wide diversity of presenting medical conditions, specific subpopulations of youth sampled, variation in CBT approach and dose, and different outcomes assessed. This review integrates the existing literature about CBT in youth with chronic physical illness to make recommendations specific to medical coping, extending beyond psychological adjustment issues. This task is accomplished by reviewing specific findings in the limited child and adolescent literature, as well as by incorporating relevant findings from the adult literature.

SPECIAL CONSIDERATIONS FOR USING CBT IN PHYSICALLY ILL YOUTH
Developmental Considerations

Developmental stages must be taken into account when providing treatment to children and adolescents with chronic physical illnesses. Emotional, cognitive, and intellectual development can be severely affected by chronic illness; youth of all ages may turn to maladaptive coping strategies in response to crises, looking to their parents to shoulder much of the burden of the chronic illness.[12] Avoidant coping, or cognitive distortions such as denial and magical thinking, can cause more stress for the family unit and often negatively affect treatment adherence.[13,14] In addition, depending on the challenges associated with a particular disease or its treatment, delayed acquisition of developmental milestones or regression to early developmental periods can occur at any age. Because younger children are typically in an earlier stage of identity development, they often adjust more easily and assimilate their chronic illness into their developing sense of self, particularly if they are nested in a supportive family environment.[15] The social stigma of chronic medical illness has typically not taken hold and therefore may not be a barrier to treatment adherence or a focus of psychological treatment among children in this age group. Nevertheless, children less than 12 years of age seem to be motivated by needs of mastery and competence, and the loss of control experienced during medical procedures threatens these basic emotional needs and may engender feelings of anxiety and helplessness.[16] Among this age group, CBT skills may be most helpful by enhancing mastery skills, increasing self-efficacy, decreasing avoidance, and instilling a sense of control and responsibility regarding their medical treatment and current situation.

Adolescence is often a challenging developmental time for youth because they begin to individuate from their parents, develop an autonomous sense of self, and increasingly turn to their peers for feedback and support.[12] In addition to these basic psychosocial changes, pubertal maturation is changing the inward and outward appearance of the developing body. During this time, adolescents tend to be resistant to parental authority and naturally rebel as they seek autonomy from their family. They also experience growth in their cognitive reasoning and abstraction abilities, [17] but often still have difficulty modulating extreme emotions, all of which can affect their decision making, coping, view of the world, and the meaning of their lives. Their desire for independence, along with embarrassing aspects of symptoms and, perhaps, a misunderstanding of their medical needs, may result in some adolescents being hesitant to discuss their illness symptoms with their parents and medical providers or be nonadherent with treatment. Collectively, these factors can have an adverse effect on disease morbidity and course.[18]

General Medical Considerations

Damaged self

Chronic physical illnesses have a considerable effect on the QoL of affected youth and families. Frequent medical appointments, procedures, and hospitalizations often limit youth's activities; increased school absences, decreased involvement in extracurricular activities, hobbies, and decreased time with friends and family are also common and result in lost social opportunities. Feelings of isolation, boredom, loss, and not belonging can be overwhelming as the youth is forced to miss social opportunities because of illness. Youths diagnosed with a chronic illness often experience grief in response to the loss of their past lifestyles, mourning the loss of the healthy self that now has new parameters required by the symptoms and treatment of their chronic illness. Anxiety and depression frequently occur as they cope with their symptoms, the changes in their life, body image, fear of disease relapse, and loss of social, familial and academic experiences. Feelings of not being in control can be overwhelming and can exacerbate the depressive state.

Chronic illness symptoms and medication side effects exert a physical and emotional toll on the patients. Diseases that are noticeably disfiguring (eg, rheumatoid arthritis) as well as conditions in which the symptoms are hidden (eg, diarrhea in IBD) may have shame and embarrassment associated with them.[19] Medication side effects can also amplify depression, anxiety, social isolation, and stigma; steroids used to treat cancer, asthma, or IBD may cause acne, facial swelling (ie, moon facies), weight gain, insomnia, irritability, moodiness, and agitation.[20] For the adolescent who is extremely concerned about their physical appearance, the physiologic effects of the disease process often affect them socially and emotionally. For example, individuals with IBD experience an inflamed bowel, which releases a complex immunologic cascade of cytokines that have been shown to induce depressive symptoms in animal models.[21] These cytokine-mediated symptoms, also called serum sickness, include anhedonia, irritability, apathy, fatigue, sleep disturbances, and anorexia. For youth with IBD, learning about IBD-induced depression decreases stigma and facilitates seeking behavioral coping therapy. Youth are also greatly affected physically and psychologically by the other model diseases to be addressed in this review. SCD can cause jaundice, shortness of breath, extreme exhaustion, and pain. Youth with type 1 diabetes may be embarrassed with the glucose checks and the insulin pump, and individuals with cancer often experience hair loss, weight loss, fatigue, and nausea when in treatment. Adolescents with IBD, SCD, and cancer often experience delays in puberty as a result of nutritional deficiencies or medication side effects. Youth with chronic illnesses may experience embarrassment centering on their experience of symptoms and feel ashamed of their need to take medications and undergo medical procedures, which often negatively affect their ego as they see themselves as damaged or not normal. For disease processes and treatments involving the central nervous system (eg, neurofibromatosis, leukemia, lymphoma, solid cancer tumors), greater neurologic involvement has been associated with increased emotional and social problems.[22,23] With these physical and emotional side effects, adolescents with chronic illnesses present differently from their peers and may appear sick, which leads to avoidance of peer interaction or being a target of bullying. This situation may result in further social isolation from their peer group. In summary, these physiologic effects of disease-related processes and accompanying psychological reactions affect adaptation and are ideal targets for a CBT approach.

Illness narratives

The thoughts and fears discussed earlier make up the youth's illness experience and perception, terms that have been collectively referred to as the illness narrative. In youth and young adults with chronic physical diseases, qualitative analysis of illness narratives have shown illness-related feelings of damaged self, embarrassment and shame about symptoms, concern about appearance, misattribution about illness causes, desire for independence, and compliance with medical treatment, highlighting the potential importance of addressing such conflicting attitudes and emotional reactions in treatment planning.[24,25] Themes that have emerged from the adult literature in the context of diabetes include illness image, meaning, integration, priority, care responsibility, and future outlook.[26] The usefulness of looking at family illness narratives, or the stories and collective understanding surrounding chronic illnesses affecting multiple generations, has received attention in cancer research and suggests that narrative methods can be helpful in facilitating psychosocial adjustment and familial communication. Family narrative methods can also be helpful because they encourage the integration of contrasting illness views within a family. This in turn may open up families to the possibility of hope and new medical advances despite a history of poor course and outcome, as well as give others permission to attempt a new life trajectory through the practice of adaptive medical and coping strategies that can lead to enhanced physical and mental health.[27]

Daily functioning
Living with a chronic illness can be extremely stressful as a result of the functional restrictions frequently imposed on the patient. For example, the daily activity of eating may be difficult to negotiate among those with chronic illness: youth with gastrointestinal issues must avoid foods that exacerbate their symptoms and youth with diabetes must monitor their sugar and carbohydrate intake. Children with cancer often experience nausea as a side effect of chemotherapy, which then decreases their appetite and causes nutritional deficiencies. Moreover, social gatherings are often centered on meals (eg, family dinners, celebratory parties, lunchtime with friends) and when dealing with the effects of chronic illness, these situations can remind youth of their illness and related limitations. The manner in which the individual handles this stress can have a considerable effect on his or her overall mood and well-being. Coinciding with this issue of eating is the reality that his or her natural growth potential may be negatively affected by nutritional deficiencies, medications, and the stress response of dealing with his or her illness. CBT interventions can target these fears, stress, and anxiety in a way to help increase treatment adherence, by improving QoL, restoring activities that boost confidence, and facilitating cognitive change to reframe treatment positively.

Grief
Often when youth are first diagnosed with a chronic illness, they have been sick for some time and may be struggling with the uncertainty of confusing symptoms, medical testing, and potential diagnoses. The relief and disappointment that follow a confirmed diagnosis can lead to anxiety, fear, anger, and sadness as the family learns what the youth will have to deal with for the rest of his or her life. Although medication may provide adequate psychological and medical relief for some, some chronic illnesses shorten the lifespan or affect daily life with an undetermined prognosis. Thus, confronting one's eventual mortality and a foreshortened future may be a concern, either because death is a real possibility or because of diagnosis misperception and catastrophic amplification. For those with cancer or SCD, the possibility of an early, perhaps sudden, death is real and may cause a host of emotional responses as the loss of the healthy self is compounded with the additional loss of their hopes, dreams, and future. With each medication side effect, active symptom, medical procedure or hospitalization, the child and family may experience anxiety and fear, not knowing if the chronic illness is reactivating or intensifying. The process of accepting a medical condition and related courses of treatment can closely mimic the grief stages identified by Kübler Ross (1972), and children may cycle through times of anxiety, depression, anger, denial, and regression.[28,29]

Family involvement
Parents experience difficulties related to the effects of the youth's illness on the family and related feelings of guilt, and how parents respond to these difficulties directly influences how the rest of the family copes. Living with a chronic physical illness often involves a host of psychosocial stressors in addition to the demands of addressing illness symptoms and medical treatment, including negotiating academic and occupational limitations, financial burden and medical coverage, communication difficulties, uncertainties about the youth's future well-being and mortality, and lack of adequate leisure-work balance.[30] Parents often focus most of their attention on the ill child, and struggle to balance their jobs, personal needs, and the needs of their other children effectively. Many studies have shown a correlation between parental adjustment and the psychosocial adjustment of the pediatric patient.[31–35] An adequate

psychosocial support network may help to alleviate these demands and facilitate more adaptive parental adjustment.[36] Clinicians have recognized that including parents and other family members can increase the effectiveness of the therapy by systemically enhancing coping skills throughout the family unit. Training parents to become CBT coaches for their children not only provides an active and constructive focus of parental energy but also may mitigate against maladaptive parental coping such as distancing, denial, and overprotection of the sick child.

Summary

CBT has been shown to improve functioning in youth with a wide variety of chronic physical illnesses.[37,38] These physical health issues affect kids and families in a variety of ways; however, the similarities are most significant for our discussion. Treatment adherence, medication compliance, pain levels, sleep disturbance, and family involvement can all have an enormous effects on the well-being of the patient and are common issues encountered across the physical illness spectrum. The following section considers several different diseases such as diabetes, IBD, cancer, and sickle cell anemia as models to demonstrate specific issues that can be addressed using CBT.

CBT FOR MODEL DISEASES
Diabetes

Childhood-onset diabetes is a chronic medical condition consisting of 2 subtypes (type 1 and type 2), both of which involve dysregulation of insulin and glucose metabolism leading to polyuria, extreme thirst, fatigue, and changes in weight. In its most severe forms, diabetic ketoacidosis may occur, leading to hospitalization, coma, and death. The management of diabetes necessitates conscientious daily care to regulate blood glucose concentrations. The regimen is often complex, including periodic blood glucose checks and insulin replacement, in addition to nutritional and exercise components. Diabetes is a manageable condition; however, mismanagement can lead to increased negative medical outcomes and poorer QoL. Thus, treatment and medication adherence is of vital importance and nonadherence is one of the most salient issues in the pediatric literature, particularly among the developing adolescent.[39,40] Social problems and acquisition of adequate coping skills to effectively dampen diabetes-related anxiety and stress management are also common problems among this population.[40,41] The role of the family unit is very important and stress emanating from this unit in the form of familial conflict, poor communication, and poor problem solving has been linked to poor diabetes control.[42] Studied interventions are frequently family based and behaviorally focused, with varying degrees of intensity and patient contact. Psychoeducation alone has not been found effective for families and youth with diabetes and poor glycemic control.[43] Similarly, behavioral interventions focused only on treatment adherence and self-management interventions show minimal treatment effects on glycemic control indices, whereas those including emotional, social, and familial components tend to have larger, more beneficial effects.[44]

The efficacy of CBT interventions has been relatively well studied in the pediatric diabetes population, with a variety of approaches being examined in RCTs (**Table 1**). Ellis and colleagues[40,45–48] have been at the forefront of this literature examining the effectiveness of multisystemic therapy (MST), a home- and community-based family intervention that addresses the multiple systems within which adolescents and families live, function and ideally thrive (eg, peer group, nuclear family, schools, health care system, and so forth). The interventions typically delivered

Table 1
RCTs evaluating the effectiveness of cognitive-behavioral interventions for comorbid physical illness in the pediatric population

Study (year)	Sample	Type of Intervention	Distress Symptoms	Medical Adherence and Outcomes	Service Utilization	Pain	Social Functioning	QoL
Liossi & Hatira,[77] 1999	Cancer (N = 30)	Individual 1. Coping skills 2. Hypnosis 3. Standard care	Improved (faces rating)	Not assessed	Not assessed	Improved (PBCL, faces rating)	Not assessed	Not assessed
Grey et al,[51] 2000	Type 1 diabetes (N = 77)	Group 1. Coping skills 2. Standard care	No effect (CDI)	Improved (SDS, IDM coping, laboratory tests)	Not assessed	Not assessed	Not assessed	Improved (DQL-Y)
Gil et al,[96] 2001	SCD (N = 46)	Individual 1. Coping skills 2. Standard care	No effect (CDI, RCMAS)	Improved (CSQ)	Improved (daily diary, interview)	No effect (pressure stimulator)	Not assessed	Improved (daily diary)
Ellis et al,[47] 2005	Type 1 diabetes (N = 31)	Family 1. Multisystemic 2. Standard care	Not assessed	Not reported	Improved (medical chart)	Not assessed	Not assessed	Not assessed
Ellis et al,[40,45,46] 2007, 2005, 2005	Type 1 diabetes (N = 127)	Family 1. Multisystemic 2. Standard care	Improved (DSQ)	Variable (blood glucose meter, laboratory tests)	Improved (medical chart)	Not assessed	Not assessed	Not assessed
Wysocki et al,[42,49,50] 2006, 2007, 2008	Diabetes (N = 104)	Family 1. Behavioral systems 2. Education 3. Standard care	Not assessed	Variable (DSMP, laboratory tests)	Not assessed	Not assessed	Variable (PARQ, DRC)	Not assessed
Szigethy et al,[6,65] 2007, 2006	IBD (N = 41)	Individuals 1. PASCET-PI 2. Standard care	Variable (K-SADS, CDI, PCSC)	Improved (PCDAI, Kozarek)	Not assessed	Not assessed	Not assessed	Improved (CGAS)
Grey et al,[52] 2009	Type 1 diabetes (N = 82)	Group 1. Coping skills 2. Education	No effect (CDI)	No effect (SDS, laboratory tests)	Not assessed	Not assessed	No effect (DFBS)	No effect (DQL-Y)
Lemanek et al,[98] 2009	Sickle cell disease (N = 34)	Family 1. Massage 2. Control	Improved (CES-D, STAIC, CDI)	Not assessed	No effect (medical chart)	Improved (PPS)	Not assessed	Improved (FS-IIR)

Abbreviations: CDI, Children's Depression Inventory; CES-D, Center for Epidemiological Studies of Depression Scale - Depression Scale; CGAS, Child Global Assessment of Functioning Scale; CSQ, Coping Strategies Questionnaire; DFBS, Diabetes Family Behavior Scale; DQL-Y, Diabetes Quality of Life - Youth; DRC, Diabetes Responsibility and Conflict Scale; DSMP, Diabetes Self-Management Profile; DSQ, Diabetes Stress Questionnaire; FS-IIR, Functional Status - II - Revised; IDM Coping, Issues in Coping with Intensive Diabetes Management Scale; K-SADS, Kiddie Schedule for Affective Disorders and Schizophrenia; Kozarek, Clinical Score of Kozarek; PARQ, Parent-Adolescent Relationship Questionnaire; PBCL, Procedure Behavioral Checklist; PCDAI, Pediatric Crohn's Disease Activity Index; PCSC, Perceived Control Scale for Children; PPS, Pediatric Pain Scale; RCMAS, Revised Children's Manifest Anxiety Scale; SDS, Self-efficacy for Diabetes Scale; STAIC, State-Trait Anxiety Inventory for Children.

through an MST approach are intensive (multiple, weekly home-based sessions) and largely behavioral, with treatment adherence being a significant target of intervention, given the diabetic adolescent population involved. More specifically, interventions included development of behavioral contingency plans for parents and adolescents, implementation of a family schedule and routine, teaching of effective communication skills, and increasing the involvement and collaboration of school, community, and peer systems to increase treatment adherence. Results from 2 trials consistently showed that adolescents with diabetes randomized to MST had improved health outcomes, including decreases in the number of inpatient admissions, significantly lower cost of medical care (direct hospital costs decreased by 68%, whereas control patient costs were approximately doubled), improved metabolic control, and increases in the frequency of blood glucose testing compared with a standard care control group.[45,47] Moreover, this research group found that metabolic control improved as a function of increased treatment adherence,[46] with the relationship between MST treatment fidelity and metabolic control being fully mediated by treatment adherence.[48] Intensive, cognitive-behavioral interventions involving family and systemic components can lead to improvements in adolescent adherence, which seem to yield improved treatment outcomes. Although some improvements of MST were not maintained over follow-up periods among specific subgroups (eg, frequency of glucose testing), decreases in inpatient admissions remained statistically significant and suggestive of beneficial treatment effects.[40] Despite the positive implications of these findings, the MST was compared with usual care and not an attentional control group, thus the effectiveness attributable specifically to MST interventions (rather than to patient contact time) needs further investigation, as well as the cost-effectiveness of such intensive treatment.

Behavioral family systems therapy geared specifically for diabetic control (BFST-D) has also shown positive treatment effects on adherence, glycemic control, and diabetes self-management.[42,49] There is much overlap between BFST-D interventions and MST, including the development of behavioral contingencies to decrease problematic diabetes-related behavior, use of other behavioral approaches, family as the treatment unit, and the extensions of therapeutic activities to domains outside of the family. Key differences include less frequent therapist contact, delivery in a treatment setting (not in the home), predominant emphasis of problem solving and communication training, and delivery of cognitive restructuring to reframe irrational and unhelpful thinking patterns. Given its treatment focus, it is not surprising that individuals receiving BFST-D also reported improvements in family conflict and adolescent-mother communication compared with standard care and educational support.[42,50] Unfortunately, these improvements were not always maintained throughout long-term follow-up. Nevertheless, indices of improved glycemic control were maintained across extended follow-up.[49]

Individual interventions targeting the youth, such as adjunct coping skills training (CST) combined with intensive diabetes management (IDM), have shown mixed results depending on the sample and point of intervention delivery. IDM is characterized by daily insulin injections or subcutaneous insulin infusion, blood glucose self-monitoring, monthly outpatient visits, and periodic telephone contacts.[51] CST targeted feelings of self-competence through facilitating the acquisition of adaptive behavioral, communication, and interpersonal patterns in adolescent CST training groups (2–3 patients). Group sessions included role playing various social situations that can be problematic to negotiate during adolescence, particularly given the additional pressures that come along with diabetes management (eg, food selection with peers present, substance-related decision making), and receiving feedback/interventions that specifically emphasized problem solving, social skills training (eg, assertive communication), and cognitive behavior modification.[51]

In the first trial, Grey and colleagues[51] examined the effectiveness of combined CST and IDM compared with the effectiveness of IDM alone among an adolescent cohort aged 12 to 20 years. Those in the CST+IDM group showed greater improvement on indices of glycemic control, increased self-efficacy as it related to diabetes and medical treatment, and less effects of diabetes on QoL at 1-year follow-up. The combination of CST+IDM was found to be particularly beneficial for the incidence of weight gain and hypoglycemia among female participants, with involvement in CST being related to significant decreases among these indices. No such associations were found among male participants. A different pattern of findings emerged when CST was examined in a sample of children (aged 8–12 years). In this RCT, CST and an attentional, educational control group did not significantly differ on outcome measures of metabolic control, QoL, depression, coping, self-efficacy, and familial functioning; both groups showed comparable improvement in psychosocial outcomes.[52] Treatment was delivered separately to patients and parents in a small group format. Lack of study significance may be attributable to low statistical power and high baseline levels of functionality (psychosocial and medical) possibly making it difficult to detect positive treatment effects.

Summary

Treatment adherence is vital in the regulation of diabetes and is a salient treatment target that often needs to be addressed in the youth population, in addition to emotional, social, and familial adjustment needs. Both psychoeducation and behavioral self-management alone are not adequate in addressing the barriers to treatment adherence, thus treatments likely need to incorporate psychosocial and familial components to increase outcomes among individuals with poor glycemic control.[44] There currently is some support for CBT-oriented treatment interventions. Of the trials covered in the present review, BFST-D has been most rigorously tested and shows the most promising outcomes compared with an educational support group. Nevertheless, long-term improvement in psychosocial outcomes as a result of BFST-D was not always maintained, although improvement in glycemic control indices was maintained. Adding on the experiential components specific to CST (eg, repeated communication and interpersonal effectiveness role plays) may be a strategy that might enhance such treatment of youth and families. Future RCTs comparing active treatments to adequate attentional control groups are necessary for any psychological standard of treatment to be established.

IBD

IBD, which includes Crohn's disease (CD) and ulcerative colitis (UC), illustrates the bidirectional relationship between stress and the gastrointestinal tract. Both CD and UC are chronic and debilitating autoimmune conditions predominantly consisting of symptoms such as abdominal pain, bloody diarrhea, and weight loss with an unpredictable course and complicated treatment. Patients with IBD have been shown to have increased rates of associated anxiety and depression, functional abdominal pain and fatigue, even when the disease is in remission, and there is a growing literature showing that stress can lead to exacerbations of IBD course.[53] With prevalence rates of IBD increasing, the negative effects that IBD can have on the life of children and families is multiplying.[54] Frequent medical procedures, multiple hospitalizations, treatments with negative side effects, pubertal and growth retardation, and fecal incontinence all affect the development of the child, physically, mentally, and socially.

Youth with IBD often miss a significant amount of school, extracurricular activities, and social time with friends. Moreover, during active IBD flares, the immune system releases proinflammatory cytokines systemically, which can influence the brain both directly and indirectly inducing depression. All of these factors create the perfect storm so that youth with IBD are found to experience depression at a much higher rate than their healthy peers and youth with other chronic conditions.[55,56] In addition to comorbid depression, patients with IBD often continue to experience functional abdominal pain in the absence of overt IBD-related inflammation.[57,58]

A multisite RCT conducted by our research group recruited depressed pediatric patients with endoscopically confirmed IBD (see **Table 1**). Participants were youth age 11 to 17 years and were randomized to either manualized CBT (modified to treat IBD-related problems) or standard care with no additional psychological intervention. The CBT was based on the Primary and Secondary Control Enhancement Training (PASCET) model developed by Weisz and colleagues[59] (1997), which postulated that depressive symptoms can be improved by teaching adolescents appropriate locus of control. Primary control is for modifiable stress factors (eg, feeling bored) so behaviors are changed to better match wishes. Secondary control is for factors that cannot be altered (eg, having IBD), thus teaching the patient how to change thinking about such factors to decrease distress. Physical illness-related modifications to the basic PASCET model included (1) focus on illness narrative (ie, perceptions and experience of having IBD), (2) hypnotherapy for pain and immune functioning, (3) psychoeducation about the relationship between IBD and depression, and (4) emphasis on IBD-related cognitions (eg, pessimism about having IBD) and behaviors (eg, medical nonadherence).[11] Modifications in structure included phone sessions and coupling face-to-face sessions with medical appointments. The resultant intervention was called PASCET-Physical Illness (PASCET-PI). The modifications in PASCET-PI were drawn from examples in the adult literature that suggest a beneficial effect of such interventions on coping with physical illness, highlighting the importance of increasing patients' knowledge of the disease process and understanding illness perception.[60,61] This can be accomplished by using narrative approaches to help patients rework pessimistic narratives and correct misattributions about the disease process.[62] The hypnotherapy was adapted from studies in adults with IBD showing positive effects of relaxation and hypnosis on IBD-related QoL and inflammation.[63,64]

Both the youth and parents worked from a PASCET-PI workbook; the youth received 9 individual sessions whereas the parents participated in 3 sessions during the 3-month intervention. CBT sessions were organized into 2 sets of skills: ACT skills for behavioral activation (primary control) and THINK skills for cognitive restructuring (secondary control). ACT skills consisted of learning to problem solve, engagement in activities that positively affect mood and provide a sense of social belonging, and learning relaxation techniques. THINK skills targeted the acquisition of adaptive thought content by challenging negative thought patterns and encouraging focus on helpful, positive thoughts and personal strengths. Not only did the PASCET-PI group show improved depressive severity and global functioning after treatment, these positive effects were maintained 1 year after treatment compared with the standard care group.[6,65] In addition, IBD severity improved in youth receiving PASCET-PI for up to 6 months after treatment.[65] Although other factors could account for these positive changes in the CBT group, collectively these results are consistent with PASCET-PI having a positive effect on both emotional and physical aspects of IBD. Moreover, youth who had more pessimistic illness narratives and received PASCET-PI showed significantly more optimistic attitudes toward IBD after treatment.[66] When comparing youth receiving CBT with normal matched controls, depressed youth with IBD showed increased metabolism in brain regions, such as the dorsolateral prefrontal cortex, that have been associated with depression in other depressed populations.[67]

Summary

CBT for the treatment of IBD is an emerging area of scientific inquiry in the pediatric population. Promising advances from adult studies are currently being applied in clinical trials with youth to facilitate the development of effective treatment interventions for this patient group. Preliminary work suggests that CBT is a viable treatment option, with results showing improved psychological well-being and QoL. Results also implicate the involvement of specific brain regions and cognitive processing that may partially explain the improvements seen among those completing CBT treatment, although these results need replication. Additional studies exploring mechanisms by which CBT may exert effects on the brain and body are also needed. Future research is necessary with long-term follow-up to examine the duration of treatment effectiveness, as well as to track these individuals as they age and mature to better understand what coping strategies are most adaptive longitudinally. This future research is particularly important in adolescents with IBD as they transition into adulthood, as IBD is incurable. The cost-effectiveness of psychological intervention for this group is also of interest and should be explored in future clinical trials.

Cancer

High rates of depression and adjustment disorders among adults with cancer have been consistently reported in the literature.[68,69] This is not unexpected given the frequent psychosocial difficulties faced by this population, including grief (eg, loss of healthy self, control, independence, time to accomplish goals) and mortality (eg, sense of a foreshortened future and fears of death, pain, isolation, and others' well-being once gone).[70] Most of these studies have been performed in adult populations, although a recent naturalistic study among pediatric patients with cancer has shown that children with tumors diagnosed in their first year of life have greater difficulties with behavioral and psychological adjustment, particularly with internalizing symptoms (ie, depression and anxiety).[71] Moreover, these individuals also showed a significantly decreased health-related QoL with social functioning and psychosocial health being most affected, compared with their healthy counterparts during childhood and adolescence.

The clinical picture of adult survivors of childhood cancer is mixed, with several studies reporting conflicting results. In response to this, the Childhood Cancer Survivor Study, a recent retrospective cohort study examining the psychological and health status of adult survivors of childhood cancer, found that a significant proportion of cancer survivors reported more symptoms of distress and poorer physical health-related QoL compared with a sibling control group.[72] Although not all survivors of childhood cancer experience clinically significant impairment, those with childhood onset of leukemia, brain tumor, neuroblastoma, and lymphoma seem to be at greater relative risk for psychological distress (eg, depression, anxiety, somatization, or fatigue) than their sibling counterparts, and in some cases, the normative population. Brain tumors, bone tumors, and sarcomas have also been linked to impaired physical health, and leukemia, specifically, to social skills deficits. Across the entire sample of childhood cancer survivors, perceived health and the presence of a major medical condition were related to reports of increased psychological distress. It becomes clear that cancer diagnosed in childhood is related to increased psychological distress and impairment in a subset of individuals. The effect of common courses of treatment (ie, neurotoxicity of chemotherapy and brain tissue resection encountered in neurosurgery), in combination with inflammation of the immune system and resulting changes in neurotransmitter availability, also seems to be a likely culprit in the increased biologic vulnerability to depression, fatigue, impaired sleep, and cognition in patients with cancer.[1]

To date, a limited number of RCTs of CBT interventions have been conducted. Of the research that has been conducted, the literature has largely focused on adult adjustment and clinical trials within the adult cancer population. A recent meta-analysis of RCTs examining the effectiveness of CBT and patient education (PE) for the treatment of psychological distress, pain, physical functioning, and QoL among adult cancer survivors identified 15 empirical studies of sufficient quality to include in a conservative test of CBT effects.[73] CBT interventions included stress management and problem solving, as well as other cognitive and behaviorally focused interventions, whereas PE reflected only educational information delivery regarding the illness and symptoms, symptom management, or discussion of treatment options. Findings indicated that cancer survivors who underwent individually administered CBT showed significant improvement on depression, anxiety, and QoL measures, whereas those who received PE and group-delivered CBT did not show significant improvements. The positive effect of individual CBT was evident for psychological distress symptoms only at short-term follow-up (<8 months), whereas improvement in QoL was maintained through long-term follow-up. However, results from this study also suggested that both CBT and PE interventions had little effect on pain and physical functioning improvement. In contrast, a RCT comparing CBT with standard care in the treatment of acute physical symptoms (ie, pain, fatigue, diarrhea, nausea, vomiting, infection) among adults diagnosed with a solid tumor undergoing their first course of chemotherapy showed that CBT helped to decrease symptom severity, specifically among those with the most severe baseline levels of physiologic distress.[74] The extant literature shows mixed support for the effectiveness of behavioral exercise interventions toward increasing physical functioning of patients with cancer, as well as psychological well-being and QoL.[75,76]

The gap between science and clinical treatment needs becomes even wider for the pediatric population specifically, with only 2 controlled trials of CBT interventions being identified. Hypnosis and cognitive-behavioral coping skills have been shown to be effective compared with no intervention in decreasing pain and pain-related anxiety among young patients with cancer undergoing bone marrow aspirations.[77] With regard to anxiety and behavioral distress, hypnosis showed a significant advantage compared with cognitive-behavioral coping skills. Although hypnotherapy is often classified as its own treatment modality distinct from CBT, there are common techniques used in both modalities (eg, relaxation and visual imagery) that are clearly within the CBT framework. In the matter of coping with acute pain, it seems that these classic hypnotherapy techniques, in addition to hypnotic suggestion, might be more advantageous when briefly intervening (ie, 2 30-minute sessions) for short-term relief of anxiety and behavioral distress related to painful medical procedures than traditional cognitive restructuring techniques (see **Table 1**). More recently, Poggi and colleagues[78] found that brain tumor survivors receiving 4 to 8 months of CBT intervention, including weekly individual and parent treatment sessions, showed significantly greater improvement in internalizing symptoms, social relationships, social skills, somatic complaints, and attentional problems than individuals receiving no psychological intervention. Both studies found support for the effectiveness of conventional CBT interventions in the acute and longer-term management of pain and somatic complaints among pediatric patients with cancer. CBT also seems beneficial in the long-term treatment of internalizing symptoms and social functioning, whereas hypnotherapy may be more advantageous for the acute treatment of anxiety and distress as it relates to painful medical procedures.

Summary

Although a clear relationship has been observed between cancer and behavioral comorbidities, including psychological adjustment and QoL issues, trials examining the effectiveness of CBT interventions that target this specific group have been limited. This is particularly true among the pediatric population; therefore, there is a strong need for RCTs to apply recent advances in CBT (and hypnotherapy) to pediatric patients who have cancer struggling with clinical and subthreshold levels of pain and distress. Such interventions seem promising for increasing psychological well-being and may potentially have a beneficial effect on medical treatment outcomes.[79] Telemedicine or providing psychiatric services remotely via technology and secure remote means may also be a fruitful avenue of future research, providing a means for efficient long-term treatment delivery, enabling health care professionals to overcome various obstacles to systematically monitor, detect, and adjust medical and psychological treatment as needed.[80,81] A recent RCT in a sample of adult patients with cancer found automated home-based symptom monitoring and centralized tele-management more effective than usual care in the treatment of cancer-related pain management and depression.[82] Similar research is also being conducted in the multiple sclerosis and IBD populations with promising patient response and treatment outcomes.[83–85]

SCD

SCD is a genetic blood disorder primarily affecting people of African and Caribbean descent. SCD is a chronic, unpredictable and life-long blood disorder that is associated with an uncertain outcome in that all patients afflicted face the threat of an early and sudden death, in addition to associated pain.[86] When people have an SCD crisis, they experience intense pain and are hospitalized for pain management and treatment, which is estimated to occur at least once annually in most patients.[87] Although SCD crises may be relatively short-lived and require acute hospitalization, there is a certain level of chronic pain that is ongoing, requiring individuals with SCD to cope with pain on a daily basis.[86] Studies do suggest that on average, youth with SCD show adequate psychosocial adjustment and do not differ from controls on measures of anxiety and depression.[88,89] Nevertheless, daily stress and negative moods do occur and have been linked to SCD adolescents' experience of increased pain, health care use, and decreased academic and social engagement, whereas positive daily mood has been related to decreased pain, health care use, and increased activity participation.[90] Pain coping strategies have also been consistently implicated in the experience of pain and related psychosocial adjustment among adults and youth with SCD.[32,91,92] Individuals with a tendency toward negative thinking (eg, catastrophizing, fear, and anger self-statements) and overreliance on medical recommendations (eg, increased fluid intake and resting) have more severe pain, experience increased levels of distress, health care use, and are less active.[32,91] Parental coping also seems related to child coping activity and perceived child adjustment.[32,33]

Because coping strategies among youth show less temporal stability, it would seem that there is opportunity to intervene during childhood and adolescence. Because coping strategies are more malleable during these stages of development, intervening to facilitate the acquisition of adaptive coping skills during this time frame seems highly warranted.[93] Chen and colleagues[94] conducted a review of the empirical literature for pain and adherence outcomes in SCD and concluded that CBT is probably efficacious in the treatment of sickle cell pain across the age spectrum. CBT is intended to help SCD patients learn how to effectively cope with the life-long presence of pain, remaining functional and active to the extent possible in their everyday lives, in addition to facilitating the development of other coping skills to help these individuals effectively manage their emotions and relationships. Following a biopsychosocial model of pain, CBT helps address the multidimensional self, not just at the biologic or medical level.[95] Interventions typically include relaxation, biofeedback, distraction, hypnosis, cognitive coping strategies, in addition to other conventional CBT techniques. Daily practice of relaxation and calming techniques alone (with minimal therapist contact) seems to yield increased functionality in daily activities and decreased health care use.[96] RCTs have also shown positive effects of CBT for the treatment of psychological distress and increased use of positive coping strategies among adults with SCD.[86,97] These positive effects seem to persist 6 months after intervention (during the same duration of maintained treatment effects) compared with attentional control and treatment-as-usual groups.[87] Massage therapy delivered by parents nightly to their children with SCD has recently been associated with lower levels of depression, anxiety, and pain compared with attentional control participants (see **Table 1**). However, this treatment was also associated with increased endorsement of parental depression and anxiety.[98]

Summary

Among the SCD population, pain seems to be the primary issue with which children and their families must learn to cope. The pain-tension-anxiety cycle is a well-accepted phenomenon that needs to be consistently addressed among the pediatric population to increase long-term treatment outcomes and use of life-long coping skills. Through CBT, children can be taught relaxation and calming skills, distraction and attentional control techniques in an effort to reduce the experience of pain. Setting realistic goals regarding pain relief and creating a plan for quick pain relief are crucial to the well-being of the child. CBT can be quite empowering for the child and family, enabling a sense of control of the situation without always needing to seek medical attention or rely on narcotic medications. Given that SCD occurs primarily in ethnic minorities, the positive effects of CBT seem to be applicable across different ethnic and cultural groups, and this also serves as a reminder to be culturally sensitive when adapting skills and approaches. Continued RCTs with positive treatment implications are needed before CBT is identified as a well-established treatment of SCD. There is more work that needs to be done to confirm the functional benefits that can be gained through CBT pain management; however, the current literature is promising.

SUMMARY AND FUTURE DIRECTIONS

The reviewed literature suggests that CBT interventions can improve treatment adherence, psychosocial adjustment, pain, and QoL of pediatric patients with chronic physical illnesses. Nevertheless, much work remains before CBT can be established as an empirically supported treatment modality for specific chronic medical conditions and related comorbidities among pediatric patients. The strongest support for CBT's effectiveness is found in the literature examining the treatment of pain management in SCD.[94] Evidence is emerging in support of the positive effects of CBT for improving medical adherence, physiologic indicators of illness, emotional adjustment, and communication skills in pediatric patients with IBD and diabetes, with limited evidence from a small number of RCTs.[6,42,49,50,65] Of the model disorders specifically examined in this review, the effectiveness of CBT for the treatment of distress, pain, and QoL in pediatric patients with cancer is particularly understudied. This is quite paradoxic given the host of major psychosocial concerns that arise throughout the course of cancer diagnosis and subsequent treatment.

Overall, CBT seems promising for the treatment of behavioral health and medical coping issues; however, continued research is needed to better understand what interventions facilitate the most improved outcomes within specific chronic physical illness subgroups. Large RCTs with adequate control groups are necessary to establish the effectiveness of CBT beyond that of other treatment modalities and supportive services affecting not just psychological outcomes but also physical illness outcomes. The pediatric population can be a difficult group to work with given the developing and complex nature of adolescence; nonetheless, an integrated psychosocial approach to medical treatment and care may be the link that is necessary to improve treatment outcomes and prognosis. It will be necessary for these future studies to examine specific treatment targets that consider developmental age, puberty, psychological adjustment, coping strategies, pertinent QoL measures, and medical adherence outcome data. In addition, the measurement of biologic markers, genetic abnormalities, and physiologic and neuroimaging outcomes will be critical in determining mechanistic mediators of treatment effect in these medical and psychiatrically comorbid populations. Familial components to treatment interventions seem to be an emerging standard of care and might equally serve as a preventative measure for future psychosocial adjustment and medical adherence issues. The course of physical illness is often unpredictable and the acquisition of positive coping skills by parents and siblings might help decrease personal burden, as well as the economic and service use burden accrued by medical service providers. Studying the effect of integrating behavioral interventions into comprehensive medical care, individualizing treatment to better target specific symptom clusters, and focusing on the effect of treatment on medical use and costs will also be important in showing the benefit that CBT may have in a medically complicated pediatric population.

REFERENCES

1. Miller AH, Ancoli-Israel S, Bower JE, et al. Neuroendocrine-immune mechanisms of behavioral comorbidities in patients with cancer. J Clin Oncol 2008;26:971–82.
2. Goodhand JR, Wahed M, Rampton DS. Management of stress in inflammatory bowel disease: a therapeutic option? Expert Rev Gastroenterol Hepatol 2009;3:661–79.
3. Holahan CJ, Pahl SA, Cronkite RC, et al. Depression and vulnerability to incident physical illness across 10 years. J Affect Disord 2010;123:222–9.
4. Beck AT, Rush AJ, Shaw BF, et al. An overview. In: Mahoney JA, editor. Cognitive therapy of depression. New York: Guilford Press; 1979. p. 1–33.
5. Butler AC, Chapman JE, Forman EM, et al. The empirical status of cognitive-behavioral therapy: a review of meta-analyses. Clin Psychol Rev 2006;26:17–31.
6. Szigethy E, Kenney E, Carpenter J, et al. Cognitive-behavioral therapy for adolescents with inflammatory bowel disease and subsyndromal depression. J Am Acad Child Adolesc Psychiatry 2007;46:1290–8.
7. van Straten A, Geraedts A, Verdonck-de Leeuw I, et al. Psychological treatment of depressive symptoms in patients with medical disorders: a meta-analysis. J Psychosom Res 2010;69:23–32.
8. Beck JS. Cognitive conceptualization. In: Cognitive therapy: basics and beyond. New York: Guilford Press; 1995. p. 13–24.
9. Beck AT. The current state of cognitive therapy: a 40-year retrospective. Arch Gen Psychiatry 2005;62:953–9.

10. Carter BD, Kronenberger WG, Baker J, et al. Inpatient pediatric consultation-liaison: a case-controlled study. J Pediatr Psychol 2003;28:423–32.
11. Szigethy E, Whitton SW, Levy-Warren A, et al. Cognitive-behavioral therapy for depression in adolescents with inflammatory bowel disease: a pilot study. J Am Acad Child Adolesc Psychiatry 2004;43:1469–77.
12. Abraham A, Silber TJ, Lyon M. Psychosocial aspects of chronic illness in adolescence. Indian J Pediatr 1999;66:447–53.
13. Friedman IM, Litt IF. Promoting adolescents' compliance with therapeutic regimens. Pediatr Clin North Am 1986;33:955–73.
14. Abbott J, Dodd M, Gee L, et al. Ways of coping with cystic fibrosis: implications for treatment adherence. Disabil Rehabil 2001;23:315–24.
15. Wood BL. Beyond the "psychosomatic family": a biobehavioral family model of pediatric illness. Fam Process 1993;32:261–78.
16. Stewart JL. Children living with chronic illness: an examination of their stressors, coping responses, and health outcomes. Annu Rev Nurs Res 2003;21:203–43.
17. Romine CB, Reynolds CR. A model of the development of frontal lobe functioning: findings from a meta-analysis. Appl Neuropsychol 2005;12:190–201.
18. Lavigne JV, Faier-Routman J. Psychological adjustment to pediatric physical disorders: a meta-analytic review. J Pediatr Psychol 1992;17:133–57.
19. Rubin DT, Dubinsky MC, Panaccione R, et al. The impact of ulcerative colitis on patients' lives compared to other chronic diseases: a patient survey. Dig Dis Sci 2010;55:1044–52.
20. Pollack VP, Ravenscroft AD. Inflammatory bowel disease. In: Jackson PL, Vessey JA, editors. Primary care of the child with a chronic condition. St Louis (MO): Mosby; 2000. p. 583–605.
21. Szigethy EM, Low C. Cytokines. In: Ingram RE, editor. International encyclopedia of depression. New York: Springer; 2009. p. 200–4.
22. Noll RB, Reiter-Purtill J, Moore BD, et al. Social, emotional, and behavioral functioning of children with NF1. Am J Med Genet A 2007;143:2261–74.
23. Vannatta K, Gerhardt CA, Wells RJ, et al. Intensity of CNS treatment for pediatric cancer: prediction of social outcomes in survivors. Pediatr Blood Cancer 2007; 49:716–22.
24. McLafferty LP, Craig A, Courtright R, et al. Qualitative narrative analysis of physical illness perceptions in depressed youth with inflammatory bowel disease [abstract 133]. In: Abstracts of the North American Society for Pediatric Gastroenterology, Hepatology, and Nutrition Annual Meeting. National Harbor, November 13, 2009, p. E59.
25. Grinyer A. Contrasting parental perspectives with those of teenagers and young adults with cancer: comparing the findings from two qualitative studies. Eur J Oncol Nurs 2009;13:200–6.
26. Hörnsten A, Sandström H, Lundman B. Personal understandings of illness among people with type 2 diabetes. J Adv Nurs 2004;47:174–82.
27. Werner-Lin A, Gardner DS. Family illness narratives of inherited cancer risk: continuity and transformation. Fam Syst Health 2009;27:201–12.
28. Kübler-Ross E, Wessler S, Avioli LV. On death and dying. JAMA 1972;221:174–9.
29. Kupst MJ. Assessment of psychoeducational and emotional functioning. In: Brown RT, editor. Cognitive aspects of chronic illness in children. New York: Guilford Press; 1997. p. 25–46.
30. Barakat LP, Kazak AE. Family issues. In: Brown RT, editor. Cognitive aspects of chronic illness in children. New York: Guilford Press; 1997. p. 333–54.

31. Daniels D, Moos RH, Billings AG, et al. Psychosocial risk and resistance factors among children with chronic illness, healthy siblings, and healthy controls. J Abnorm Child Psychol 1987;15:295–308.

32. Gil KM, Williams DA, Thompson RJ, et al. Sickle cell disease in children and adolescents: the relation of child and parent pain coping strategies to adjustment. J Pediatr Psychol 1991;16:643–63.

33. Thompson RJ, Gil KM, Burbach DJ, et al. Role of child and maternal processes in the psychological adjustment of children with sickle cell disease. J Consult Clin Psychol 1993;61:468–74.

34. Drotar D. Relating parent and family functioning to the psychological adjustment of children with chronic health conditions: what have we learned? What do we need to know? J Pediatr Psychol 1997;22:149–65.

35. Jobe-Shields L, Alderfer MA, Barrera M, et al. Parental depression and family environment predict distress in children before stem cell transplantation. J Dev Behav Pediatr 2009;30:140–6.

36. Stancin T, Wade SL, Walz NC, et al. Family adaptation 18 months after traumatic brain injury in early childhood. J Dev Behav Pediatr 2010;31:317–25.

37. Walco GA, Ilowite NT. Cognitive-behavioral intervention for juvenile primary fibromyalgia syndrome. J Rheumatol 1992;19:1617–9.

38. McQuaid EL, Nassau JH. Empirically supported treatments of disease-related symptoms in pediatric psychology: asthma, diabetes, and cancer. J Pediatr Psychol 1999;24:305–28.

39. Wysocki T. Behavioral assessment and intervention in pediatric diabetes. Behav Modif 2006;30:72–92.

40. Ellis DA, Templin T, Naar-King S, et al. Multisystemic therapy for adolescents with poorly controlled type 1 diabetes: stability of treatment effects in a randomized controlled trial. J Consult Clin Psychol 2007;75:168–74.

41. White K, Kolman ML, Wexler P, et al. Unstable diabetes and unstable families: a psychosocial evaluation of diabetic children with recurrent ketoacidosis. Pediatrics 1984;73:749–55.

42. Wysocki T, Harris MA, Buckloh LM, et al. Effects of behavioral family systems therapy for diabetes on adolescents' family relationships, treatment adherence, and metabolic control. J Pediatr Psychol 2006;31:928–38.

43. Murphy HR, Rayman G, Skinner TC. Psycho-educational interventions for children and young people with type 1 diabetes. Diabet Med 2006;23:935–43.

44. Hood KK, Rohan JM, Peterson CM, et al. Interventions with adherence-promoting components in pediatric type 1 diabetes: meta-analysis of their impact on glycemic control. Diabetes Care 2010;33:1658–64.

45. Ellis DA, Frey MA, Naar-King S, et al. Use of multisystemic therapy to improve regimen adherence among adolescents with type 1 diabetes in chronic poor metabolic control. Diabetes Care 2005;28:1604–10.

46. Ellis DA, Frey MA, Naar-King S, et al. The effects of multisystemic therapy on diabetes stress among adolescents with chronically poorly controlled type 1 diabetes: findings from a randomized, controlled trial. Pediatrics 2005;116: 826–32.

47. Ellis DA, Naar-King S, Frey M, et al. Multisystemic treatment of poorly controlled type 1 diabetes: effects of medical resource utilization. J Pediatr Psychol 2005; 30:656–66.

48. Ellis DA, Naar-King S, Templin T, et al. Improving health outcomes among youth with poorly controlled type 1 diabetes: the role of treatment fidelity in a randomized clinical trial of multisystemic therapy. J Fam Psychol 2007;21:363–71.

49. Wysocki T, Harris MA, Buckloh LM, et al. Randomized trial of behavioral family systems therapy for diabetes. Diabetes Care 2007;30:555–60.
50. Wysocki T, Harris MA, Buckloh LM, et al. Randomized, controlled trial of behavioral family systems therapy for diabetes: maintenance and generalization of effects on parent-adolescent communication. Behav Ther 2008;39:33–46.
51. Grey M, Boland EA, Davidson M, et al. Coping skills training for youth with diabetes mellitus has long-lasting effects on metabolic control and quality of life. J Pediatr 2000;137:107–13.
52. Grey M, Whittemore R, Jaser S, et al. Effects of coping skills training in school-age children with type 1 diabetes. Res Nurs Health 2009;32:405–18.
53. Tang Y, Preuss F, Turek FW, et al. Sleep deprivation worsens inflammation and delays recovery in a mouse model of colitis. Sleep Med 2009;10:597–603.
54. Baldassano RN, Piccoli DA. Inflammatory bowel disease in pediatric and adolescent patients. Gastroenterol Clin North Am 1999;28:445–58.
55. Szigethy E, Levy-Warren A, Whitton S, et al. Depressive symptoms and inflammatory bowel disease in children and adolescents: a cross-sectional study. J Pediatr Gastroenterol Nutr 2004;39:395–403.
56. Burke P, Meyer V, Kocoshis S, et al. Depression and anxiety in pediatric inflammatory bowel disease and cystic fibrosis. J Am Acad Child Adolesc Psychiatry 1989;28:948–51.
57. Minderhoud IM, Oldenburg B, Wismeijer JA, et al. IBS-like symptoms in patients with inflammatory bowel disease in remission; relationships with quality of life and coping behavior. Dig Dis Sci 2004;49:469–74.
58. Farrokhyar F, Marshall JK, Easterbrook B, et al. Functional gastrointestinal disorders and mood disorders in patients with inactive inflammatory bowel disease: prevalence and impact on health. Inflamm Bowel Dis 2006;12:38–46.
59. Weisz JR, Thurber CA, Sweeney L, et al. Brief treatment of mild-to-moderate child depression using Primary and Secondary Control Enhancement Training. J Consult Clin Psychol 1997;65:703–7.
60. Barlow C, Cooke D, Mulligan K, et al. A critical review of self-management and education interventions in inflammatory bowel disease. Gastroenterol Nurs 2010;33:11–8.
61. Bernstein KI, Promislow S, Carr R, et al. Information needs and preferences of recently diagnosed patients with inflammatory bowel disease. Inflamm Bowel Dis 2011;17(2):590–8.
62. Pennebaker JW, Seagal JD. Forming a story: the health benefits of narrative. J Clin Psychol 1999;55:1243–54.
63. Mawdsley JE, Jenkins DG, Macey MG, et al. The effect of hypnosis on systemic and rectal mucosal measures of inflammation in ulcerative colitis. Am J Gastroenterol 2008;103:1460–9.
64. Miller V, Whorwell PJ. Treatment of inflammatory bowel disease: a role for hypnotherapy? Int J Clin Exp Hypn 2008;56:306–17.
65. Szigethy E, Hardy D, Kenney E, et al. Longitudinal effects of cognitive behavioral therapy for depressed adolescents with inflammatory bowel disease [abstract P-0086]. In: Abstracts from the CCFA National Research and Clinical Conference, 5th Annual Advances in the Inflammatory Bowel Diseases. Miami (FL), 2006. p. 673–4.
66. McLafferty L, Craig A, Levine A, et al. Thematic analysis of physical illness perceptions in depressed youth with inflammatory bowel disease. Paper presented at: 57th Annual Meeting of the American Academy of Child & Adolescent Psychiatry. New York, October 28, 2010.

67. Szigethy EM, Jones NP, Silk J, et al. Brain Processing of illness perception in depressed adolescents with inflammatory bowel disease. Paper presented at: 6th Annual NIH Director's Pioneer Award Symposium. Bethesda (MD), October 1, 2010.
68. Sellick SM, Crooks DL. Depression and cancer: an appraisal of the literature for prevalence, detection, and practice guideline development for psychological interventions. Psychooncology 1999;8:315–33.
69. Pirl WF. Evidence report on the occurrence, assessment, and treatment of depression in cancer patients. J Natl Cancer Inst Monogr 2004;32:32–9.
70. Szigethy E, Noll RB. Individual psychotherapy. In: Shaw RJ, DeMaso DR, editors. Textbook of pediatric psychosomatic medicine. Arlington (TX): American Psychiatric Publishing; 2010. p. 423–38.
71. Gerber NU, Zehnder D, Zuzak TJ, et al. Outcome in children with brain tumours diagnosed in the first year of life: long-term complications and quality of life. Arch Dis Child 2008;93:582–9.
72. Zeltzer LK, Recklitis C, Buchbinder D, et al. Psychological status in childhood cancer survivors: a report from the Childhood Cancer Survivor Study. J Clin Oncol 2009;27:2396–404.
73. Osborn RL, Demoncada AC, Feuerstein M. Psychosocial interventions for depression, anxiety, and quality of life in cancer survivors: meta-analyses. Int J Psychiatry Med 2006;36:13–34.
74. Given C, Given B, Rahbar M, et al. Effect of a cognitive behavioral intervention on reducing symptom severity during chemotherapy. J Clin Oncol 2004;22: 507–16.
75. Conn VS, Hafdahl AR, Porock DC, et al. A meta-analysis of exercise interventions among people treated for cancer. Support Care Cancer 2006;14:699–712.
76. Jacobsen PB, Donovan KA, Vadaparampil ST, et al. Systemic review and meta-analysis of psychological and activity-based interventions for cancer-related fatigue. Health Psychol 2007;26:660–7.
77. Liossi C, Hatira P. Clinical hypnosis versus cognitive behavioral training for pain management with pediatric cancer patients undergoing bone marrow aspirations. Int J Clin Exp Hypn 1999;47:104–16.
78. Poggi G, Liscio M, Pastore V, et al. Psychological intervention in young brain tumor survivors: the efficacy of the cognitive behavioural approach. Disabil Rehabil 2009;31:1066–73.
79. Manne SL, Andrykowski MA. Are psychological interventions effective and accepted by cancer patients? II. Using empirically supported therapy guidelines to decide. Ann Behav Med 2006;32:98–103.
80. Myers K, Cain S. Practice parameters for telepsychiatry with children and adolescents. J Am Acad Child Adolesc Psychiatry 2008;47:1468–83.
81. Kroenke K, Theobald D, Norton K, et al. The Indiana Cancer Pain and Depression (INCPAD) trial design of a telecare management intervention for cancer-related symptoms and baseline characteristics of study participants. Gen Hosp Psychiatry 2009;31:240–53.
82. Kroenke K, Theobald D, Wu J, et al. Effect of telecare management on pain and depression in patients with cancer: a randomized trial. JAMA 2010;304: 163–71.
83. Cross RK, Arora M, Finkelstein J. Acceptance of telemanagment is high in patients with inflammatory bowel disease. J Clin Gastroenterol 2006;40:200–8.
84. Cha E, Castro HK, Provance P, et al. Acceptance of home telemanagement is high in patients with multiple sclerosis. AMIA Annu Symp Proc 2007;893.

85. Cross RK, Cheevers N, Finkelstein J. Home telemanagement for patients with ulcerative colitis (UC HAT). Dig Dis Sci 2009;54:2463–72.
86. Thomas VN, Wilson-Barnett J, Goodhart F. The role of cognitive-behavioural therapy in the management of pain in patients with sickle cell disease. J Adv Nurs 1998;27:1002–9.
87. Thomas VJ, Gruen R, Shu S. Cognitive-behavioural therapy for the management of sickle cell disease pain: identification and assessment of costs. Ethn Health 2001;6:59–67.
88. Midence K, McManus C, Fuggle P, et al. Psychological adjustment and family functioning in a group of British children with sickle cell disease: preliminary empirical findings and a meta-analysis. Br J Clin Psychol 1996;35:439–50.
89. Noll RB, Vannatta K, Koontz K, et al. Peer relationships and emotional well-being of youngsters with sickle cell disease. Child Dev 1996;67:423–36.
90. Gil KM, Carson JW, Porter LS, et al. Daily stress and mood and their association with pain, health-care use, and school activity in adolescents with sickle cell disease. J Pediatr Psychol 2003;28:363–73.
91. Gil KM, Abrams MR, Phillips G, et al. Sickle cell disease pain: relation of coping strategies to adjustment. J Consult Clin Psychol 1989;57:725–31.
92. Barakat LP, Schwartz LA, Simon K, et al. Negative thinking as a coping strategy mediator of pain and internalizing symptoms in adolescents with sickle cell disease. J Behav Med 2007;30:199–208.
93. Gil KM, Wilson JJ, Edens JL. The stability of pain coping strategies in young children, adolescents, and adults with sickle cell disease over an 18-month period. Clin J Pain 1997;13:110–5.
94. Chen E, Cole SW, Kato PM. A review of empirically supported psychosocial interventions for pain and adherence outcomes in sickle cell disease. J Pediatr Psychol 2004;29:197–209.
95. Thomas VJ. Cognitive behavioural therapy in pain management for sickle cell disease. Int J Palliat Nurs 2000;6:434–42.
96. Gil KM, Anthony KK, Carson JW, et al. Daily coping practice predicts treatment effects in children with sickle cell disease. J Pediatr Psychol 2001;26:163–73.
97. Thomas VJ, Dixon AL, Milligan P. Cognitive-behaviour therapy for the management of sickle cell disease pain. Br J Health Psychol 1999;4:209–29.
98. Lemanek KL, Ranalli M, Lukens C. A randomized controlled trial of massage therapy in children with sickle cell disease. J Pediatr Psychol 2009;34:1091–6.

Applying Cognitive-Behavioral Therapy for Anxiety to the Younger Child

Dina R. Hirshfeld-Becker, PhD[a,b,c,*], Jamie A. Micco, PhD[a,b,c],
Heather Mazursky, MA[b], Lindsey Bruett, BA[b], Aude Henin, PhD[a,b,c]

KEYWORDS

• Cognitive-behavioral therapy • Anxiety • Preschool-age
• Young children

THE NEED TO TREAT ANXIETY IN YOUNGER CHILDREN

Anxiety disorders in older children and adolescents have long been recognized as common,[1] impairing,[2,3] persistent, and predictive of subsequent anxiety and mood disorders.[4] By contrast, anxiety symptoms in preschoolers and younger children have until recently been regarded as transient difficulties falling within developmentally normative parameters. Mounting evidence suggests, however, that anxiety disorders in younger children are as common, impairing, and persistent as those in older children. In a community sample of 2- to 5-year-olds, the prevalence of anxiety disorders was 9.5%, and affected children showed significantly greater impairment.[5] Factor analytical studies[6,7] have shown that symptoms in preschoolers closely parallel those in older children, reflecting fears, obsessive-compulsive symptoms, and social, separation, and general anxiety. With regard to persistence, anxiety symptoms in an epidemiologic sample of first-graders predicted anxiety symptoms and academic impairment in the fifth grade.[8] In untreated control groups followed over time, 82% of children aged 4 to 7 years with anxiety disorders still had anxiety disorders 6 months later,[9] and 63.5% of behaviorally inhibited children aged 3 to 5 years (approximately

Financial disclosures: See last page of article.
[a] Child Cognitive-Behavioral Therapy Program, Department of Psychiatry, Massachusetts General Hospital (MGH), 55 Fruit Street, Boston, MA 02114, USA
[b] Clinical and Research Program in Pediatric Psychopharmacology, MGH, 185 Alewife Brook Parkway, Suite 2000, Cambridge, MA 02138, USA
[c] Harvard Medical School, Boston, MA, USA
* Corresponding author. Clinical and Research Program in Pediatric Psychopharmacology, MGH, 185 Alewife Brook Parkway, Suite 2000, Cambridge, MA 02138.
E-mail address: dhirshfeld@partners.org

Child Adolesc Psychiatric Clin N Am 20 (2011) 349–368
doi:10.1016/j.chc.2011.01.008
1056-4993/11/$ – see front matter © 2011 Elsevier Inc. All rights reserved.

childpsych.theclinics.com

91.5% of whom had anxiety disorders at baseline) still had anxiety disorders at 12-month follow-up.[10] Even separation anxiety disorder, which has lower persistence rates than other disorders,[9–12] is associated with subsequent onset of new anxiety and mood disorders.[13] It is clear that anxiety disorders in younger children are important targets for intervention.

COGNITIVE-BEHAVIORAL THERAPY FOR CHILDHOOD ANXIETY DISORDERS

The number of cognitive-behavioral interventions for anxiety disorders in older children and adolescents has grown dramatically over the past two decades,[14–17] and cognitive-behavioral therapy (CBT) has demonstrated efficacy for childhood anxiety disorders, including obsessive-compulsive disorder (OCD)[17,18] and posttraumatic stress disorder (PTSD),[19,20] whether offered in individual or group format.[16] CBT shows benefit whether offered to the child only or family,[21] or alone or in combination with sertraline.[22] However, until very recently the majority of these CBT protocols have been aimed at older school-age children or adolescents, targeting mainly children age 8 years or older. Although some studies extended their inclusion range down to age 5 or 6,[23–27] they tended to include relatively low numbers of the youngest children, with mean ages significantly higher (ranging from 7.8 to 11.03 years), and did not report results separately for the youngest children.

In the past 5 years, a burgeoning number of researchers have begun testing CBT programs for younger children with anxiety. In the sections that follow, the authors discuss the developmental modifications for conducting CBT with younger children and review the studies conducted to date. The article concludes with a discussion of future directions needed in this area of research.

ADAPTING CBT FOR YOUNGER CHILDREN

CBT protocols for anxiety disorders in older children tend to combine coping skills with hierarchical exposure to feared situations (with response prevention in the case of OCD). Coping skills include relaxation methods, strategies for addressing anxious cognitions, and tools for quantifying anxiety and observing its decrease. The coping skills serve to facilitate participation in exposure, which is considered the most essential element of treatment. Other treatment components may include psychoeducation about anxiety, modeling of exposure, and contingent reinforcement for exposure or skills practice. For OCD, a common additional approach is to differentiate the child from the anxiety symptoms, that is, to externalize the OCD as separate from the child.[28]

HOW THESE ELEMENTS CAN BE ADAPTED FOR YOUNGER CHILDREN
Training in Coping Skills

Early studies addressing specific fears and phobia analogs in young children are important "proofs-of-concept" demonstrating how coping techniques, such as relaxation and self-instruction, may fruitfully be applied with young children. In one study,[29] 42 preschoolers aged 3 to 5 years with no previous dental treatment were randomly assigned to 1 of 3 treatment conditions administered half an hour before having a cavity filled. Children in the coping skills condition were taught general relaxation, which involved deep breathing with the cue words "calm" and "nice" and imagery about a pleasant scene or favorite place, and were instructed to repeat the phrase "I will be all right in just a little while. Everything is going to be all right." Children in a sensory information condition were given a description of the basic procedures, sensations, sights, and sounds they would experience (reframed with terms like "sleepy water," or "a pinch"). Controls were read a chapter from *Winnie the Pooh*. Children in both the coping skills and information conditions were blindly rated by dentists as less disruptive, more cooperative, and less anxious than controls, and showed less distress to the injection and lower pulses after the procedure. Children who had been taught relaxation also had lower pulses going into the procedure. This study suggests that coping skills, and in particular relaxation, may be used effectively by preschoolers. Similarly, a controlled study of 45 nonreferred kindergarteners with mild to moderate fear of darkness showed that teaching children to rehearse positive self-descriptions about coping with darkness (eg, " I am a brave boy. I am able to take care of myself in the dark") lengthened the time the children tolerated darkness exposure.[30] This study demonstrates that self-instruction can be a useful anxiety management strategy for young children.

Modeling

Three early studies suggested that modeling can improve preschoolers' willingness to approach a feared animal.[31–33] Preschoolers with dog fears who watched peers approach dogs, either live or on film, were more likely to approach the dog than controls who viewed the dog without modeling.[31–33]

Exposure

Exposure-based approaches found efficacious in treating animal or water fears in 3- to 6-year-olds include systematic desensitization[34] and contingency management or reinforced practice.[35–37] In fact, reinforced practice may be considered a "well-established" treatment for fears in this age range,[14] because it has been shown to be superior to a nontreatment condition[35] and to 2 other active treatments: verbal coping skills[37] and live modeling.[36]

Exposure exercises with young children are modified in several ways. First, it is often necessary to move more slowly and incrementally than with older children, beginning with very brief exposures on the order of seconds, and giving parents concrete instructions as to how to implement exposures at home.[38] Second, these exercises often incorporate fun and games, in addition to contingent reinforcement. For example, Kuroda[34] had frog-fearing 3- to 5-year-olds participate in songs, stories, and games during exposure to frogs. In an open trial with 15 4- to 8-year-old children with phobias of the dark and loud noises, Mendez and Garcia[39] incorporated treasure-hunting games and dramatic play in exposure exercises. In an open trial with 9 anxious 4- to 7-year-olds, Hirshfeld-Becker and colleagues[40] used treasure-hunting games to practice separating from parents, "survey" games (asking questions, noting eye color) to practice social interaction, and humorous use of role-play of mistakes or rule-breaking behaviors for children with perfectionistic worries.

Addressing Anxious Cognitions

Some investigators have argued that because preschoolers and young children tend to think prelogically and to be influenced more by perception than logic, they ought not to be able to engage in the cognitive aspects of cognitive therapy.[41] However, studies suggest that although young children cannot engage as readily as adolescents or adults in meta-cognition (eg, recognizing and cognitively challenging automatic thoughts), they can engage in some basic elements of cognitive therapy. For example, a study of 72 5- to 7-year-olds with average IQ from a community sample found that most children in this age range could generate alternative explanations for why an ambiguous social event occurred, name and recognize emotions, and logically link thoughts to feelings using cartoon drawings with thought bubbles.[42] With developmental adaptations such as use of concrete picture and stories, children may be able to understand basic cognitive therapy concepts.[41] For example, the authors have found clinically[40] that when 4- to 7-year-olds are presented with hypothetical future situations by means of role-play or puppet-play, they can choose between possible thoughts that might make them feel more brave or less brave.

Other clinicians have implemented these techniques more formally. For example, in their downward adaptation of the FRIENDS program, a CBT protocol for treating and preventing anxiety disorders in children, Pahl and Barrett[43] trained 4- to 6-year-olds to distinguish "red thoughts" (negative cognitions) and "green thoughts" (positive cognitions) and to generate "green thoughts," reinforced with the use of colored puppets. Similarly, in cognitive-behavioral play therapy developed for 2.5- to 6-year-olds, therapists modeled coping strategies through play and used puppets to model positive coping statements.[44] The kinds of narrative paradigms used to treat OCD in older children (eg, March's approach of teaching the child to "run OCD off my land") can be adapted fruitfully for use with younger children as well.[45] Moreover, through stories, cartoons, and basic explanations, young children can internalize ideas such as reframing anxiety from a cue to escape to a cue to remain and practice coping, and learn to respond to feared situations with coping self-statements such as "It's scary at first, but if you stay, you'll have fun."[40]

Inclusion of Parents as Active Participants

Inclusion of parents is crucial for several reasons.[46] Beyond logistical reasons (ie, parents' involvement in children's daily activities, management of contingencies, and oversight of homework assignments), parents may be unskilled at helping young children in managing anxiety, and may inadvertently reinforce anxious behaviors, for example by exhibiting attitudes of overprotection, restricting autonomy, or facilitating avoidance.[47] In addition, parents of anxious children are very likely to be anxious themselves.[48] A recent study has suggested that training parents in managing their own anxious thoughts and behaviors and reinforcing their child's adaptive coping maintains long-term remission of anxiety in children treated with CBT.[49] Including parents as coaches or facilitators in CBT for young children ensures that they gain experience in helping their child overcome fears, strategies that they may use again if symptoms recur.

Several cognitive-behavioral skills are important to include in parent training approaches.[46] It is helpful to provide parents with an understanding of the basic principles of anxiety management and good coping, both for themselves and their child, to enable them to distinguish helpful versus unhelpful approaches to their child's anxiety (including reinforcing brave behaviors and extinguishing fearful ones), and to teach them to plan and implement graded exposure exercises with reinforcement. It is also useful to help parents modify their view of the child from one who is vulnerable and in need of protection to one who can be brave and learn to cope well. Finally, parents should gain skills that they can implement if symptoms recur, and should understand when further professional help may be necessary.

Other Useful Adaptations

Because young children are unable to give subjective units of distress (SUDs) ratings or to understand the "fear thermometers" used with older children, it can be useful to introduce simpler pictorial means of rating anxiety.[9,50] Because very young children cannot necessarily read, the mnemonics developed to cue older children to remember coping steps (eg, F-E-A-R[51]; S-T-O-P[24]) may need to be modified to include picture cues or rhymes.[40] Similarly, although older children can wait to accumulate points toward rewards, very young children may need to be reinforced after each exposure practice.

NEW DEVELOPMENTALLY APPROPRIATE CBT PROTOCOLS FOR YOUNG CHILDREN

If the approaches discussed can address specific fears and phobias in young children, they should also be applicable to more severe anxiety disorders. **Table 1** summarizes chronologically the published research reports to date. In addition to the open trials reported here, the authors know of at least 6 others that are under development. Seven groups to date have published randomized clinical trials (RCTs). The various approaches have included parent training in the implementation of CBT; CBT offered directly to the child in combination with parent training; and primary parenting skills training, modified to include anxiety-relevant strategies. The authors discuss these first with regard to anxiety disorders in general, and then discuss specific adaptations for OCD and PTSD.

Parent Education on Implementing CBT for Children with Anxiety

One approach to applying CBT to young children is to teach parents anxiety management skills to implement at home. In 2 RCTs, Rapee and colleagues[10,12,52] tested this approach as a preventive intervention for children with behavioral inhibition (BI), a temperamental tendency to be quiet, restrained, and reticent in novel or unfamiliar settings[53] that has been shown to confer risk for anxiety disorders, particularly social phobia.[54] In the first study,[10] 146 3- to 5-year-old preschoolers were screened for BI using both a parent temperament questionnaire and a laboratory observation. More than 90% of the children with BI met criteria for anxiety disorders at baseline on the parent report version of the Anxiety Disorders Interview Schedule for Children [ADIS-IV-C/P]. Families were randomized to parent education groups or yearly monitoring. The groups, offered to 6 parents each (mostly mothers), consisted of 6 90-minute sessions covering the nature of anxiety and its development; basic principles of parent management, with emphasis on reducing overprotection; principles and application of exposure hierarchies; application of cognitive restructuring to the parent's own worries, with encouragement to apply cognitive techniques to the child's thoughts as he matured; and the importance of high-risk transition periods. Children were followed up by clinicians who were blind to condition, using yearly parent-administered ADIS and BI assessments. Although BI was not affected, the intervention reduced the number of anxiety disorders at 1-year follow-up; however, a significant number of children were still affected (50% intervention vs 63.5% controls). At 2- and 3-year follow-up,[12] levels of BI still did not differ, but the children from the intervention condition had lower frequency and severity of anxiety disorders. By mean age 7 years, rates of anxiety disorders were 40% (intervention) versus 69% (controls). These data suggest that a relatively low-intensity parent-administered CBT intervention can modify the trajectory of anxiety symptoms among preschoolers at risk.

In the second study,[52] seventy one 3- to 4-year-olds were selected on the basis of high risk for anxiety, defined as both extreme BI (>2 SDs above the mean) and a parent with a DSM-IV (*Diagnostic and Statistical Manual of Mental Disorders* Fourth Edition, Text Revised) anxiety diagnosis, and randomized to the parent intervention or to a 6-month wait-list control condition. All children also met criteria for at least one if not multiple anxiety disorders, and all but one child had primary social phobia. The parent intervention was modified to include eight 90-minute sessions and a telephone follow-up session. Added content included exposure for the parents' own fears,

Table 1
Studies adapting CBT for anxiety for use with younger children

Study Citation	Anxiety Disorder	Ages	N	Approach Used, Number of Sessions	Results
Case Series or Small Open Trials					
Waldrop and de Arellano,[71] 2004	PTSD (physical abuse)	5 y	1	Individual CBT (22 sessions)	Decreased CBCL internalizing and PTSD arousal symptoms
Choate et al,[62] 2005	Separation anxiety disorder	5–8 y	3	PCIT (child- and parent-directed interaction modules), 10 wk	All 3 children showed declines in fear, avoidance, and separation anxiety behaviors
Pincus et al,[63,64] 2005	Separation anxiety disorder	4–8 y	10	PCIT (child- and parent-directed interaction modules), 10 wk	Slight decrease in severity of disorder, but no improvement to nonclinical levels
Scheeringa et al,[70] 2007	PTSD (motor vehicle accident, hurricane)	4 y	2	Cognitive-behavioral therapy, with parent, 12 wk	Decrease in number of PTSD symptoms for both children
Cartwright-Hatton et al,[61] 2005	Children referred for anxiety (above CBCL internalizing cutoff)	4–9 y	11	Parenting skills training plus cognitive restructuring, fostering a confident cognitive style in the child, handling worry, and conducting hierarchical exposure, 10 wk	CBCL internalizing scales decreased
Hirshfeld-Becker et al,[40] 2008	Anxiety disorders in children at high risk	4–7 y	9	Cognitive-behavioral therapy (7 parent-only sessions, plus 8–13 child-parent sessions), mean of 17 wk	8/9 children showed much or very much improvement; significant improvement in no. of anxiety diagnoses and coping
Larger Open or Nonrandomized Trials (or Preliminary Reports of Randomized Trials)					
Cartwright-Hatton et al,[50] 2005	Internalizing symptoms in children with externalizing behaviors	2–4 y	43	"Parent survival course": parent groups teaching parenting skills (praise, limit-setting, contingent reinforcement), 8 wk	CBCL internalizing scores normalized and remained so at 6-month follow-up

Pahl and Barrett,[43] 2007	Universal prevention protocol (no diagnoses necessary)	4–6 y	70	"Fun FRIENDS," a CBT child group offered in school, with parent information sessions and workbook, 10 sessions	Preschool Anxiety Scale ratings decreased for girls
Pincus et al,[64] 2008	Separation anxiety disorder	4–8 y	34	PCIT (child-directed, "bravery-directed"—ie, 3 sessions of parent teaching and child exposure and parent-directed interaction modules). 9–11 wk	Children receiving modified PCIT had mean severity scores which decreased markedly to nonclinical range
Monga et al,[56] 2009	Anxiety disorders (social, separation, GAD, selective mutism)	5–7 y	43	Concurrent parent and child group CBT, 12 wk	72% of children had at least one anxiety disorder resolve, and 44% had all resolve. Significant improvement on SCARED and GAS scores
Randomized Clinical Trials					
Cohen and Mannarino,[68] 1996	PTSD symptoms (sexual abuse)	2–7 y	67	Group CBT versus nondirective supportive therapy	CBT group had greater reductions in internalizing and externalizing symptoms and sexual behaviors
Deblinger et al,[69] 2001	PTSD symptoms (sexual abuse)	2–8 y	54	Separate parent and child group CBT versus supportive group therapy, 11 sessions	Mothers in CBT had greater decreases in intrusive thoughts and negative emotional reactions; children had improved body safety skills
Rapee et al,[10,12] 2005	Anxiety disorders in children with BI (prevention trial)	3–5 y	146	Six 90-min parent group sessions teaching CBT principles for child anxiety versus monitoring only (with outcome measured at 1, 2, and 3 y)	Significant reduction in anxiety disorders at 12, 24, and 36 mo, and anxiety severity at 24 and 36 mo
Santacruz et al,[38] 2006	Specific phobia of darkness	4–8 y	78	Five 45-min parent training sessions of 2 approaches to graduated exposure using play or no treatment	Children receiving both therapies showed improvement in symptoms compared with controls, with effects maintained at 12 mo

(continued on next page)

Table 1
(continued)

Study Citation	Anxiety Disorder	Ages	N	Approach Used, Number of Sessions	Results
Kennedy et al,[52] 2009	Anxiety disorders in high-risk children with BI plus parental anxiety	3–4 y	71	8 parent group sessions teaching CBT principles for child and parent anxiety versus 6-month wait-list	46.7% of treated versus 6.7% of controls had no anxiety disorders at 6-month follow-up
Freeman et al,[75] 2008	Obsessive-compulsive disorder	5–8 y	42	Family-based CBT (compared with family-based relaxation training), 12 sessions	Completers showed significantly lower C-YBOCS scores, with 69% versus 20% showing remission on the C-YBOCS
Waters et al,[57] 2009	Anxiety disorders (specific phobia, social phobia, GAD, or separation anxiety disorder)	4–8 y	80	Parent group CBT versus parent-group + child group CBT, 10 sessions, versus a wait-list control group	84%, 74%, and 18% of children respectively no longer met criteria for their primary diagnosis and 61%, 60%, and 9% lost all anxiety diagnoses. Gains maintained to 1 y
Hirshfeld-Becker et al,[9] 2010	Anxiety disorders in children at high risk (separation, social phobia, GAD, specific phobia)	4–7 y	64	Cognitive-behavioral therapy (7 parent-only sessions, plus 8–13 child-parent sessions) versus a wait-list control group	At 6 mo, 69% versus 33% of completers showed much or very much improvement; 59% versus 18% had all anxiety disorders resolve. Gains maintained at 1 y

Abbreviations: BI, behavioral inhibition; CBCL, Child Behavior Checklist; CBT, cognitive-behavioral therapy; C-YBOCS, Child Yale-Brown Obsessive-Compulsive Scale; GAD, generalized anxiety disorder; GAS, global assessment scale; PCIT, Parent-Child Interaction Therapy; PTSD, posttraumatic stress disorder; SCARED, Self-report for Childhood Anxiety-Related Disorders.

information on the development and enhancement of social skills, and summary of anxiety management skills and coping plans for children. This intervention significantly reduced BI as well as anxiety disorders (with anxiety-free rates of 46.7% in the intervention group vs 6.7% in controls), decreased anxiety severity, and reduced interference with family functioning. Parents' anxiety symptoms did not decrease. The differences between this study and the prior one may stem from the higher risk status of the children (reducing change in the untreated children), the more intensive intervention, or the shorter follow-up time. This study suggests that a parent-education CBT-based intervention can be helpful in treating anxiety in young children, although again, a substantial proportion of children persisted with anxiety disorders after treatment (more than 53%).

Another approach to parent-orchestrated CBT is to teach the parents to implement exposure. Santacruz and colleagues[38] compared 2 interventions in an RCT enrolling seventy eight 4- to 8-year-olds with specific phobia of darkness, recruited through a school system. The treatments, offered to parents in 5 weekly 45-minute sessions, taught parents to implement exposure games using modeling, role-playing, positive reinforcement, and feedback, with written instructions provided. The first treatment, "bibliotherapy and games," was based on a program developed by Mikulas and Coffman, which involved reading the child book chapters about a boy who learns from his uncle how to overcome darkness fears, and playing games reinforcing the strategies used in the chapters. Parents provided social and material reinforcement and taught the children to use happy thoughts to face darkness. The second treatment, an "emotive performance" game called "Olympiad of Braves" had the child role-play a brave or heroic character and beat successive darkness exposure records. The exposures were conducted while the child lay in bed, with the parent announcing each bravery trial, and awarding, in an Olympic medal ceremony, super-tokens for perfect performances or smaller tokens for performances that need parental coaching or support. If a child needed help, parents could coach the child in the use of bravery statements. Friends or siblings acted as models. Both groups showed significant reduction of bedtime fears and improvement on darkness behaviors compared with controls and continued improvement at 12-months, with gains greatest for the emotive performance condition. This study suggests that parents can implement playful exposure activities with children.

CBT Offered Directly to the Child

Direct intervention with young children has been tried in both group and individual formats. One approach under development is the "Fun FRIENDS" program,[43] an adaptation by Barrett of the Australian "FRIENDS" program,[55] which has been used both for treatment and universal prevention. "Fun FRIENDS," geared to children aged 4 to 6 years, includes ten 60- to 90-minute sessions, offered in a classroom setting, that teach children skills to cope with anxiety and other emotions. The program includes general socioemotional skills, addresses interpersonal challenges and family and peer support, and also teaches strategies helpful for anxiety reduction, including coping skills and graduated exposure to fears. Principles are reinforced via repetition through dramatic play, puppet play, games, storytelling, songs, and crafts activities. Whereas the content is taught directly to the children, parents are introduced to the skills during several information sessions and are provided with a workbook with skills-building exercises to try at home. Although no published data are available on this program's effects on anxiety disorders, preliminary data from an open universal prevention trial with 70 nonreferred preschoolers showed significant decreases in Preschool Anxiety Scale scores from pre- to post-intervention (mean of 22.09, SD 12.29 to mean of 18.67, SD 10.81; t = 3.45, P<.001), evident mainly in girls (25.61, 12.53 to 19.19, 12.01; t = 4.43, P<.0005).

Monga and colleagues[56] conducted an open trial of concurrent child and parent group CBT for children aged 5 to 7 years with anxiety disorders (including social phobia, separation anxiety disorder, generalized anxiety disorder [GAD], and selective mutism, with 63.5% having more than one). The program (called "Taming Sneaky Fears") consisted of 12 1-hour sessions, with 5 to 8 children per group. The child sessions used stories, puppets, crafts, games, and activities, with each session reviewing content of the previous one. Content included recognizing and labeling feeling states; relaxation strategies; and cognitive strategies, such as talking to adults, ignoring scary thoughts, and generating alternative "brave thoughts." Parent sessions included psychoeducation, parent-management and behavioral strategies, and relaxation exercises and desensitization strategies to help the child confront fears. The group format enabled parents to obtain support and problem-solve together. Parent ratings on the generalized anxiety, separation anxiety, social anxiety, and school refusal scales of the SCARED (Self-report for Childhood Anxiety-Related Disorders) were significantly reduced at posttreatment, as were ratings on the anxious/shy and psychosomatic subscales of the Conners' Parent Rating Scale-R: L. ADIS severity scores for the primary anxiety disorder decreased significantly to the nonclinical range, with 71.9% of children losing at least one anxiety disorder and 43.8% losing all anxiety disorders.

Hirshfeld-Becker and colleagues[40] combined parent education sessions and child CBT to treat DSM-IV anxiety disorders in 4- to 7-year-old children. The intervention (called "Being Brave"), offered individually to each family, consisted of 6 parent sessions, 8 or more child-parent sessions, and a final parent-only relapse prevention session. The parent-only sessions covered psychoeducation about anxiety and the factors maintaining it; observing the child's anxious responses and their antecedents and consequences; restructuring parents' anxious thoughts; identifying helpful and unhelpful responses to child anxiety; modeling adaptive coping; playing with the child in a nondirective way; learning to protect the child from danger rather than anxiety; using praise to reinforce adaptive coping; and planning and implementing graduated exposure. The child-parent sessions were loosely adapted from Kendall's "Coping Cat," and included teaching the child (a) a model for working on "being even more brave"; (b) basic coping skills; and (c) the use of a coping plan to face feared situations; as well as planning, rehearsing, and performing exposure exercises, often introduced as games, and conducted with immediate reinforcement. At the end of treatment, each child made a final book, poster/collage, or short video teaching other children how to "be brave," and treatment ended with a party celebrating the child's gains. In an open pilot study, 9 children aged 4 to 7 years selected on the basis of elevated risk for anxiety disorder (ie, having BI [n = 6], parental anxiety disorder history plus elevated Child Behavior Checklist [CBCL] anxiety symptoms [n = 8], and/or an anxiety disorder [n = 8]) were treated. After a mean of 17 sessions, 8 of 9 were rated as "much" or "very much improved" on a Clinical Global Impression—Improvement (CGI-I) scale, with significant reduction of anxiety diagnoses and improvement on parent-rated ability to cope with the most feared situations.

In a subsequent RCT,[9] 64 4- to 7-year-old children with DSM-IV anxiety disorders (including 67% with social phobia, 44% with separation anxiety disorder, 44% with GAD, 48% with specific phobia, and 36% with agoraphobia) were randomized either to the "Being Brave" intervention or to a 6-month wait-list control condition. Seventy-seven percent had more than one anxiety disorder, 63% had BI, and 73% had parental history of anxiety disorder. At posttreatment, 69% of completers of CBT versus 32%

of controls were rated by clinicians blind to treatment assignment as "much" or "very much" improved on the CGI-I scale (59% vs 30% in intent-to-treat [ITT] analysis), with 59% versus 18% of completers free of all anxiety disorders. Children in CBT were rated as significantly more improved than controls on social and separation anxiety disorder and specific phobia (using the CGI), as well as on a laboratory indicator of BI, and on their ability to cope with their most feared situations. Gains were maintained at 1-year follow-up.

One study to date has directly compared parent-only with parent plus child group CBT for anxiety disorders in 4- to 8-year-old children.[57] In this study, 80 children (mean age 6.8 years) were randomized to receive a 10-session parent group CBT (training parents to facilitate CBT with their child; n = 24/31 completers), parent group CBT plus child group CBT (25/38 completers, with 7–11 children per group), or a wait-list control condition (11/11 completers). The most common primary diagnosis was specific phobia (41% of participants), but more than 80% of children had more than one anxiety disorder, including GAD, separation anxiety disorder, and social phobia. The treatment (called the "Take ACTION" program) taught children 6 steps for managing anxiety, including psychoeducation about anxiety and bodily reactions, training in relaxation, identifying anxious self-talk and substituting coping statements or calm thoughts, graded exposure exercises, using problem-solving skills and identifying a support team, and social skills training to develop confident and assertive behaviors. Parent groups covered psychoeducation about child anxiety, parent strategies for managing child anxiety and improving parent-child relationships, introduction of the child "Take ACTION" steps and parent strategies for helping the children, promotion of positive parent coping, and training in communication and problem-solving skills. Both treatment conditions included booster sessions 8 weeks after the end of treatment to review progress and reinforce strategies.

Although the postintervention interviews were conducted by the primary therapist of both groups and therefore were not independent or blind, children in both treatments improved significantly compared with controls, with rates of recovery from the primary anxiety disorder among completers of the parent + child, parent-only, and wait-list conditions 74%, 84%, and 18%, respectively (ITT: 54.8%, 55.3%, and 18.2%). Rates of recovery from all anxiety disorders were 61%, 60%, and 9% (ITT: 54.8%, 44.7%, and 18%). Severity ratings in both CBT conditions declined significantly. At 6- and 12-month follow-up, progress continued for both groups. Although further research using blind outcome assessment is needed, this study suggests that it may be possible to successfully treat children in this age range using only parent groups, particularly if the groups are of relatively long duration and provide parents with week-by-week material to introduce to the children. Alternatively, as the investigators suggest, parents in the parent + child condition who knew the therapist was also working with their child may have taken less responsibility for working with the child than parents in the parent-only condition, who were solely responsible for introducing the material to their child. It is interesting also to note that this child CBT intervention, geared originally to older youth and using a workbook and a complicated acronym with difficult vocabulary, was able to be applied successfully with these younger children.

Parenting Skills Training Approaches

Another type of intervention offered to parents of young anxious children derives from the long tradition of general parenting skills training. Several well-studied parent training approaches have been developed and implemented successfully with parents of young children with disruptive behavior disorders, including The Incredible Years[58] and Parent-Child Interaction Therapy (PCIT).[59] Common elements in these programs include enhancement of the parent-child relationship through child-directed play, positive discipline (specific praise, positive attention, rewards), extinction of unwanted behaviors through inattention, effective limit-setting, and strategies for improving compliance.

These approaches, even when unmodified, have shown some efficacy for the treatment of anxiety symptoms as well. For example, Cartwright-Hatton and colleagues[60] openly implemented a parenting skills training group for 43 parents of 2- to 4-year-old children referred for moderate to severe externalizing behaviors, living in neighborhoods with high social and economic deprivation. The 8-week "parent survival course" was offered in weekly 90-minute sessions to groups of 6 to 8 parents, and was based on the program developed by Webster-Stratton and Reid.[58] Parents were taught to give positive attention through play, to use selective attention to increase good behavior and reduce inappropriate behavior, to use specific labeled praise and frequent small rewards, to give effective age-appropriate directives, and to use "time-out" for dangerous or destructive behaviors. At postintervention and 6-month follow-up, CBCL-rated internalizing symptoms decreased with an effect size (0.44) equivalent to that of externalizing symptoms (0.41). The percentage of children with clinically elevated internalizing symptoms decreased from 40% to 5% (and 9% at 6-month follow-up).

In a subsequent study, Cartwright-Hatton and colleagues[61] piloted a 10-week parenting skills intervention adapted to address anxiety symptoms directly. In addition to the components of the previous intervention, this program was "cognitively enhanced." That is, techniques were socratically guided rather than taught, and cognitive obstacles to using the strategies were challenged with cognitive therapy techniques. In addition, parents were encouraged to engender a "confident cognitive style," by generating a list of 7 cognitive thoughts a confident child might have about the world, other people, and the child's ability to cope with negative events. Strategies were introduced for countering the child's anxious thoughts and fostering confident ones. Parents were also encouraged to praise and reinforce brave behaviors and discourage fearful ones, to avoid modeling anxiety, and to understand children's anxious symptoms cognitive-behaviorally, and were given a session on strategies for dealing with worry and a session on how to use graded hierarchies to help children face fears. Open treatment of 11 children aged 4 to 9 years referred for anxiety led to significant decrease in CBCL internalizing scores, with continued improvement at 3-month follow-up.

In similar fashion, Pincus and colleagues[62–64] adapted Eyberg's PCIT for the treatment of young children (aged 4–8 years) with separation anxiety disorder (SAD). In PCIT, children participate in "coaching" sessions during which parents practice new skills and receive ongoing feedback from their therapist who watches the interaction through a one-way mirror. During Child-Directed Interaction (CDI), parents learn to increase warmth and responsiveness during playtime with their children and to differentially reinforce their children's desired behavior. In Parent-Directed Interaction (PDI), parents learn behavior-modification strategies, such as giving clear directives, rewarding positive child behaviors, and applying consequences to acting out behaviors. In a multiple baseline case series with 3 children aged 5 to 8 years, PCIT was associated with reduction in SAD for all 3 children.[62] PCIT was also associated with reduction in SAD severity in 10 children aged 4 to 8 years in an open pilot study[63,64]; however, the children did not reach nonclinical levels of severity. Pincus and colleagues[63,64] are currently conducting an RCT versus a wait-list control condition of a PCIT program modified to include a Bravery-Directed Interaction (BDI). BDI includes parental psychoeducation about child anxiety, as well as the child's gradual exposure to feared situations, during which parents are taught to use skills learned in CDI, such as labeled praise and differential reinforcement (without live coaching). Although final results are not yet published, the results of the first 34 children in the RCT suggest that the ADIS severity ratings of the children receiving modified PCIT decreased to below clinical levels.[64]

Treatment of OCD

Freeman and colleagues[45] developed a treatment program for OCD specifically tailored to young children aged 5 to 8 years and their families. The adaptations they used included the use of specific, concrete, and child-friendly examples for explaining the rationale for exposure with response prevention (ERP), differentiating obsessional from other nonintrusive repetitive cognitions, and understanding the associations between obsessions and compulsions (eg, an obsession is like a "worry monster" that tells you to do things it wants you to do). Parents were included in treatment and trained as coaches to facilitate adherence outside of sessions, to address tendencies to accommodate the child's OCD behaviors, and to learn to tolerate their own distress to child exposure exercises. The treatment also included two 90-minute parent sessions to address the impact of the child's diagnosis and logistical issues related to homework, and to provide a clear rationale for the treatment. The child-parent sessions included a clear rationale for treatment (learning to be the "boss" of OCD), taught with the use of visual imagery, metaphors, and developmentally relevant examples. For example, the child was encouraged (as in manuals for older children) to nickname and draw a picture of his OCD; and exposures could be performed playfully, for example, pretending to be "Oscar the Grouch" when practicing exposure to dirt or germs.[65] Parents were taught to use differential attention, modeling, and scaffolding (ie, coaching the child to try to "boss back" or resist OCD compulsions as they arise in daily life). In a pilot RCT, 42 children were randomized to receive either family-based CBT or family-based relaxation training in 12 sessions. Among completers, 69% of children receiving CBT achieved clinical remission on the Child Yale-Brown Obsessive-Compulsive Scale compared with 20% of those receiving relaxation (P<.01; ITT rates were 50% vs 20%, P<.05). This promising protocol is now being tested in a larger RCT.

Treatment of PTSD

Parents usually play a large role in CBT for children and adolescents with PTSD diagnoses or symptoms. Standard parent treatment components include psychoeducation about trauma and posttraumatic stress in children, correction of distorted cognitions about the child's abuse (eg, "I should have known something was wrong"), child behavior management skills including contingent reinforcement of adaptive behaviors, active ignoring, and time out, and exposure to traumatic memories and associated situations and learning to practice exposures with children. As detailed by Dorsey, Briggs, and Woods elsewhere in this issue, the treatments offered to children commonly include affective education; coping skills training; gradual exposure to memories of the traumatic event(s) and associated situations (eg, through drawings, writing, or imagery); body safety awareness and assertiveness training (for sexually abused children); and relapse prevention.[66,67]

Several groups have adapted these approaches for preschool-age children.[68–71] For example, Waldrop and De Arellano[71] modified a manualized CBT for older children who had been physically abused to treat a 5-year-old boy with PTSD. Sessions were conducted individually with the boy, but his mother was included for portions of most sessions. Skills were taught in the context of games or fun activities.

Exposure exercises were facilitated using hypothetical stories about other children and role plays using puppets. After 22 sessions, the boy showed substantial improvement on CBCL internalizing symptoms (particularly withdrawn and anxious/depressed subscales). Similarly, Scheeringa and colleagues[70] demonstrated the feasibility and effectiveness of CBT for the treatment of 2 preschoolers with PTSD. In particular, these investigators showed that young children are able to engage in structured sessions, practice relaxation exercises, and cooperate with exposure practices.

To date, there have been only 2 RCTs of CBT for preschoolers with symptoms of PTSD. Cohen and Mannarino[68] randomized 67 sexually abused preschoolers (aged 2–7 years) and their nonoffending parents to CBT (12 sessions) or nondirected supportive therapy (NST). Children did not have to meet criteria for PTSD for inclusion in the trial, although they had to have at least mild symptoms of post-traumatic stress or at least one sexually inappropriate behavior. For both modalities, weekly sessions lasted 90 minutes, 50 with the parent and 40 with the child. Parent CBT sessions targeted thoughts and attributions regarding the child's abuse, how to support the child's emotional needs and manage inappropriate child behavior, and parental anxiety management. Child sessions focused on safety and personal boundaries, assertiveness, ambivalent feelings about the abuser, inappropriate behaviors, and anxiety. In NST, the therapist provided emotional support and encouraged children and parents to express their feelings, to control for nonspecific therapeutic factors. At posttreatment, children in the CBT condition showed a greater reduction on CBCL internalizing and externalizing scales, reductions in proportions scoring in the clinical ranges on these scales, and fewer inappropriate sexual behaviors. Treatment gains were maintained at 1 year[72] and were mediated by higher levels of emotional support given to and provided by mothers,[73] highlighting the importance of including parents in treatment.

Deblinger and colleagues[69] randomized 67 children aged 2 to 8 years and their mothers to 11 sessions of group CBT or supportive therapy; there were separate groups for mothers and children. The parent CBT group included modules on psychoeducation and coping skills; parent-child communication, modeling, gradual exposure for parents' fears; and behavior management skills. Parent supportive therapy groups were nondirective, with parents selecting topics of conversation. Both the supportive and CBT child groups covered affective education, communication skills, and body safety awareness, but children in the CBT group learned skills in an interactive format that involved a workbook, role plays, and skills rehearsal, whereas therapists in the supportive group used a more didactic format (presenting pictures and stories). Of note, exposure was not a component of the child CBT groups. Of the 67 dyads enrolled, 54 completed at least 3 sessions and 44 completed treatment. At posttreatment, mothers in the CBT condition had greater reductions in intrusive thoughts about the abuse and lower emotional distress, and children showed improved body safety skills. Children in both groups experienced symptom reductions, although the effect for the CBT group was larger.

In summary, there is evidence that CBT can reduce emotional and behavioral symptoms in traumatized preschoolers. However, neither RCT required that children meet criteria for PTSD, and one did not include exposure, which may have limited the comparative efficacy of CBT. Additional studies including more severely affected preschoolers who meet criteria for PTSD are warranted. In addition, dismantling studies that examine the degree to which exposure exercises add to the efficacy of CBT for PTSD will help clinicians better understand how best to treat these young children and their parents.

FUTURE DIRECTIONS

The growing number of studies addressing the developmental adaptation of CBT for anxiety disorders in children younger than 8 years is very encouraging, given the great need in this previously neglected population. In particular, 2 treatments for PTSD,[68,69] 1 for OCD,[45] and 4 for anxiety disorders in general[9,10,52,57] (including 2 preventive studies[10,52]) have demonstrated efficacy in RCTs. Parents, pediatricians, preschool teachers, and other caregivers seeking to refer young children for treatment of anxiety now have several CBT-based approaches and modalities to choose from.

However, several areas for further research can be identified. First, with few exceptions,[45,68,69] most treatments to date have been tested only against wait-list control conditions. To best understand the active elements of treatment, it is necessary to test them against attention-control or non-CBT treatment conditions. Second, although one study to date has suggested that parent treatment alone may be as beneficial as treatment that includes the child, the question of whether intervening directly with the child can increase the benefit of treatment, or better buffer children against future disorder, needs further research. In addition, there may be subsets of young children (eg, older children) for whom child intervention may be more important and subsets of children (eg, younger preschoolers or toddlers) for whom parent intervention might be sufficient. Similarly, studies are needed to compare the benefits of individualized versus group treatment. Although the studies reviewed suggest that group interventions have higher drop-out rates,[57,69] it is not known whether some children (eg, those with more or less severe comorbid presentations) may benefit more from individual parent-child treatment or from group treatment. It could also be important to distinguish whether specific strategies are better suited to particular clinical presentations. For example, anxious children with comorbid externalizing disorders may be better treated with an approach such as that by Cartwright-Hatton and colleagues,[60] which also specifically addresses externalizing behaviors. Large-scale studies comparing parent-only with parent-child treatment using blinded evaluation of outcome, as well as large-scale studies comparing group with individual (parent-child) CBT, or CBT-based parent groups versus parenting skills groups modified to include some CBT strategies are needed to answer these questions.

As we have seen, a wide variety of interventions have been included in each of the protocols reviewed. Dismantling studies examining the relative importance of general parenting skills, child coping skills, and progressive exposure could be helpful. Another question, given the difficulty of implementing some cognitive strategies with young children, is to understand the degree to which recovery from anxiety in this age group is mediated by reduction in anxious cognitions, regardless of whether the cognitions are the target of the intervention, because exposure might also operate through experientially disproving anxious cognitions. To study this issue, it would be important to measure cognitive processes such as attentional or interpretative biases to threat and to examine these constructs as mediators of change in young children.

It can be challenging with this age group to find developmentally appropriate measures of anxiety. For several reasons, youngsters age 6 and under are not reliable reporters of anxiety symptoms. Children this young have an undeveloped sense of time and are unable to report on frequencies or durations of symptoms. In addition, they are frequently hesitant to admit to fears or worries, and often do not understand the importance of accurate reporting. Therefore, it is important to use other informants, including parents, teachers, and other caregivers. Although some preschool-specific structured interviews have been developed (such as the Preschool-Age Psychiatric Assessment]), the recognition that young children present with the same disorders as older children has led many investigators to use parent reports on the ADIS-IV or K-SADS-E (Schedule for Affective Disorders and Schizophrenia for School-Aged Children) anxiety modules, with reasonable reliability and sensitivity to change. These reports are usually supplemented with parent or teacher questionnaires normed on younger children (eg, CBCL; Preschool Anxiety Scale). However, it would also be useful to include more objective measures such as direct behavioral assessments, similar to those used to assess BI.

In addition, more data are needed about predictors of treatment response in this age group, an area explored in only a few studies to date. For example, Hirshfeld-Becker[74] found that child age and parental anxiety disorder did not moderate response to CBT, but that BI was a negative predictor of treatment response. In their study, children without BI showed a global improvement rate of 94% compared with only 63% for those with BI, and the rate of remission of all anxiety disorders was significantly lower for children with BI. This finding may in part explain the relatively low rates of remission from anxiety among children with BI in other studies, and may also partly explain the relatively low recovery rates in general for childhood anxiety disorders, because many anxious children also have BI, and may suggest that children with BI need longer or more intensive treatments. Finally, it will be important to evaluate the effectiveness of these treatments as they are disseminated from research settings to broader community and school settings, and to more diverse cultural and socioeconomic groups of children.

FINANCIAL DISCLOSURES

Drs Hirshfeld-Becker and Henin have received honoraria from Reed Medical Education (a logistics collaborator for the MGH Psychiatry Academy). The education programs conducted by the MGH Psychiatry Academy were supported, in part, through independent medical education grants from pharmaceutical companies, including AstraZeneca, Bristol-Myers Squibb, Forest Laboratories Inc, Janssen, Lilly, McNeil Pediatrics, Pfizer, Pharmacia, the Prechter Foundation, Sanofi Aventis, Shire, the Stanley Foundation, UCB Pharma Inc, and Wyeth. In addition, in the past 12 months, Dr Henin has been a consultant for Concordant Rater Systems and Pfizer. She receives royalties from Oxford University Press. Dr Micco serves as a paid consultant to Concordant Rating Systems Inc. Drs Hirshfeld-Becker, Henin, and Micco are funded by research grants from the National Institutes of Health. The other authors have nothing to disclose.

REFERENCES

1. Costello EJ, Mustillo S, Erkanli A, et al. Prevalence and development of psychiatric disorders in childhood and adolescence. Arch Gen Psychiatry 2003;60: 837–44.
2. Essau CA, Conradt J, Petermann F. Frequency, comorbidity, and psychosocial impairment of anxiety disorders in German adolescents. J Anxiety Disord 2000; 14:263–79.
3. Ezpeleta L, Keeler G, Erkanli A, et al. Epidemiology of psychiatric disability in childhood and adolescence. J Child Psychol Psychiatry 2001;42:901–14.
4. Hirshfeld-Becker DR, Micco JA, Simoes NA, et al. High risk studies and developmental antecedents of anxiety disorders. Am J Med Genet C Semin Med Genet 2008;148C:99–117.

5. Egger HL, Angold A. Common emotional and behavioral disorders in preschool children: presentation, nosology, and epidemiology. J Child Psychol Psychiatry 2006;47:313–37.
6. Spence SH, Rapee RM, McDonald C, et al. The structure of anxiety symptoms among preschoolers. Behav Res Ther 2001;39:1293–316.
7. Eley TC, Bolton D, O'Connor TG, et al. A twin study of anxiety-related behaviours in pre-school children. J Child Psychol Psychiatry 2003;44:945–60.
8. Ialongo N, Edelsohn G, Werthamer-Larsson L, et al. The significance of self-reported anxious symptoms in first-grade children: prediction to anxious symptoms and adaptive functioning in fifth grade. J Child Psychol Psychiatry 1995; 36:427–37.
9. Hirshfeld-Becker DR, Masek B, Henin A, et al. Cognitive-behavioral therapy for 4–7-year-old children with anxiety: a randomized clinical trial. J Consult Clin Psychol 2010;78:498–510.
10. Rapee RM, Kennedy S, Ingram M, et al. Prevention and early intervention of anxiety disorders in inhibited preschool children. J Consult Clin Psychol 2005; 73:488–97.
11. Kearney CA, Sims KE, Pursell CR, et al. Separation anxiety disorder in young children: a longitudinal and family analysis. J Clin Child Adolesc Psychol 2003;32: 593–8.
12. Rapee RM, Kennedy SJ, Ingram M, et al. Altering the trajectory of anxiety in at-risk young children. Am J Psychiatry 2010;167(12):1518–25.
13. Biederman J, Petty C, Hirshfeld-Becker DR, et al. Developmental trajectories of anxiety disorders in offspring at high risk for panic disorder and major depression. Psychiatry Res 2007;153:245–52.
14. Ollendick TH, King NJ. Empirically supported treatments for children with phobic and anxiety disorders: current status. J Clin Child Psychol 1998;27:156–67.
15. James A, Soler A, Weatherall R. Cognitive behavioural therapy for anxiety disorders in children and adolescents. Cochrane Database Syst Rev 2005;4:CD004690.
16. Silverman WK, Pina AA, Viswesvaran C. Evidence-based psychosocial treatments for phobic and anxiety disorders in children and adolescents. J Clin Child Adolesc Psychol 2008;37:105–30.
17. Barrett PM, Farrell L, Pina AA, et al. Evidence-based psychosocial treatments for child and adolescent obsessive-compulsive disorder. J Clin Child Adolesc Psychol 2008;37:131–55.
18. Watson HJ, Rees CS. Meta-analysis of randomized, controlled treatment trials for pediatric obsessive-compulsive disorder. J Child Psychol Psychiatry 2008;49: 489–98.
19. Dagleish T, Meiser-Stedman R, Smith P. Cognitive aspects of posttraumatic stress reactions and their treatment in children and adolescents: an empirical review and some recommendations. Behav Cogn Psychother 2005;33:459–86.
20. Cohen JA. Treating traumatized children: current status and future directions. J Trauma Dissociation 2005;6:109–21.
21. Kendall PC, Hudson JL, Gosch E, et al. Cognitive-behavioral therapy for anxiety disordered youth: a randomized clinical trial evaluating child and family modalities. J Consult Clin Psychol 2008;76:282–97.
22. Walkup JT, Albano AM, Piacentini J, et al. Cognitive behavioral therapy, sertraline, or a combination in childhood anxiety. N Engl J Med 2008;359:2753–66.
23. King NJ, Tonge BJ, Heyne D, et al. Cognitive-behavioral treatment of school refusing children: a controlled evaluation. J Am Acad Child Adolesc Psychiatry 1998;37:395–403.

24. Silverman WK, Kurtines WM, Ginsburg GS, et al. Treating anxiety disorders in children with group cognitive-behavioral therapy: a randomized clinical trial. J Consult Clin Psychol 1999;67:995–1003.
25. Silverman WK, Kurtines WM, Ginsburg GS, et al. Contingency management, self-control, and education support in the treatment of childhood phobic disorders: a randomized clinical trial. J Consult Clin Psychol 1999;67:675–87.
26. Shortt AL, Barrett PM, Fox TL. Evaluating the FRIENDS program: a cognitive-behavioral group treatment for anxious children and their parents. J Clin Child Psychol 2001;30:525–35.
27. Rapee RM, Abbott MJ, Lyneham HJ. Bibliotherapy for children with anxiety disorders using written materials for parents: a randomized controlled trial. J Consult Clin Psychol 2006;74:436–44.
28. March JS, Mulle K. OCD in children and adolescents: a cognitive-behavioral treatment manual. New York: Guilford Press; 1998.
29. McMurray NE, Lucas JO, Arbes-Duprey V, et al. The effects of mastery and coping models on dental stress in young children. Aust J Psychol 1985;37:65–70.
30. Kanfer F, Karoly P, Newman A. Reduction of children's fear of the dark by competence-related and situational threat-related verbal cues. J Consult Clin Psychol 1975;43:251–8.
31. Bandura A, Grusec JE, Menlove FL. Vicarious extinction of avoidance behavior. J Pers Soc Psychol 1967;5:16–23.
32. Bandura A, Menlove FL. Factors determining vicarious extinction of avoidance behavior through symbolic modeling. J Pers Soc Psychol 1968;8:99–108.
33. Hill JH, Liebert RM, Mott DE. Vicarious extinction of avoidance behavior through films: an initial test. Behav Ther 1968;20:499–508.
34. Kuroda J. Elimination of children's fears of animals by the method of experimental desensitization: an application of learning theory to child psychology. Psychologia 1969;12:161–5.
35. Leitenberg H, Callahan E. Reinforced practice and reduction of different kinds of fears in adults and children. Behav Res Ther 1973;11:19–30.
36. Menzies RG, Clarke JC. A comparison of in vivo and vicarious exposure in the treatment of childhood water phobia. Behav Res Ther 1993;31:9–15.
37. Sheslow DV, Bondy AS, Nelson RO. A comparison of graduated exposure, verbal coping skills, and their combination in the treatment of children's fear of the dark. Child Fam Behav Ther 1983;4:33–45.
38. Santacruz I, Mendez FJ, Sanchez-Meca J. Play therapy applied by parents for children with darkness phobia: comparison of two programmes. Child Fam Behav Ther 2006;28:19–35.
39. Mendez F, Garcia M. Emotive performances: a treatment package for children's phobias. Child Fam Behav Ther 1996;18:19–34.
40. Hirshfeld-Becker DR, Masek B, Henin A, et al. Cognitive-behavioral intervention with young anxious children. Harv Rev Psychiatry 2008;16:113–25.
41. Grave J, Blissett J. Is cognitive behavior therapy developmentally appropriate for young children: a critical review of the evidence. Clin Psychol Rev 2004;24:399–420.
42. Doherr L, Reynolds S, Wetherly J, et al. Young children's ability to engage in cognitive therapy tasks: association with age and educational experience. Behav Cogn Psychother 2005;33:201–15.
43. Pahl KM, Barrett PM. The development of social-emotional competence in preschool-aged children: an introduction to the Fun FRIENDS program. Aust J Guid Counsell 2007;17:81–90.

44. Knell S. Cognitive-behavioral play therapy. Northvale (NJ): Jason Aronson Inc; 1993.
45. Freeman JB, Choate-Summers ML, Moore PS, et al. Cognitive behavioral treatment for young children with obsessive-compulsive disorder. Biol Psychiatry 2007;61:337–43.
46. Hirshfeld-Becker DR, Biederman J. Rationale and principles for early intervention with young children at risk for anxiety disorders. Clin Child Fam Psychol Rev 2002;5:161–72.
47. Rapee RM, Schniering CA, Hudson JL. Anxiety disorders during childhood and adolescence: origins and treatment. Annu Rev Clin Psychol 2009;5:311–41.
48. Last CG, Hersen M, Kazdin AE, et al. Anxiety disorders in children and their families. Arch Gen Psychiatry 1991;48:928–34.
49. Cobham VE, Dadds MR, Spence SH, et al. Parental anxiety in the treatment of childhood anxiety: a different story three years later. J Clin Child Adolesc Psychol 2010;39:410–20.
50. Freeman JB, Garcia AM. Family based treatment for young children with OCD: therapist guide (treatments that work). New York: Oxford University Press; 2009.
51. Kendall P, Kane M, Howard B, et al. Cognitive-behavioral therapy for anxious children: therapist manual. Ardmore (OK): Workbook Publishing; 1992.
52. Kennedy SJ, Rapee RM, Edwards SL. A selective intervention program for inhibited preschool-aged children of parents with an anxiety disorder: effects on current anxiety disorders and temperament. J Am Acad Child Adolesc Psychiatry 2009;48:602–9.
53. Kagan J, Reznick JS, Snidman N. Biological bases of childhood shyness. Science 1988;240:167–71.
54. Hirshfeld-Becker DR, Micco J, Henin A, et al. Behavioral inhibition. Depress Anxiety 2008;25:357–67.
55. Barrett PM. Evaluation of cognitive-behavioral group treatments for childhood anxiety disorders. J Clin Child Psychol 1998;27:459–68.
56. Monga S, Young A, Owens M. Evaluating a cognitive behavioral therapy group program for anxious five to seven year old children: a pilot study. Depress Anxiety 2009;26:243–50.
57. Waters AM, Ford LA, Wharton TA, et al. Cognitive-behavioral therapy for young children with anxiety disorders: comparison of a child + parent condition versus a parent only condition. Behav Res Ther 2009;47:654–62.
58. Webster-Stratton C, Reid MJ. The incredible years parents, teachers and children training series: a multifaceted treatment approach for young children with conduct problems. In: Weisz J, Kazdin A, editors. Evidence–based psychotherapies for children and adolescents. 2nd edition. New York: Guildford; 2010. p. 194–210.
59. Eyberg SM, Boggs S, Algina J. Parent-child interaction therapy: a psychosocial model for the treatment of young children with conduct problem behavior and their families. Psychopharmacol Bull 1995;31:83–91.
60. Cartwright-Hatton S, McNally D, White C, et al. Parenting skills training: an effective intervention for internalizing symptoms in younger children? J Child Adolesc Psychiatr Nurs 2005;18:45–52.
61. Cartwright-Hatton S, McNally D, White C. A new cognitive behavioural parenting intervention for families of young anxious children: a pilot study. Behav Cogn Psychother 2005;33:243–7.
62. Choate ML, Pincus DB, Eyberg SM, et al. Parent-child interaction therapy for treatment of separation anxiety disorder in young children: a pilot study. Cogn Behav Pract 2005;12:126–35.

63. Pincus DB, Eyberg SM, Choate ML. Adapting parent-child interaction therapy for young children with separation anxiety disorder. Educ Treat Children 2005;28: 163–81.

64. Pincus DB, Santucci LC, Ehrenreich JT, et al. The implementation of modified parent-child interaction therapy for youth with separation anxiety disorder. Cogn Behav Pract 2008;15:118–25.

65. Freeman JB, Garcia AM. Family based treatment of early childhood OCD. Presented at the World congress on behavioral and cognitive therapy. Boston (MA), June, 2010.

66. Deblinger E, McLeer SV, Henry D. Cognitive behavioral treatment for sexually abused children suffering post-traumatic stress: preliminary findings. J Am Acad Child Adolesc Psychiatry 1990;29:747–52.

67. Cohen JA, Mannarino AP, Berliner L, et al. Trauma-focused cognitive behavioral therapy for children and adolescents. J Interpers Violence 2000;15:1202–23.

68. Cohen JA, Mannarino AP. A treatment outcome study for sexually abused preschool children: initial findings. J Am Acad Child Adolesc Psychiatry 1996; 35:42–50.

69. Deblinger E, Stauffer LB, Steer RA, et al. Comparative efficacies of supportive and cognitive behavioral group therapies for young children who have been sexually abused and their nonoffending mothers. Child Maltreat 2001;6:332–43.

70. Scheeringa MS, Salloum A, Arnberger RA, et al. Feasibility and effectiveness of cognitive-behavioral therapy for posttraumatic stress disorder in preschool children: two case reports. J Trauma Stress 2007;20:631–6.

71. Waldrop AE, de Arellano MA. Manualized cognitive behavioral treatment for physical abuse-related PTSD in an African American child: a case example. Cogn Behav Pract 2004;11:343–52.

72. Cohen JA, Mannarino AP. A treatment study for sexually abused preschool children: outcome during a one-year follow-up. J Am Acad Child Adolesc Psychiatry 1997;36:1228–35.

73. Cohen JA, Mannarino AP. Factors that mediate treatment outcome of sexually abused preschool children: six- and 12-month follow-up. J Am Acad Child Adolesc Psychiatry 1998;37:44–51.

74. Hirshfeld-Becker DR. Familial and temperamental risk factors for social anxiety disorder. In: Gazelle H, Rubin KH, editors. Social anxiety in childhood: bridging developmental and clinical perspectives: directions for child and adolescent development. San Francisco (CA): Jossey-Bass; 2010. p. 51–65, 127.

75. Freeman JB, Garcia AM, Coyne L, et al. Early childhood OCD: preliminary findings from a family-based cognitive-behavioral approach. J Am Acad Child Adolesc Psychiatry 2008;47:593–602.

Core Principles in Cognitive Therapy with Youth

Robert D. Friedberg, PhD, ABPP[a],*, Gina M. Brelsford, PhD[b]

KEYWORDS

- Cognitive therapy • Adolescence • Children
- Session structure

Cognitive therapy (CT), once a treatment considered only for circumscribed adult disorders, is currently applied to a variety of clinical conditions. Child psychiatry is recognizing its value and embracing the approach. March[1(p174)] emphasized that "psychiatry will move to a unified cognitive behavioral intervention model, that is housed within neurosciences medicine." Moreover, cognitive behavior therapy is a polymorphous treatment system. Because there are many forms of the psychotherapy, confusion about the approach can erupt. Accordingly, in this article, the authors adopt Aaron T. Beck's[2] CT as a particular focus. Beck's CT is seen as a theoretically robust and clinically flexible treatment model, which has been conceptualized as *the* integrative psychotherapy.[3] Several recent texts have specifically applied Beck's paradigm to children and adolescents,[4,5] and many other treatment packages borrow heavily from the Beck tradition.

This article begins with an overview of cardinal principles, practices, and processes associated with CT with children. A brief overview of the CT model is presented, and case conceptualization in CT is emphasized. Further, therapeutic stance variables such as collaborative empiricism and guided discovery are discussed. The importance of the therapeutic alliance is explained, and the role of empiricism and transparency in treatment is described. Valuing experiential learning to bring the head and heart to consensus concludes the first section. These rudiments are then followed by a description of the classic session structure used with children. Accordingly, mood check-ins, homework review, agenda setting, processing session content, homework assignment, and eliciting feedback are spelled out.

Disclosures: Friedberg: Guilford Publications (Royalties), Routledge Publications (Royalties), Wiley Publication (Royalties), and Professional Resource Press (Royalties). Brelsford: None.
[a] Division of Child Psychiatry, Penn State Milton Hershey Medical Center/College of Medicine, 22 NE Drive, Hershey, PA 17033, USA
[b] School of Behavioral Sciences and Education, Penn State University-Harrisburg, W311 Olmsted, 777 West Harrisburg Pike, Middletown, PA 17057, USA
* Corresponding author.
E-mail address: rfriedberg@psu.edu

Child Adolesc Psychiatric Clin N Am 20 (2011) 369–378
doi:10.1016/j.chc.2011.01.009
1056-4993/11/$ – see front matter © 2011 Elsevier Inc. All rights reserved.

CARDINAL PRINCIPLES, PRACTICES, AND PROCESSES
Brief Overview

Many clinicians naive to the Beck's CT believe that the approach holds that thoughts cause feelings. However, Beck[6] clearly articulated that when people are distressed, 4 interrelated systems are energized (physiological, emotional, behavioral, and cognitive systems). These spheres reciprocally influence each other, and no one domain is primary. In addition, Beck noted that intervening in any one of these systems is legitimate (eg, medication as an intervention at the physiologic level, gestalt therapy as an intervention at the emotional level) but proposed that intervening at the behavioral and cognitive spheres is the most effective treatment strategy.

CT is a dynamic information processing system that is rooted in operant, classical, and social learning theory. Accordingly, the manner in which youngsters interpret their experiences and form conclusions about themselves, others, and the future represents a clinical centerpiece. Young people wrap strong emotions around these mental parcels. This cognitive packaging carries a powerful affective punch as children and adolescents actively fashion their explanations via a selective encoding process.

The personal views of children and adolescents are self-maintaining. According to CT, people work to preserve their homeostasis and avoid disruptions in the information flow. Therefore, they selectively attend to experiences that confirm their assumptions and relatively neglect disconfirming evidence. Liotti[7(p93)] parsimoniously explained that in this assimilation process, "the new is actively reduced to what is already known." Therefore, children and their therapists need to design powerful cognitive, emotional, and behavioral experiments to provide disconfirming data.

Focus on Case Conceptualization

The straightforward nature of CT is often deceiving. Casual observers may mistakenly assume that the approach is purely technical and see it as a bag of tricks. However, CT with children is governed by a firm reliance on case conceptualization.[4,8,9] Readers should not mistake CT as a treatment paradigm that can be applied without a grasp of learning theory and information processing models.

Bieling and Kuyken[10] suggested that theory is fundamental to case formulation and, in turn, case formulation is essential to evidence-based practice. Indeed, case conceptualization is the medium that translates general findings from empirically based treatment research and applies them to individual patients. Kendall and colleagues[11] emphasized that case conceptualization breathes life into a manual.

An in-depth discussion of the case formulation process is beyond the scope of this article. Nonetheless, in their case formulation model, Friedberg and McClure[4] integrated developmental history, cultural context, behavioral antecedents and consequences, cognitive structures, and presenting problems into a dynamic system. All these variables exert a bidirectional influence on each other. For instance, presenting problems such as separation anxiety influence antecedents (eg, mother not encouraging play with peers), consequences (reduction of avoidance), developmental history (eg, separations at school, being invited to birthday parties) and cognitions (eg, "I'm not safe unless I am close to my mom"). In turn, these cognitions, behavioral antecedents/consequences and historical factors work to exacerbate and maintain presenting problems. A clinical approach driven by a case formulation is well equipped to address comorbidity, contextual variations, and cultural/ethnic differences. For a complete explanation of case conceptualization, the reader is referred to other sources on the topic.[4,8,9,12]

Modular Components: Beyond Alphabet Soup

CT's roots lie in applying specific techniques to particular disorders (eg, depression, anxiety, posttraumatic stress disorder [PTSD], obsessive-compulsive disorder [OCD]). Typically, this stance involves a manual approach. Consequently, a plethora of discrete manuals for specific disorders yields a veritable alphabet soup (eg, CT for GAD, CT for OCD, CT for SAD, CT for PTSD). Manuals clearly offer working clinicians valuable treatment options. They offer precise content, replicable procedures, and spelled-out treatment plans. However, there is a movement to a more transdiagnostic approach.[13] A transdiagnostic approach advocates core treatments that provide general applicability to a variety of clinical conditions. This paradigm emphasizes modules over manuals.

Modules are constructed by grouping techniques according to their common theoretical basis and practice elements.[14–16] Modules cull various procedures from manuals and integrate them into unifying conceptual categories. Simply, modules appear to offer the best of both possible worlds. Empirically supported procedures are synthesized, which allows for clinical flexibility guided by case conceptualization. In this way, clinicians can remain both faithful to the CT model as well as flexible in their approach.[17]

Psychoeducation, self-monitoring, behavioral interventions, cognitive restructuring, rational analysis, and performance attainment are common modules. Psychoeducation gives patients and their families a schema for treatment, including information on diagnosis, treatment options, and coping skills. Self-monitoring paves the road to self-directed change by providing tools to track physiologic, behavioral, emotional, interpersonal, and cognitive data. The behavioral module contains basic skill training sets such as social skills, contingency contracting, relaxation, systematic desensitization, and habit reversal training. The first cognitive module deals with simpler cognitive restructuring, self-instruction, and problem solving. Generally, these techniques focus on changing thought content. Rational analysis methods are more sophisticated procedures and target thought processes by teaching patients to ask better questions of themselves. Performance attainment emphasizes behavioral enactment and includes experiments/exposures. Performance attainment makes use of many experiential learning exercises and stresses action over discussion.

Collaboration and Guided Discovery

CT rests firmly on the notions of collaboration and guided discovery. Dattilio and Padesky[18(p5)] explained that "emphasis is placed on the collaborative aspect of the approach, on the assumption that people learn to change their thinking more readily if the rationale for changes comes from their own insights rather than from the therapist." The therapeutic enterprise in CT is not seen as a prescriptive one. Procedures are not done *to* children but rather they are done *with* them. Pedantry is out of place in CT with children and adolescents. Salkovskis[19(p50)] urged, "...there is no place in the theory or therapy for the idea of therapist-defined wrong thinking which is inappropriately judgmental." Thoughts are tested and behavioral experiments are assigned via mutual agreement.

Guided discovery involves the clinical application of the scientific method.[20] Perris[21] stated that guided discovery encouraged a hypothesis-testing approach to managing emotional distress. Hypotheses (automatic thoughts) are elicited; an experimental method is used to test the accuracy of the hypothesis; results are observed, recorded, and analyzed; and finally, reasonable conclusions are drawn.

The goal of guided discovery is to cast a doubt on rather than absolutely refute or dispute youngsters' thinking.[22,23] Cognitive therapists are well advised not to interrogate youngsters until their assumptions wilt under hot lights. The idea is to gently guide patients through multiple angles and perspectives. Guided discovery and collaboration spark the necessary curiosity in treatment sessions.[24] Fresh perspectives are born out of a Socratic dialogue, which invites young patients to examine their interpretations, conclusions, and judgments. In the seminal CT text, Beck and colleagues[22(p154)] wrote, "analysis of meaning and attitudes express the unreasonableness and self-defeating nature of the attitudes."

Importance of Therapeutic Alliance

Many professionals erroneously assume that the treatment alliance is unimportant in CT. However, building strong treatment relationships has always been a pivotal clinical task.[22] More recently, the treatment relationship is receiving renewed interest.[25,26]

Emotional closeness and interpersonal liking characterize successful treatment relationships.[27] In addition, Creed and Kendall[27] found that collaboration was essential in establishing a strong working alliance. Therapists should be seen as advocates rather than adversaries by their young patients. Ronen[28] noted that effective cognitive therapists are flexible, creative, and engaging.

Traditionally, the treatment relationship is seen as a dimensional construct in CT.[29] CT therapists readily recognize that treatment takes place in an interpersonal context.[30] This interpersonal relationship is highly valued and necessary for successful treatment. However, a good relationship itself is not sufficient for treatment progress. Therefore, skill building and alliance coexist on a balanced platform. Friedberg and McClure[4] concluded that the treatment relationship and interventions are not independent of each other. Rather, they are contemporaneous. Essentially, effective procedures increase treatment alliances, and good working alliances promote application of procedures.

Empiricism and Transparency in Practice

Empiricism and transparency reduce the mysterious nature of therapy. These concepts reflect the model's phenomenological roots.[3,31] Children's subjective experiences are honored, and data come directly from them. Empiricism and transparency ignite the guided discovery process. Empiricism steers clinicians away from the reflexive stance that assumes that children's negative automatic thoughts are distorted and inaccurate.

Progress is tracked via objective measures. Patient feedback is directly elicited. Homework assignments and behavioral experiments are recorded and evaluated. The reliance on empiricism allows both clinicians and patients to analyze the levels of progress. Empiricism drives accountability in CT. When the data indicate that interventions are not working, changes in the treatment strategy are made.

Transparency in CT refers to clinicians and patients being on the same page. Although power differentials are inevitable in any psychotherapy, they are explicitly addressed and processed in CT. Case conceptualizations, assessment measures, treatment rationale, treatment plans, and descriptions of procedures are shared with patients in a clear, common sense language. This transparency facilitates genuine informed consent.

Bringing Head and Heart to Consensus

CT is an action-based, goal-oriented approach. Although insight is appreciated, it is rarely sufficient without associated behavioral action. Waller[32] warned that both patients and therapists can become too complacent with purely verbal interventions and avoid the challenge of helping patients to act differently. Accordingly, emphasis is placed on young patients and their families experimenting with new behaviors and assumptions. The long-standing importance of patients enacting new behavioral patterns is well documented.[33]

CT with children is an emotionally evocative approach. The treatment process is far from a mechanistic, emotionally sterile approach. Rather, CT is best applied in the context of negative emotional arousal.[34] Indeed, recent affective neuroscience findings underscore this point.[35]

Essential CT "brings the head and heart to consensus."[36] Experiential learning facilitates this crucial alignment of rational and emotional domains. Samoilov and Goldfried[37] emphasized the importance of in-session arousal in launching cognitive, emotional, and behavioral change.

Safran and Muran[38] explained that experiential learning energizes generalization. They argued that if coping skills are learned in negatively emotional contexts similar to the ones where they are required, they are more likely to be applied and generalized in real life circumstances. Moreover, by emphasizing action over talk, experiential exercises forge the genuine mastery necessary for on-going behavioral change. In his early writing, Beck[2(p214)] advocated for experiential learning, stating, "the experiential approach exposes the patient to experiences that are in themselves powerful enough to change misconceptions."

SESSION STRUCTURE

CT emphasizes the use of a session structure when working with patients. Session structure provides a template for moving through sessions that is predictable and well organized but remains tailored to the individual needs of the patient.[4] This clinical approach emphasizes the need for consistency between sessions to assuage anxiety in the therapeutic setting. Patients, both adults and children, may attend therapy sessions with trepidation and unfamiliarity. Providing session structure dissipates this anxiety about therapy and allows the patient to become a collaborator in the therapy.[39] Indeed, the external structure soothes chaotic inner worlds. Through providing session structure, the patient may feel there is a safe and predicable space to explore paths to wellness.[40]

A typical session within a CT framework includes the following components: (1) mood check-in, (2) homework review, (3) agenda setting, (4) processing session content, (5) assigning homework, and (6) providing a summary of the session with client feedback.[4] Each component of CT is reviewed in the following sections.

Mood Check-in and Use of Objective Measures

As the first component of most sessions, mood check-in tends to be brief, but nonetheless salient. For adults or older children, a mood check-in involves soliciting verbal reports of mood states coupled with using objective test scores to determine if there is consistency between the 2 methods of reporting.[8] If a discrepancy is detected between verbal reports and objective measures, this is presented to the patient as a point of discussion. With younger children or less-verbal adolescents, use of verbal mood check-in may be replaced or supplemented with asking the child to draw a face indicating how they are feeling. Most children find this an engaging activity that eventually allows for expansion of their feeling word vocabulary.[4] Children's reports of feeling states can be supplemented with objective caregiver reports. Multiple reporters provide valuable information from the different perspectives of teachers, parents, and children. This comparison of data can yield beneficial results for moving forward in the therapeutic hour.[5]

Objective measures frequently used to assess mood and anxiety disorders in the initial session with children younger than 14 years include the Child Depression Inventory (CDI)[41] or the Screen for Child Anxiety Related Emotional Disorders (SCARED).[42] For older patients, use of the Beck Depression Inventory-II (BDI-II)[43] and the Multidimensional Anxiety Scale for Children (MASC)[44] are recommended. To allow for comparison of symptom reports, it is recommended to also gather caregiver reports on the SCARED and the CDI.

The CDI is an easy tool to complete and score, which assesses childhood depression, providing a total score with a raw score cutoff of 13.[41] There are also CDI factor scores, all of which can be converted to standard scores. Factor scores on the CDI consist of negative mood, interpersonal difficulties, anhedonia, ineffectiveness, and negative self-esteem.[5,41] The BDI-II is another measure of depression, with scores of 20 or more indicating serious levels of depressive symptoms and scores of 13 to 19 suggesting dysphoria to moderate depressive symptoms.[43] In addition, items 2 and 9 on both the CDI and the BDI-II provide direct assessment of hopelessness and suicidality.[5]

The SCARED is also simple to complete and score. It provides an overall score for anxiety (raw score of 25 or above) coupled with 5 factor scores.[42] The factor scores include a measure of generalized anxiety, somatic/pain symptoms, separation anxiety, school avoidance, and social anxiety. Both children and their parents can complete the SCARED, which allows for comparison of reports.[5] The MASC is a slightly more complex instrument used to assess anxiety than the SCARED. It also provides a full anxiety score coupled with factor scores related to separation anxiety, social anxiety, harm reduction, and physiologic symptoms.[44] However, the MASC also breaks down the factor scores into perfectionism, anxious coping, restlessness, and humiliation/rejection, coupled with providing an inconsistency scale and an anxiety disorder index.[5] Both of these measures are found to be useful, and it is up to the therapist to determine which would be best used.

When there are reports of attention-deficit/hyperactivity disorder (ADHD) symptoms, the use of the Conners Parent Rating Scales-Revised (CPRS-R)[45] or the Swanson, Nolan, and Pelham Rating Scale-IV (SNAP-IV)[46] are recommended.[5] The CPRS-R, which also has a version used for teachers (CTRS), are behavior-rating scales for children presenting with ADHD symptoms. The parent version provides 7 factor scores including inattention, anxious-shy, perfectionism, social problems, psychosomatic problems, and hyperactive-impulsive indices.[5,45] The SNAP-IV is also used to assess ADHD but can also measure oppositional defiant disorder and aggression in children between 6 and 18 years of age. The SNAP-IV is based on the *Diagnostic and Statistical Manual of Mental Disorders* (Fourth Edition) criteria and provides subset scores.[5,46]

All of these measures can be provided as a baseline assessment of mood, anxiety, and behavior at the outset of treatment, but many (eg, CDI) can also be used at the beginning of each session to check on current mood states.

Homework Review

Session homework may be rephrased as weekly projects, helping sheets, or experiments to decrease anxiety that some patients may feel when the word homework is mentioned.[4] A consistent review of homework from the previous session reinforces the importance of what occurred in the session and the need to generalize it to time between sessions.[8] Homework administration also involves the patient in deciding what the next steps are in handling their current difficulties, which encourages engagement and investment in the therapeutic process. The review of homework also reinforces the therapeutic relationship by conveying the therapist's interest in the child's current emotional and cognitive states.[5] Young children may present with different needs related to homework review, including brevity, creativity, and fun, whereas older children and adolescents may need to be engaged in the process such that they feel it is worthwhile to complete.[5]

Setting an Agenda

Setting an agenda is integral in the therapeutic process and serves a variety of purposes. One purpose includes providing structure and predictability to the therapeutic process.[4] Children and adolescents may find that their lives are driven by chaos, which they expect to continue in therapy. Presenting a concise plan for each session alleviates this chaos and allows the young patient to partake in deciding what will be discussed during each session. This provides boundaries, predictability, and a role for the child or adolescent in the therapeutic process, thereby increasing their investment in therapy.[4,8] Agenda setting is also a clever way to intertwine goals for therapy, providing information on key therapeutic techniques, allowing a space to practice these techniques, and elucidating a path for homework planning between the current and next session.[8]

For example, when an adolescent decides to put an argument with the mother on the agenda, the therapist may begin to explore the patient's automatic thoughts about these disagreements. These automatic thoughts set the stage for negative emotions that are evident to the patient.[8] However, the patient is not aware of the automatic thoughts that facilitate these negative emotions. Awareness of these thoughts and practice detecting, writing down, and challenging these thoughts all become part of the therapeutic process. As a result, the patient's use of homework, stemming from this agenda item, could focus on awareness of these thoughts to reduce their powerful role in the parent-child conflict.

Processing the Session

There is a balancing act between session content, process, and structure in CT. The session structure tends to remain uniform for most sessions, in which therapeutic tasks such as games, homework, and thought records are used. However, session content and process are different for each patient.[4] Session content encompasses the thoughts, feelings, and behavior elicited via therapeutic procedures.[4] The content of therapy is processed via the therapists' use of many techniques, including Socratic questioning, empathy, and behavioral experiments, with the purpose of increasing the therapeutic alliance, providing symptom relief, and problem solving.[4,8] These techniques influence skill acquisition and generalization to the real world.

However, when working with young children and adolescents, the content of each session is largely influenced by their developmental and motivational levels. Although it is not possible to modify the developmental level of the patient, the therapist can encourage involvement and motivation in the session by remaining dynamic and using creative activities to engage the child.[4]

Finally, session process is the way in which a patient goes about completing tasks during therapy or responding to questions posed.[4,8] Some children and adolescents complete thought records with sincerity, and others may refuse to engage in the therapeutic task. To increase engagement in the process of each session, once again use of creativity and empowerment are essential in moving the patient toward meeting therapeutic goals.[4] This effort may involve playing games, journaling, or using artistic endeavors to aid in skill generalization to outside the session.[8] The use of charts and reward systems may also engage youth in session by encouraging their participation in the therapeutic process. The use of rewards systems, including token economies and reward charts, could also allow for generalization of work in session to behavior and functioning outside of sessions.

Assigning Homework

Homework stems directly from session content.[4] Interlacing the content of each session with homework between the end of session and the next meeting reinforces what occurs in the session and moves the patient toward completing their therapeutic goals. Further, deciding on homework is a collaborative process between the therapist and patient. Instead of "assigning homework," it is essential to work with children in determining what type of assignment might be helpful, which reduces resistance and increases likelihood of completion.

Gathering Feedback and Summarizing

The final component of CT is summarizing and requesting feedback from the patient. This is another essential component of therapy to solidify the therapeutic alliance.[4] The process of summarizing gives the patient time to hear what has been discussed and make decisions if they agree with the therapist's summary.[8] Summarizing can also present major points made in the session that are moving the patient toward goal completion. This positive spin on what was discussed can be powerful and empower the patient in the therapeutic process.

Children or adolescents are rarely asked for feedback about how something should occur in their lives. When youth are asked to provide feedback, they may provide stock responses either praising the adult or unabashedly berating the adult. In therapy, when young patients are asked for how the therapy session is going for them, it provides an honest space for them to investigate how this particular adult will react to their response. Many children need assistance with constructive feedback when presented with gathering feedback. If this is the case, the therapist may need to directly ask what was annoying or not helpful about the session.[4] Other times, when therapists have difficulty seeking feedback, it may be because of their own automatic thoughts about their abilities as a therapist, which hinders the process. So, as with the clients, attacking and testing those automatic thoughts often disarms their weight, allowing for therapists to move into gathering helpful feedback.[4,8]

SUMMARY

CT created a revolution in psychotherapy circles in the 1970s. In the twenty-first century, the approach is no longer a young sensation but a mature treatment approach embraced by many professionals from varied disciplines. CT has enjoyed a 40-year career, augmented by rigorous research and widening clinical practice. CT continued to evolve and further expand its scope. The cardinal principles, practice and processes, as well as its trademark session structure, equip clinicians and researchers for the future challenge of new frontiers.

REFERENCES

1. March JS. The future of psychotherapy for mentally ill children and adolescents. J Child Psychol Psychiatry 2009;50:170–9.
2. Beck AT. Cognitive therapy and the emotional disorders. New York: International Universities Press; 1976.

3. Alford BA, Beck AT. The integrative power of cognitive therapy. New York: Guilford; 1997.
4. Friedberg RD, McClure JM. Clinical practice of cognitive therapy with children and adolescents: the nuts and bolts. New York: Guilford; 2002.
5. Friedberg RD, McClure JM, Garcia JH. Cognitive therapy techniques for children and adolescents: tools for enhancing practice. New York: Guilford; 2009.
6. Beck AT. Cognitive therapy, behavior therapy, psychoanalysis, and pharmacotherapy: a cognitive continuum. In: Mahoney MJ, Freeman A, editors. Cognition and psychotherapy. New York: Plenum; 1985. p. 325–47.
7. Liotti G. The resistance to change of cognitive structures. J Cognit Psychother 1987;1:87–104.
8. Beck JS. Cognitive therapy: basics and beyond. New York: Guilford; 1995.
9. Kuyken W, Padesky CA, Dudley R. Collaborative case conceptualization: working effectively with clients in cognitive behavior therapy. New York: Guilford; 2008.
10. Bieling PJ, Kuyken W. Is cognitive case formulation science or science fiction. Clin Psychol Sci Pract 2003;10:892–902.
11. Kendall PC, Chu B, Gifford A, et al. Breathing life into a manual. Cognit Behav Pract 1998;5:89–104.
12. Persons JB. The case formulation approach to cognitive-behavioral psychotherapy. New York: Guilford; 2008.
13. Ehrenreich JT, Goldstein CM, Wright LR, et al. Development of a unified protocol for the treatment of emotional disorders in youth. Child Fam Behav Ther 2009;31: 20–37.
14. Chorpita BF. Modular cognitive behavioral therapy for childhood anxiety disorders. New York: Guilford; 2006.
15. Chorpita BF, Daleiden EL, Weisz JR. Identifying and selecting the common elements of evidence based interventions: a distillation and matching model. Ment Health Serv Res 2005;7:5–20.
16. Chorpita BF, Daleiden EL, Weisz JR. Modularity in the design and application of therapeutic interventions. Appl Prev Psychol 2005;11:141–56.
17. Kendall PC, Gosch E, Furr, et al. Flexibility within fidelity. J Am Acad Child Adolesc Psychiatry 2008;47:987–93.
18. Dattilio FM, Padesky CA. Cognitive therapy for couples. Sarasota (FL): Professional Resource Press; 1990.
19. Salkovskis PM. The cognitive approach to anxiety, threat beliefs, safety-seeking behavior and the special case of health anxiety and obsessions. In: Salkovskis PM, editor. Frontiers in cognitive therapy. New York: Guilford; 1996. p. 48–74.
20. Padesky CA. Developing cognitive therapist competency: teaching and supervision models. In: Salkovskis PM, editor. Frontiers in cognitive therapy. New York: Guilford; 1996. p. 266–92.
21. Perris C. Cognitive therapy with schizophrenic patients. New York: Guilford; 1989.
22. Beck AT, Rush AJ, Shaw BF, et al. Cognitive therapy of depression. New York: Guilford; 1979.
23. Padesky CA. Intensive training course in cognitive therapy. Newport Beach (CA): Center for Cognitive Therapy; 1988.
24. Padesky CA, Greenberg DP. Clinician's guide to mind over mood. New York: Guilford; 1995.
25. Chu BC, Suveg C, Creed TA, et al. Involvement shifts, alliance ruptures, and managing over therapy. In: Castro-Blanco D, Karver MS, editors. Elusive alliance: treatment engagement strategies with high risk adolescents. Washington, DC: American Psychological Association; 2010. p. 95–122.

26. Kendall PC, Comer JS, Marker CD, et al. In session exposure tasks and therapeutic alliance across the treatment of anxiety disorders. J Consult Clin Psychol 2009;77:517–25.

27. Creed TA, Kendall PC. Therapist alliance building within a cognitive behavioral treatment for anxiety in youth. J Consult Clin Psychol 2005;10:498–505.

28. Ronen T. Cognitive constructionist psychotherapy with children and adolescents. New York: Kluwer/Plenum; 2003.

29. Waddington L. The therapy relationship in cognitive therapy: a review. Behav Cognit Psychother 2002;30:179–91.

30. Southam-Gerow M. Some reasons that mental health treatments are not technologies: toward treatment development and adaptation outside labs. Clin Psychol Sci Pract 2004;11:186–9.

31. Pretzer JL, Beck AT. A cognitive theory of personality disorders. In: Clarkin JF, Lenzenweger MF, editors. Major theories of personality disorder. New York: Guilford; 1996. p. 36–105.

32. Waller G. Evidence based treatment and therapist drift. Behav Res Ther 2009;47:119–27.

33. Bandura AB. Social learning theory. Englewood Cliffs (NJ): Prentice-Hall; 1977.

34. Robins CJ, Hayes AM. An appraisal of cognitive therapy. J Consult Clin Psychol 1993;61:205–14.

35. Illardi SS, Feldman D. The cognitive neuroscience paradigm: a unifying meta-theoretical framework for the science and practice of clinical psychology. J Clin Psychol 2001;57:1067–88.

36. Padesky CA. Behavioral experiments. In: Bennett-Levy J, Butler G, Fenell M, et al, editors. Oxford guide to behavioral experiments in cognitive therapy. Oxford (UK): Oxford University Press; 2004. p. 433–8.

37. Samoilov A, Goldfried MR. The role of emotion in cognitive behavior therapy. Clin Psychol Sci Pract 2000;7:373–85.

38. Safran JD, Muran JC. Resolving therapeutic alliance ruptures: diversity and integration. J Clin Psychol 2001;56:233–43.

39. Wills F. Beck's cognitive therapy. London: Routledge; 2009.

40. Wright JH, Basco MR, Thase ME. Learning cognitive therapy. Washington, DC: American Psychiatric Publishing Inc; 2006.

41. Kovacs M. Children's depression inventory. North Tonawanda (NY): Multi-Health Systems; 1992.

42. Birmaher B, Khetarpal S, Brent D, et al. The Screen for Child Aanxiety Related Emotional Disorders (SCARED): scale construction and psychometric characteristics. J Am Acad Child Adolesc Psychiatry 1997;36:545–53.

43. Beck AT. Beck depression inventory-II. San Antonio (TX): Pearson; 1996.

44. March JS. Multidimensional Anxiety Scale for Children (MASC). Toronto: Multi-Health Systems; 1997.

45. Conners CK. Conner's Rating Scales–revised. North Tonawanda (NY): Multi-Health Systems; 1997.

46. Swanson JM, Sandman CA, Deutsch C, et al. Methylphenidate hydrochloride given with or before breakfast: I. Behavioral, cognitive, and electrophysiological effects. Pediatrics 1983;72:49–55.

Acceptance and Commitment Therapy (ACT): Advances and Applications with Children, Adolescents, and Families

Lisa W. Coyne, PhD[a],*, Louise McHugh, PhD[b],
Evan R. Martinez, BA[c]

KEYWORDS

- Acceptance and commitment therapy • Acceptance
- Commitment • Behavior therapy • Children • Parents

THE CONCEPTUAL FRAMEWORK OF ACCEPTANCE AND COMMITMENT THERAPY

Acceptance and commitment therapy (ACT; pronounced "act," not A-C-T) is a "third-wave" behavioral therapy that has attracted a great deal of empirical attention in its use with adults. A growing body of literature has supported its effectiveness across a broad array of psychiatric disorders and behavioral health issues. A recent meta-analysis[1] summarizes domains in which ACT has been shown to be useful, although the literature is still young.[2] Although this literature is rapidly expanding, in concert with other acceptance and mindfulness-based approaches, work with children, teens, and families is still in its infancy. Thus, herein the authors provide an overview of ACT and its theoretical underpinnings, describe assessment, therapy, and its adaptations with children, and provide a review of its evidence base to date.

ACT AND THE COGNITIVE-BEHAVIORAL TRADITION

ACT is a part of the cognitive-behavioral tradition, and yet is distinct from it in several ways. To appreciate those differences, it is important to consider how

The authors have nothing to disclose.
[a] Psychology Department, Early Childhood Research Clinic, Suffolk University, 41 Temple Street, Boston, MA 02114, USA
[b] School of Human and Health Sciences, Swansea University, Swansea SA2 8PP, UK
[c] Psychology Department, Suffolk University, 41 Temple Street, Boston, MA 02114, USA
* Corresponding author.
E-mail address: lcoyne@suffolk.edu

both ACT and cognitive-behavioral therapy (CBT) developed. ACT and other third-wave approaches, such as functional analytical psychotherapy (FAP),[3,4] dialectical behavior therapy (DBT),[5] and mindfulness-based stress reduction (MBSR)[6] arose in part out of a fundamental gap between the heuristic value of "second-wave" CBT approaches and their links to basic cognitive science.[1] CBT, in turn, was a response to a behavioral analytical perspective that did not adequately address human cognition in its theory of psychopathology, nor in its technology for behavior change. Thus, CBT was born of the clinical literature as a means to account for cognitive variables as treatment targets to foster symptom reduction in specific diagnostic entities such as major depressive disorder.[7] CBT models posit that behavioral change follows cognitive change, and treats thoughts as causal agents. Techniques that arose clinically (rather than empirically), such as addressing cognition through appealing to logic, cognitive restructuring, thought stopping, and using Socratic questioning, became tools in the therapeutic armamentarium. Symptom reduction, or helping individuals *feel* better through reduction of anxiety, depression, anger, and other intense, sustained emotions, as well as their related cognitions and behaviors, are explicit treatment goals.

While CBT makes conceptual sense, some argue that it has two major shortcomings. First, the links between CBT's therapeutic techniques with basic cognitive science are tenuous, at best.[1] Second, the tenet that cognitive change is necessary for behavioral change has garnered little support, at least in terms of treatment targeting depression.[8–10] Although CBT has a robust empirical base and has been shown to be efficacious in treating a variety of psychiatric disorders both in children and adults, treatment components targeting cognition explain little variance in outcomes over and above those targeting behavior.[9,11] Thus, it is not clear what cognitive techniques add over and above behavior therapy.[12,13] Moreover, it is not clear what the mechanisms of action may be, separate from purely traditional behavioral treatment components.

ACT differs from CBT in terms of its underlying philosophy of science and its scientific goals, as well as its theoretical and conceptual links to basic science of language and cognition. At its heart, ACT constitutes what has been called a "functional contextual" approach to human behavior. Whereas cognitive-behavioral models are mechanistic (stimuli enter, behavior ensues, consequences arise, and the cycle repeats), a core assumption of ACT's philosophy is that psychological events are ongoing, and best viewed within a situational and historical context. Said another way, it is meaningless (not to mention impossible) to isolate a behavior (including cognition) outside of its context. Thus, ACT assumes that (1) behaviors can have different functions for an individual in different domains, (2) different behaviors can belong to similar functional classes, and (3) behavioral change is best accomplished through manipulation of contextual factors that contain it. Contextual "meaning" that organizes behavior arises from one's learning history, and more specifically, language processes, described later.

ACT's core scientific goal is to provide an account of human behavior, including private events, linked with a technology of prediction and change. Thus, ACT uses a pragmatic, rather than ontological truth criterion—that is, it is more interested in how behavioral responses "work" for an individual rather than addressing behaviors as a symptom of a diagnostic entity. Moreover, thoughts and emotions are understood and addressed differently than in CBT: ACT is more interested in the contextual events that regulate and organize cognitions and link them with one another, than in the nature and development of cognitions themselves.[1] Because behavior is thought to be a function of its contingencies, one can change behavior through direct manipulation of maintaining contextual factors.

Similarly, with regard to cognition, an ACT therapist tends to be more interested in its *process,* or *function* (ie, how it *works* for an individual) rather than its *content* (ie, the *nature* of one's thoughts). An excellent example of this involves the work by Borkovec and colleagues[14] on worry. These investigators argued that the process of worry had particular functions for individuals with generalized anxiety disorder, namely the short-term avoidance of unpleasant physiological responses.[15] In the longer term, however, engagement in worry precluded exposure to and emotional processing of unwanted psychological events, and may prevent individuals from developing clear, concrete plans for coping with their stressors. The *content* of the worry (ie, *what* people worry about) was far less relevant than the *process* of worrying. Thus, an ACT therapist might explore how a particular stream of thought might work for an individual, and address this in functional analytical terms (eg, what does an individual gain or lose from engaging in this behavior? What function does this behavior serve?).

As one might guess, this philosophical framework has implications for the conceptualization and assessment of psychopathology. Primarily, as mentioned above, ACT focuses on the function of behavior rather than its topography. However, in considering what "works" for a given person, one must also ask the question, "for what?" In other words, ACT is most interested in what individuals value, and how effectively their behaviors support those values. Symptom reduction is not necessarily a goal from an ACT perspective. Or said another way, ACT is more interested in helping individuals lead valued lives than in helping individuals feel less anxious, depressed, and so forth. Symptom reduction is a side effect that is often observed once individuals start to progress through treatment and do things that matter to them. Thus, the metric by which psychological health is judged is broadened from symptom reduction to include how the individual as a whole organism is functioning with respect to valued domains. This may sound like a radical idea, until we begin to consider questions such as, "When you are less depressed, what would you be *doing*? How would things be different?" Progress, then, is measured in terms of how well one is living the life that one wants.

To summarize, the ACT model of behavioral change involves the manipulation of contextual variables on which behavior it depends. This idea is not a new one. In fact, it harkens to the very beginnings of behaviorism and applied behavior analysis. What is new is that ACT is deeply rooted in a basic science of language and cognition, or relational frame theory (RFT).

THE ROLE OF RFT AND LANGUAGE LEARNING PROCESSES IN BEHAVIOR

Possibly the most important feature of ACT is that it is grounded in a theory of language and cognition, RFT.[16] RFT is a functional analytical approach that accounts for the development of language and higher cognition in terms of learned generalized patterns of relational responding referred to as arbitrarily applicable relational responding (AARR). The simplest example of an arbitrary relation is the relation of coordination between words and their referents, which children begin to learn at around the age of 2 years. RFT proposes that AARR is acquired on the basis of a unique history of reinforcement, often provided by the human verbal community. Continued exposure to the socioverbal environment produces increasingly complex patterns of AARR including more extensive relations of coordination as well as relational patterns other than coordination including distinction, opposition, comparison, and so forth.[17]

The earliest and simplest form of AARR that is learned is the ability to respond to the symmetrical relations between words and objects. For example, a child may be taught to orient toward a particular object in the presence of a novel word in the context of an interaction, such as the following. A mother might say, "Where is the fire truck?" When the child looks at the fire truck, the mother responds, "Good boy!" This interaction may be represented as follows: Hear Name A—Orient toward Object B. The child may also be taught to produce the name or an approximation of the name in the presence of the object: [Fire truck shown to Child] "What is this?" [Child: "Fire truck"], "Good boy!" (See Object B—Produce Name A). Initially, the child must be explicitly taught each such symmetrical relation (ie, A–B; B–A). However, according to RFT, after a child has received a sufficient number of exemplars of bidirectional training in this relational response, eventually generalization occurs, so that contextual cues, such as "is" or the object-naming context itself, become sufficient to instantiate derived symmetrical relational responding with novel word-object combinations. In other words, at this point in time the child need be taught in only one direction (ie, either "name-object", or "object-name") and can then derive in the other direction (ie, "object-name", or "name-object", respectively). To build on this example, a toddler might learn that the spoken words "fire truck" refers to a photo of a fire truck, and then derive that the printed words "fire truck" refer to the photo and the spoken words. Thus, the earliest and most basic form of AARR is also the earliest and most basic form of language (ie, reference).

RFT research has also identified, and investigated, several other forms of arbitrarily applicable relations, or relational frames, in addition to the relations of coordination. These relations include those of "opposition",[18–21] "distinction",[19] "comparison" (eg, more than, less than),[22,23] "hierarchy",[24] "analogy",[25,26] "temporal relations",[23,27] and "deictic relations".[27]

According to RFT, all examples of this phenomenon possess the following 3 characteristics: mutual entailment (ie, the fundamental bidirectionality of relational responding), combinatorial entailment (ie, to a derived stimulus relation whereby 2 or more stimulus relations mutually combine), and transformation of stimulus functions, which refers to the transformation of psychologically relevant functions of a stimulus in accordance with the underlying derived relation in a given context.[16] The last of these 3 is particularly important from a psychological point of view, as it explains the power of language to change the meaning of stimuli. For instance, on hearing the words "fire truck," or seeing a photo of a fire truck, a child might experience a mental image of a fire truck speeding down the street, and some of the associated excitement.

In addition to these 3 main properties, AARR is always in accordance with relations between stimuli, which are determined, not by the physical characteristics of the stimuli involved but by additional, arbitrary contextual cues. Said another way, the meanings and psychological functions of elements in a particular relational frame are conferred by the context in which they are learned and, as such, are arbitrary. Contextual cues themselves are those features of the environment that predict reinforcement for a certain form of AARR.[28–30]

According to RFT, AARR and the transformation of stimulus functions provide us with a behavioral model of human language and cognition. Language and cognitive processes are associated with many psychopathologies,[31] and RFT provides an account of how these processes are learned. The contextually controlled relational nature of language as articulated by RFT suggests that rather than attempting to change aversive content, we should instead attempt to change the context in which aversive content occurs. ACT is a treatment package that has been designed to directly break down the literal hold that AARR has on human behavior.

THE ACT/RFT MODEL OF PSYCHOPATHOLOGY

An ACT/RFT model of psychopathology assumes that humans encounter pain, trauma, and loss, and that these experiences are part of life. However, *suffering* arises through the interaction of language processes with direct contingencies that create an unhelpful persistence and singular focus on managing or minimizing pain that precludes engagement in behavior toward valued domains. This end result is called psychological inflexibility, and is thought to arise from weak, ineffective contextual control over associative learning processes. As such, the ACT model of psychopathology is bound tightly to the processes described by RFT.

To illustrate these processes, consider a child who wants to feel less anxious. His peers and his parents may tell him not to worry about things, or that he's a "baby," when he shows fear. Thus he comes to understand, through a social context, that anxiety is bad, and should go away. Consequently, he begins to work very hard at not being anxious. He avoids situations that are anxiety-provoking, although it constrains his behavior and limits his opportunities to approach and thus extinguish his anxiety. However, the anxious thoughts persist. Next, perhaps he tries to not think about them, or to distract himself from them, or to replace them with coping thoughts. At the same time, he continues to attend to and struggle with those thoughts, which, through language learning processes, come to be related with the perceived effectiveness of his cognitive coping strategies. He attends more and more selectively and intensely to routing them out. However, after that fails to work, he begins to wonder what is wrong with himself that he cannot make them go away—and begins to think he might be broken, flawed, and a failure. Thus his anxiety is intensified.

This process so described illustrates two elements that ACT posits are central to the development and maintenance of psychopathology. The first is cognitive fusion, which in technical terms refers to "excessive or improper regulation of behavior by verbal processes"; specifically, derived relational networks.[1,32] In more general terms, this refers to the tendency to experience one's own thoughts and beliefs as literal or true. For example, a teen who misperceives an unintentional slight as having hostile intent might experience the thought, "I am a loser," as an accurate reflection of his or her own self-worth. When fused with one's own cognitive content, an individual is unable to contact *actual* environmental contingencies, and consequently is less likely to respond in effective, adaptive ways. Because verbal or cognitive elements are treated as *real*, an individual may become engaged in a pervasive pattern of avoidance of such elements.

Attempts to change, minimize, or otherwise control unwanted psychological experiences is termed experiential avoidance, and is the second element targeted by ACT.[33,34] This avoidance, in limited doses or used in the short term without excessive personal costs, is not a problem in and of itself. For example, children who use distraction to help tolerate immunizations may benefit from this strategy.[35] However, when individuals demonstrate excessive reliance on managing cognitive or verbal experiences, this is thought to contribute to the development of maladaptive behavioral repertoires. Exclusive reliance on experiential avoidance draws attention inward, toward the goals of managing unmanageable psychological events, and thus precluding attention to other, more meaningful pursuits. In this way, it may contribute to functional impairment across a broad range of diagnostic entities.

ACCEPTANCE AND COMMITMENT THERAPY COMPONENTS

The overarching goal of ACT is to foster psychological flexibility so that individuals may pursue goals in meaningful or valued domains. ACT targets experiential avoidance and cognitive fusion as toxic processes, and empowers individuals to engage in valued behaviors. Said simply, the core question in ACT is as follows: given a distinction between you and the things you are struggling with and trying to change, are you willing to experience those things, fully and without defense? Toward this end, ACT targets 6 psychological processes that it seeks to strengthen, and these may be divided into acceptance and mindfulness-based and behavior change processes (**Fig. 1**).[1]

Acceptance and Mindfulness Processes

Cognitive defusion can be conceptualized as deliteralization of thoughts; in other words, it refers to the process through which an individual comes to understand that his thoughts are merely verbal events rather than actual events. In contrast to CBT, which attempts to alter the *content* of one's thoughts, ACT attempts to alter the *function* of one's thoughts through changing how an individual interacts with them. For example, rather than a thought being perceived as a literal truth and serving as antecedents to avoidance, an individual might say, "I am having the thought that...." Experienced in this way, an individual might gain flexibility in choosing from a broader range of behaviors, even in the presence of a previously feared or avoided thought. Although cognitive defusion approaches address the context in which the thought is experienced, the experience of thoughts may change nonetheless. If certain cognitions are attached to physiological arousal or emotional discomfort, some of those functions may be diminished (although this is not an explicit therapeutic goal). This makes sense, given that data show that we cannot *unlearn* what we have learned. Some useful tools used for defusion include Titchner's repetition exercise, which involves the repetition of a word until the speaker experiences it as simply an auditory

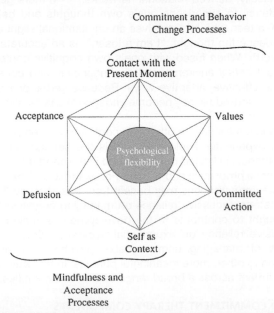

Fig. 1. The hexaflex model of the psychological processes ACT targets. (*From* Hayes S, Luoma J, Bond F, et al. Acceptance and commitment therapy: model, processes and outcomes. Behav Res Ther 2006;44:1–25; with permission.)

experience—a jumble of sounds—rather than experiencing its meaning.[36] Other tools that may be useful with children and teens are described elsewhere.[37,38]

Acceptance is an alternative to experiential avoidance, and comprises awareness and compassionate acceptance of unpleasant material without any attempts to alter or avoid it. In the case of chronic physical pain, an ACT therapist might draw a client's attention to it, or ask her to deliberately notice its quality, rather than distracting herself from it. This approach differs from a CBT model in that psychological health is concep-tualized as effective or appropriate emotion regulation, and that symptom reduction must occur in order for individuals to attain better psychosocial functioning. That being said, some cognitive-behavioral models appear to have shifted in a direction similar to ACT. In a parallel literature that has grown from emotion science, some have begun to posit emotion avoidance as a core process in anxiety and depression.[39–42] Generally speaking, in this model anxiety is conceptualized as "anxious apprehension," which is evoked by "cues or propositions" that may or may not be within an individual's aware-ness. Anxious apprehension results in a shift to an "internal, self-evaluative state," as an attempt to manage or cope with unpleasant affect.[39] Thus, anxious and depressed individuals are thought to have difficulties with emotion regulation, and thus newer treatment models, such as the Unified Protocol for Youth,[42] seek to foster better emotion regulation as an explicit treatment goal. However, ACT differs in that it attempts to foster acceptance in the context of pursuing valued ends, rather than for emotion regulation (or symptom reduction) in and of itself.

Present moment awareness is defined as ongoing, nonevaluative awareness of psychological and environmental events as they occur on a moment-to-moment basis. Rather than individuals rely on experiential avoidance and try to dismiss or mini-mize particular experiences, the goal of present moment awareness is that individuals be in direct, continuous contact with their worlds. This approach is thought to foster more behavioral flexibility, and thus more effective responses to actual, rather than internal, events. CBT approaches do not explicitly address or target this component. Within an ACT treatment package, therapists use exercises in which children are taught to focus their attention on particular aspects of situations. Another useful clin-ical tool involves discrimination training, in which children and teens are taught to discern when they are "in the moment," versus when they have become "hooked" by their thoughts and are "in their heads."

Self as context refers to the awareness that the self is distinct from and more than the sum total of thoughts. The self is experienced as a constant, unchanging perspec-tive from which one can observe thoughts, emotions, and external experiences as they come and go. RFT accounts for the development of perspective taking theory of mind and empathy in terms of deictic relations (ie, I-YOU, HERE-THERE, and NOW-THEN).[1,43] Understanding the self as a "context" through which thoughts, emotions, and physiological responses arise and ultimately pass gives some distance and perspective, reduces attachment to one's experiences, and promotes behavioral flex-ibility. CBT does not necessarily target these processes, although one could argue that cognitive restructuring techniques presuppose a stable self separate from the content of one's thoughts. Tools commonly used to promote self as context include experiential exercises. For example, a therapist might ask a child to imagine himself in a safe place, noticing strong emotions as they pass like storm clouds.

Values refer to domains of importance to individuals. Values are not goals that can be attained, but are rather guiding principles that are thought to motivate sustained and complex chains of behavior.[44] Because behaviors are enacted in the service of values, these behaviors themselves may come to have some of the rewarding psycho-logical properties of the valued domain. For example, a child may value "being a good soccer player." The nature of "being a good soccer player" may change across situations—perhaps the child makes a good pass during one game, or a few goals in another, or is integral in defending the goal. Behaviors that might lead to these include practice, attending to one's team mates, following the coach's directions, or showing bravery in the face of bigger, rougher, more aggressive children on the field. However, the child will not necessarily achieve the goal of "being a good soccer player" and simply disengage from these behaviors.

CBT does not focus explicitly on valued or meaningful domains, but does address engaging in pleasurable activities or events, yet still within the rubric of symptom reduction. Reduction of functional impairment is an explicit goal, but differs from the goals of ACT in that therapeutic "work" is targeted to remove an aversive outcome (eg, anxiety, depression) rather than to gain a desired outcome (eg, playing soccer well). This notion makes sense, as behavioral literature has demonstrated better sustainability in behaviors that are emitted in the service of earning rewards rather than avoiding unpleasant experiences.

Contextual functional analysis, in which children and teens explore what they care about, and how effectively they engage in "valuing" with respect to those domains, is a key ACT technique. Young people can also be taught to identify behaviors that move them in valued directions versus away from these directions. Also, it can be very useful in tailoring treatment to individual children to write specific behaviors from their own repertoires on cards, and ask children to sort them into separate piles of leading toward or leading away from a valued domain. Of course, it is important to highlight to children that different behaviors can have different functions across different contexts, so sorting should be revisited so children learn to understand how their behaviors "work" in particular settings.

ACT is also very explicit in its goal of fostering *committed action* in the service of one's valued goals. This is consistent with some forms of CBT that focus more exclusively on behavior, for example, behavioral activation.[45] Fostering committed action is a broad grouping of techniques that can include skills acquisition, exposure, shaping, goal setting, and so forth. Of importance, children are asked to commit to these behavioral goals—in other words, to "say yes and mean it." When individuals engage in committed action in the service of their values, they are typically brought into contact with previously avoided psychological experiences. To make a "commitment" to continued engagement in these behaviors implies willingness to have those experiences, and to persist in one's behaviors, even in the face of psychological discomfort. This is a cornerstone of the ACT model of psychological flexibility—to continue to pursue valued ends in the face of discomfort. It also lies at the heart of the difference between ACT and CBT, which holds that reduction of psychological discomfort is the primary goal, and is necessary to reduce functional impairment. CBT addresses this from a somewhat different perspective, namely, in terms of maintenance and relapse prevention. Specific therapeutic tools include making behavioral contracts, making public commitments (within and outside the context of therapy), and engaging others as a "team" to support the child or teen in his or her commitment to engage in valuing.

More recent work has simplified the ACT "hexaflex" conceptual model to a "triflex" model,[46] which is somewhat more streamlined and can help aid young people in understanding these processes and how they work together to form a whole. In this model, children and teens are invited to "open up, be present, and do what matters." One common misconception about ACT is that it is esoteric, and too complex to use with children. On the contrary, because ACT therapists rely more on experiential techniques and metaphors than on psychoeducation and rational arguments, it may actually be more readily used with children—even younger children—than CBT (**Fig. 2**).[46] However, the research base of ACT with children, teens, and families is still emerging.

RESEARCH BASE OF ACT WITH CHILDREN, TEENS, AND FAMILIES

Recent work has explored the role of experiential acceptance, mindfulness, and emotion awareness with adolescents.[47–49] In a year-long longitudinal study with a sample of 776 10th graders, prosocial tendencies were positively associated with "Acting with Awareness" (engaging fully in one's current activity with undivided attention), emotional awareness, and experiential acceptance, and all 3 variables uniquely predicted increases in well-being over the year, suggesting that these variables play a causal role in adolescent well-being.[47] In a study of 85 gay, lesbian, and bisexual youth in the 6th to 11th grades, psychological inflexibility and self-criticism jointly mediated the relationship between victimization, specifically verbal abuse and symptoms of depression.[48] This suggests that psychological inflexibility, in concert with self-critical thoughts, may help explain how verbal abuse confers risk of depression in lesbian, gay, bisexual, and transgender teens. McCracken and colleagues[49] found that greater self-reported acceptance was associated with less distress and disability, although not lower pain ratings, in a sample of 122 adolescents with severe chronic pain. Acceptance accounted for unique variance in distress, disability, and developmental and family functioning. Taken together, these studies suggest that the ACT-based constructs experiential avoidance, acceptance, and mindfulness are potentially important in adolescent well-being.

There has also been some indirect support that child or teen reliance on experiential avoidance, conceptualized as avoidant coping, has been linked with poor

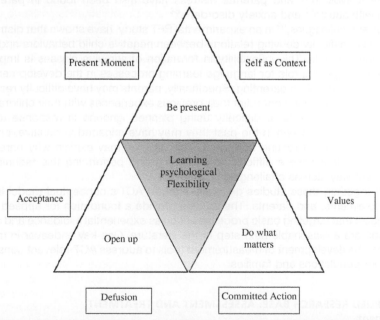

Fig. 2. Core ACT processes expressed as a triflex. (*From* Harris R. ACT made simple: an easy-to-read primer on acceptance and commitment therapy. Oakland (CA): New Harbinger Publications; 2009. p. 13; with permission.)

outcomes.[50–55] Strategies to cope with traumatic thoughts or memories have been associated with increased posttraumatic stress symptoms in urban children.[56] In addition, experiential avoidance has been linked with particular disorders. For example, in adult survivors of childhood sexual abuse, experiential avoidance mediated the relationship of childhood abuse and psychological distress[57] and substance abuse[58] in adulthood. Data from adolescents on worry,[59] chronic health issues,[60] and parent-child interaction showed that anxious children[61] with avoidance of thoughts or emotions was linked with poor psychological health. One recent theoretical article described the role of experiential avoidance in the development of childhood anxiety disorders.[41]

There is actually a small but robust literature on experiential avoidance in parents, and links with both parent and child emotional and behavioral functioning. In a sample of mothers with infants in a neonatal intensive care unit (NICU), experiential avoidance partially mediated the relationship between NICU-related stress and adjustment difficulties.[62] In mothers of preschool-aged children, as maternal empathic awareness decreased so did behaviorally measured parenting sensitivity, while mothers reported higher levels of depression and child behavior problems.[63] In a high-risk sample of 145 low-income, diverse, urban mothers, experiential avoidance was associated with maternal distress, maladaptive parenting practices, and child behavior problems. Further, experiential avoidance mediated the relationship between maternal depression and parenting stress.[64] In a similar sample (N = 74), mothers reporting higher levels of experiential avoidance also reported more depression, feeling less control in their parenting role, and describing more internalizing problems in their preschoolers.[65] In parents of adolescents, parental experiential avoidance significantly predicted inconsistent discipline, poor monitoring, and parental involvement, which in turn predicted adolescent behavior problems.[66] Links between parental experiential avoidance and parental distress have also been found in parents of children with autism[67] and anxiety disorders.[68]

Murrell and colleagues,[69] in an experimental RFT study, have shown that distressed parents have difficulty deriving relations between negative child behaviors and positive parenting words. This inflexibility in formation of stimulus classes is important because it suggests a role for language learning processes in the development and maintenance of impaired parenting. Specifically, parents may have difficulty responding to contingencies that contradict their previous experiences with their children. For example, parents may have difficulty using planned ignoring in response to mild disruptive behaviors, when in the past they may have engaged in punitive, or alternately, acquiescent parenting behaviors. This, in turn, may explain why parents of disruptive children have a difficult time learning and performing this technique in a consistent way, across challenging situations.

Taken together, these studies generally support ACT's conceptual model in children, adolescents, and parents. The studies provide a foundation for applied work, and suggest that targeting basic processes such as experiential avoidance and cognitive fusion are a reasonable next step in the literature. One key endeavor in moving forward is the development of measurement tools to address ACT-relevant constructs in younger populations and families.

ACT APPLIED RESEARCH BASE: ASSESSMENT AND TREATMENT
Assessment

Although there is significant research to support the assessment of ACT-based constructs such as experiential avoidance, fusion, and mindfulness in adults, work with children and adolescents is still emerging. Given that acceptance, mindfulness, and experiential avoidance are complex constructs, efforts to adapt extant measures, as well as create developmentally appropriate and sensitive measures for use with children, have lagged behind the adult literature. However, a small but growing body of literature has identified assessment tools that have shown some promise. Although a thorough review of recent work on assessment has been published elsewhere,[70] a handful of measures with the strongest empirical base for children and adolescents are briefly described here. Although these measures are promising, replication across samples, as well as testing these with diverse samples, are necessary next steps.

Measures of Acceptance and Mindfulness

The Child Acceptance and Mindfulness Measure (CAMM)[71] is a measure of children's awareness and acceptance of their own private events or internal experiences. The CAMM uses a Likert scale with higher scores linked to greater levels of awareness, attention, and acceptance. Evaluation for the CAMM was implemented with 606 public middle-school students as participants. The mean age of participants was 12.8 years with 62% of the population made up of girls. Empirical analysis of the results found that the CAMM has robust internal consistency ($\alpha = 0.82$) and acceptable concurrent validity.[70,71]

The Mindful Thinking and Action Scale for Adolescents (MTASA) (West A, Sbraga T, Poole D. Measuring mindfulness in youth: development of the mindful thinking and action scale for adolescents. Central Michigan University; unpublished data) was initially implemented in a sample made up of 163 children and adolescents with a mean age of 15.7 years and ranging in age from 11 to 19. The MTASA is a measure consisting of 32 items designed to assess mindful awareness in child and adolescent populations ranging in age from 11 to 19 years. Factor analysis yielded data on 4 factors: healthy self-regulation, active attention, awareness and observation, and accepting experience; and internal consistency ranged from 0.63 to 0.85 across the subscales. Strengths of this measure include its accessibility to younger populations, as well as inpatient or incarcerated youths.

The Chronic Pain Acceptance Questionnaire (adolescent version CPAQ[49]) was adapted from the Chronic Pain Acceptance Questionnaire,[72] an established measure used to assess willingness to experience chronic pain in adults. It is a 20-item measure composed of 2 subscales, pain willingness and activity engagement, and was initially implemented in a sample of 122 youths aged 10 to 18 years (mean 15.2 years) referred for pain management services at a tertiary care pain treatment center in the United Kingdom. "Pain willingness" comprises items tapping tendency to avoid or suppress pain, and "activity engagement" includes items measuring activity despite the experience of pain. Items are designed with a Likert-type scale of 0 to 4. Internal consistency was adequate (subscale αs = 0.86 for activity engagement, and 0.75 for pain willingness; 0.87 total score). Validity analyses suggest good psychometric properties.[49]

Values

Valuing is a core component of ACT, and involves engaging in behaviors that are consistent with domains of importance. The Personal Values Questionnaire (PVQ)[73] and Social Values Survey (SVS)[74] assess effectiveness in the pursuit of personal goals in child and adolescent populations. The PVQ evaluates valued domains in adolescents and adults across 9 areas: social relationships/friendships, family relationships, romantic relationships, recreation/leisure/sport, spirituality/religion, work/career, physical health, and community involvement. Respondents rate items on a 1 to 5 Likert scale regarding how important each domain is, how successful they are at pursuing their values, why pursuit of these values are important (eg, to avoid undesired outcomes, or to work toward desired outcomes), how personally meaningful the domain is, and how strong is their desire to improve adherence to their valued pursuits. The SVS is similar, but focuses more on intrinsic versus extrinsic motivations for interpersonal relationships. Although not yet published, preliminary data suggest that youths reporting more intrinsic motivations experience more joy and less sadness, whereas those reporting more extrinsic motivations experience more hostility.[75]

Experiential Avoidance/Psychological Inflexibility

The Avoidance and Fusion Questionnaire for Youths (AFQ-Y)[76] is a 17-item self-report measure developed for use with children, and modeled after the Acceptance and Action Questionnaire (AAQ),[34] to assess psychological inflexibility.[77] The questionnaire identifies psychological inflexibility as the presence of experiential avoidance, cognitive fusion, and behavioral ineffectiveness when faced with unpleasant emotions and situations. Respondents rate items on a Likert scale with low scores indicating greater psychological flexibility. The AFQ-Y was administered to 1369 children divided across 5 samples, with ages ranging from 9 to 17 years. Population was made up of approximately 45% boys and 55% girls with 80% identifying as Caucasian. Analysis found that both versions of AFQ-Y had good internal consistency ($\alpha = 0.90$–0.93) and convergent validity.[77]

Experiential Avoidance in Parents

The Parental Acceptance and Action Questionnaire (PAAQ)[78] was also developed based on the AAQ, and evaluates parents' experiential acceptance, and action tendencies in the context of their relationship with their children. It is a 15-item measure and, like previous measures, listed has been adapted from the AAQ.[34,79] Items use a 7-point Likert scale, and respondents rate how much each item describes them. The PAAQ was investigated using 154 children (90 females, 64 males) who were diagnosed with anxiety disorders based on DSM (*Diagnostic and Statistical Manual of Mental Disorders*) criteria and their parents (148 mothers, 119 fathers) as participants. The test was administered to parents along with other self-report measures designed to target adult experiential avoidance, psychopathology in the parent, affective expression, and parental control behaviors. Factor analysis of the PAAQ resulted in a two-factor solution broken into Inaction and Unwillingness. The PAAQ possessed a moderate temporal stability, $r = 0.68$–0.74, with fair internal consistency across the subscales ($\alpha = 0.64$–0.65). The clinical application of PAAQ was also supported by the measures ability to predict a significant amount of variance in the rated levels of child anxiety between the parent and the clinician.[68]

Treatment

Despite the accruing evidence from ACT/RFT research on basic processes, as well as the development of several measures for use with children, treatment adaptations with children have lagged behind. Most are single-case or small-sample, uncontrolled studies, although recent work has included some larger, randomized controlled trials. Given the developing state of this literature, any inferences regarding the efficacy of ACT with children and teens are premature. However, the results of these studies are generally consistent, and suggest that ACT is a feasible and acceptable treatment for young people that may offer an alternative to strictly behavioral and cognitive treatment models.[80] Moreover, due to ACT's attention to context and because it is based on principles rather than being bound to particular diagnostic entities, it may serve as a flexible intervention applied across a host of issues germane to children, teens, and families. It is certainly an exciting approach that merits further research.

Anxiety and Depression

There are 2 published case studies describing ACT for children with clinically significant anxiety. Heffner and colleagues[81] report using ACT to successfully reduce school refusal, maintained at 2-year follow up, of an 11-year-old male. Using an ACT protocol of 8 individual and 4 family sessions, Morris and Greco[82] reported a reduction of social anxiety and increased school attendance. With regard to nonclinical populations, one recent study reports the use of ACT with an 18-year-old moderately mentally retarded female experiencing obsessive thoughts and symptoms of anxiety.[83] After 17 sessions of ACT adapted for her developmental level, the client reported less experiential avoidance and more social confidence, and returned to school. In addition, her parents reported that she was calmer, and that her anxiety "episodes" were shorter in duration. Gains were maintained at 4-month follow-up. The investigators note that adapting ACT for individuals with disabilities was challenging, although results from this case study suggest their potential feasibility. In one group design in an open trial, ACT was shown to reduce anxiety associated with chess performance in a nonclinical population of adolescents.[84]

In a recent randomized controlled trial with 38 clinically referred adolescents of mean age 14.9 years (SD = 2.55), with 73.6% in the clinical range for depression, compared an ACT treatment adapted for teens with a treatment as usual (TAU) condition (Hayes L, Boyd CP, Sewell J. Acceptance and commitment therapy for the treatment of adolescent depression: a pilot study in a psychiatric setting. Under review.). Participants in the ACT condition reported significantly lower depression levels than those in the TAU group, and actually showed some further improvement from posttreatment to 3-month follow up. Both groups showed significant improvement in global functioning, although on clinical measures only the ACT group made gains. The investigators caution that small sample size limited inferences that may be drawn from this study, although they suggest that results support a larger, more rigorous clinical trial with clinically depressed teens.

Chronic Pain

Wicksell and colleagues[85] used an ACT protocol in a case study with a 14-year-old girl who was diagnosed with idiopathic generalized pain, and who had missed all 60 days of school in the 2 months before treatment. Treatment included 10 individual sessions, resulting in a reduction in emotional avoidance and marked gains in school attendance, with no absences through the 6-month follow up. Functional disability and pain were reduced at posttreatment and eliminated at 6-month follow-up. In a later uncontrolled pilot study using ACT for teens with chronic pain,[86] improvements in functional ability, school attendance, catastrophizing, and pain were observed and retained at both the 3- and 6-month follow-up. Greco[87] used an ACT protocol for 15 teens with functional abdominal pain recruited from a pediatric gastroenterology clinic. Treatment consisted of 12 to 14 sessions with the adolescents, and 2 to 5 parenting sessions. Participants reported significant increases in quality of life, and significantly decreased functional disability posttreatment and at 1-month follow-up. In addition, adolescents reported reduced somatic complaints and internalizing symptoms at 1-month follow-up.

In a small randomized controlled trial with 32 adolescents severely disabled by chronic pain, Wiksell and colleagues[88] compared the efficacy of ACT to a multidisciplinary treatment (MDT) including the use of amitriptyline. In 10 sessions, the ACT treatment focused on reducing functional impairment and enhancing quality of life through fostering participants' ability to engage in valued activities in the context of chronic pain and associated distress. Results suggested that teens in the ACT condition had significantly improved functioning compared with the MDT group, and that these gains were maintained at 3.5- and 6.5-month follow-up. Specifically, compared with MDT participants, ACT participants reported significantly improved functional ability, fear of reinjury, pain interference, and quality of life. These preliminary findings suggest that ACT may be a useful approach for youth with severe chronic pain conditions.

Anorexia Nervosa

To date, there is only one published case study describing ACT with eating disorders in adolescents. Heffner and colleagues[81] integrated ACT with traditional CBT and family interventions to treat a young 15-year-old Caucasian girl with anorexia. Over the course of the 14-session therapy and 4 follow-up sessions, the investigators note a reduction in anorectic symptoms and drive for thinness. In addition, the client increased to normal weight range over the course of treatment and follow-up. However, despite her gains on other measures she still displayed clinical levels of body dissatisfaction at termination.

Merwin and colleagues[89] have developed an ACT-based family intervention for anorexia nervosa. The intervention targets families with high expressed emotion, as these tend not to fare well in traditional CBT for anorexia. Treatment consists of 20 sessions, 16 of which separate parents and teens, and 4 that are conjoint. Teens participate in an ACT protocol, while parents are taught skills from an ACT-based perspective to help extinguish their children's anorectic behaviors and reinforce alternatives. To date, a feasibility study and small open trial are under way, and preliminary data are promising.

Psychosis

There is one case study published in Spanish, describing the use of ACT with a 17-year-old male diagnosed with schizophrenia and experiencing ego-dystonic auditory hallucinations.[90,91] Although the client was receiving antipsychotic medication, there was no reduction in auditory hallucinations. He was treated with ACT twice per week for 9 weeks. At posttreatment, the investigators reported a 40% reduction in hallucinations, and therefore reduced his antipsychotic medication. He maintained gains until 7 months posttreatment, at which point he experienced a personal crisis and his dosage of antipsychotic medication increased.

Parenting Interventions

Coyne and Wilson[92] described ACT used in conjunction with Parent-Child Interaction Therapy (PCIT)[93,94] for a 6-year-old male with severe aggression and noncompliance that had resulted in an extended suspension from school. PCIT is an in vivo parent training protocol used to teach parents appropriate child-directed behavior, as well as to teach effective behavior management skills for children with externalizing difficulties. ACT components were used as a way to reduce the psychological barriers that would restrict new skill acquisition. For example, mindfulness and defusion procedures were incorporated with the planned ignoring and other components of the PCIT. Treatment continued for approximately 3 months. At both termination and 1-year follow-up, overt behavioral outcomes included a decrease in the child's levels of aggression and noncompliant behavior and an increase in his mother's appropriate management behavior, as well as her own pursuit of valued activities. The mother also reported better relationship quality and greater competence in her parenting skill.

In a small open trial, Blackledge and Hayes[67] designed a 2-day, 14-hour group experiential ACT workshop for 20 parents of children with autism. These investigators observed a significant, but modest, decrease in parent distress at 3-month follow-up, with larger gains in parents reporting clinical levels of symptomatology. Avoidance and fusion were similarly reduced from baseline to follow-up, and results suggested that fusion mediated the relationship between treatment and symptom reduction. To date, the authors are aware of at least 3 other ongoing studies in very early stages exploring the use of ACT with parents of young children (preschool-aged) and elementary school–aged children.

At-Risk Youth: Prevention

There is only one reported study describing the use of ACT for prevention. Metzler and colleagues[95] conducted a randomized controlled trial for adolescents to prevent sexually transmitted diseases (STDs). Three hundred and thirty-nine diverse adolescents (aged 15–19 years) were recruited from STD clinics and randomized into treatment and "usual care" control conditions. The treatment group received a 5-session intervention that integrated ACT components into a social-cognitive approach targeting safe sex skills and responsible decision making in that domain. At 6-month follow-up, there were no differences across the 2 groups in terms of frequency of STD infections. However, the treatment group reported significantly fewer risky sexual behaviors (ie, sexual contacts with strangers, nonmonogamous partners, use of alcohol or marijuana before engaging in intercourse), and more acceptance of emotions. In addition, those in the treatment group were able to suggest more safe-sex alternatives than the control group in response to a video-taped sexual situation role play.

SUMMARY

ACT is a third-wave CBT that targets experiential avoidance and cognitive fusion as core elements of psychopathology. ACT harnesses several therapeutic techniques that specifically target these processes, and as its overarching treatment goal seeks to promote psychological flexibility in the pursuit of a meaningful, valued life, in the presence of psychological or physical pain. Although ACT is a part of the cognitive-behavioral tradition, it constitutes an extension to this literature in terms of its philosophy (functional contextualist vs mechanistic), in how it addresses cognition (changing the context giving rise to cognitions rather than the content of cognitions), and in its evidence base (links of hypothesized processes contributing to psychopathology as well as its treatment techniques to basic cognitive science; namely, RFT). In addition, it differs in terms of its tendency to rely on experiential rather than didactic therapeutic tools, and its more holistic view of psychological health as effectively engaging in behaviors consistent with values, even in the presence of great pain, rather than focusing on reduction of symptoms and functional impairment. As such, ACT constitutes an important advance in cognitive-behavioral treatment, and holds promise as a potentially useful treatment for youth populations.

ACT has several strengths, and its evidence base with adults is rapidly expanding. Across several studies and with a variety of clinical issues, ACT has performed as well as, if not better than, comparison treatments, including CBT. In addition, there are several studies suggesting that the proposed mechanisms of treatment—reduction in experiential avoidance and cognitive fusion—account for variance in treatment gains. With regard to children, there are several studies linking these constructs with psychosocial outcomes in children, teens, and parents; this is exciting given the relative age of this literature. However, there are clear areas for growth in applications with children, adolescents, and families.

First, as with any emerging treatment literature, the rigor of applied studies with youth populations varies: other than a handful of single-case studies, some small-sample open trials, and a few preliminary randomized controlled trials, ACT with youth is still a work in progress. Larger samples, randomized controlled trials that compare ACT with gold standard treatments, as well as careful investigation of mediators, moderators, and mechanisms of treatment, are much needed. In addition, very few reported studies—both in the adult and the child literature—specifically investigate ACT with diverse, underserved samples. Work exploring the feasibility and acceptability of ACT, as well as its efficacy, would strengthen its evidence base. Although several measures tapping ACT constructs have been developed for adults and children, replication across different samples would strengthen this body of work.

In recent years there has been unparalleled growth in the area of developmental psychopathology, and cognitive and affective neuroscience. Specifically, several constructs similar to those addressed in ACT, namely, emotion regulation and emotional intelligence, have begun to garner empirical attention. In addition, clearer links between child development and ACT treatment techniques would facilitate tailoring this approach to younger children. Translational work linking ACT with the developmental psychopathology literature would be an exciting avenue to explore.

ACKNOWLEDGMENTS

The authors would like to acknowledge Steven Hayes, Amy Murrell, and Rhonda Merwin for their helpful comments and suggestions on the manuscript.

REFERENCES

1. Hayes S, Luoma J, Bond F, et al. Acceptance and commitment therapy: model, processes and outcomes. Behav Res Ther 2006;44:1–25.
2. Ost L. Efficacy of the third wave of behavioral therapies: a systematic review and meta-analysis. Behav Res Ther 2008;48:296–321.
3. Kanter J, Tsai M, Kohlenberg R. The practice of functional analytic psychotherapy. New York: Springer Science + Business Media; 2010. p. 272.
4. Kohlenberg R, Tsai M. Functional analytic psychotherapy: creating intense and curative therapeutic relationships. New York: Plenum Press; 1991. p. 217.
5. Linehan M. Cognitive-behavioral treatment of borderline personality disorder. New York: Guilford Press; 1993. p. 558.
6. Segal Z, Williams M, Teasdale J. Mindfulness-based cognitive therapy for depression: a new approach to preventing relapse. New York: Guilford Press; 2002. p. 351.
7. Beck A, Rush A, Shaw B, et al. Cognitive therapy for depression. New York: Guilford Press; 1979. p. 425.
8. Gortner E, Gollan J, Dobson K, et al. Cognitive-behavioral treatment for depression: relapse prevention. J Consult Clin Psychol 1998;66:377–84.
9. Jacobson N, Dobson K, Truax P, et al. A component analysis of cognitive-behavioral treatment for depression. J Consult Clin Psychol 1996;64:295–304.
10. Zettle R, Hayes S. Component and process analysis of cognitive therapy. Psychol Rep 1987;61:939–53.

11. Dimidjian S, Hollon S, Dobson K, et al. Randomized trial of behavioral activation, cognitive therapy, and antidepressant medication in the acute treatment of adults with major depression. J Consult Clin Psychol 2006;74:658–70.
12. Dobson K, Khatri N. Cognitive therapy: looking backward, looking forward. J Clin Psychol 2000;56:907–23.
13. Ilardi S, Craighead E. 1994 The role of nonspecific factors in cognitive-behavior therapy for depression. Clin Psychol Sci Pract 1994;1:138–56.
14. Borkovec T, Ray W, Stober J. Worry: a cognitive phenomenon intimately linked to affective, physiological, and interpersonal behavioral processes. Cognit Ther Res 1998;22:561–76.
15. Borkovec T, Hu S. The effect of worry on cardiovascular response to phobic imagery. Behav Res Ther 1990;8:69–73.
16. Hayes S, Barnes-Holmes D, Roche B. Relational frame theory: a post-skinnerian account of human language and cognition. New York: Kluwer Academic/Plenum Publishers; 2001. p. 285.
17. Whelan R, Barnes D. The transformation of consequential functions in accordance with the relational frames of same and opposite. J Exp Anal Behav 2004;82:177–95.
18. Dymond S, Barnes D. Behavior analytic approaches to self-awareness. Psychol Rec 1997;47:181–200.
19. Roche B, Barnes D. Arbitrarily applicable relational responding and human sexual categorization: a critical test of the derived difference relation. Psychol Rec 1996;46:451–75.
20. Roche B, Barnes D. A transformation of respondently conditioned stimulus function in accordance with arbitrarily applicable relations. J Exp Anal Behav 1997;67: 275–300.
21. Steele D, Hayes S. Stimulus equivalence and arbitrarily applicable relational responding. J Exp Anal Behav 1991;56:519–55.
22. Dymond S, Barnes D. A transformation of self-discrimination response functions in accordance with the arbitrarily applicable relations of sameness, more-than, and less-than. J Exp Anal Behav 1995;64:163–84.
23. O'Hora D, Roche B, Barnes-Holmes D, et al. Response latencies to multiple derived stimulus relations: testing two predictions of relational frame theory. Psychol Rec 2002;52:51–76.
24. Griffee K, Dougher M. Contextual control of stimulus generalization and stimulus equivalence in hierarchical categorization. J Exp Anal Behav 2002;78:433–47.
25. Barnes D, Hegarty N, Smeets P. Relating equivalence relations to equivalence relations: a relational framing model of complex human functioning. The Analysis of Verbal Behavior 1997;14:1–27.
26. Stewart I, Barnes-Holmes D, Roche B. A functional-analytic model of analogy using the relational evaluation procedure. Psychol Rec 2004;54:531–52.
27. O'Hora D, Barnes-Holmes D, Roche B, et al. Derived relational networks and control by novel instructions: a possible model of generative verbal responding. Psychol Rec 2004;54:437–60.
28. Bush K, Sidman M, de Rose T. Contextual control of emergent equivalence relations. J Exp Anal Behav 1989;51:29–46.
29. Kennedy C, Laitinen R. Second-order conditional control of symmetric and transitive stimulus relations: the influence of order effects. Psychol Rec 1988;38: 437–46.
30. Wulfert E, Hayes S. Transfer of a conditional ordering response through conditional equivalence classes. J Exp Anal Behav 1988;50:125–44.

31. Williams C. Overcoming depression: a five areas approach. London: Arnold; 2001.
32. Hayes S, Wilson K, Strosahl K. Acceptance and commitment therapy: an experiential approach to behavior change. New York: Guilford Press; 1999. p. 304.
33. Hayes S, Wilson K, Gifford E, et al. Experiential avoidance and behavioral disorders: a functional dimensional approach to diagnosis and treatment. J Consult Clin Psychol 1996;64:1152–68.
34. Hayes S, Wilson K, Strosahl K, et al. Measuring experiential avoidance: a preliminary test of a working model. Psychol Rec 2004;54:553–78.
35. Cohen L, Bernard R, Greco L, et al. Using a child-focused intervention to manage procedural pain: are parent and nurse coaches necessary? J Pediatr Psychol 2002;27:749–57.
36. Masuda A, Hayes S, Sackett C, et al. Cognitive defusion and self-relevant negative thoughts: examining the impact of a ninety year old technique. Behav Res Ther 2004;42:477–85.
37. Greco L, Barnett E, Blomquist K, et al. Acceptance, body image, and health in adolescence. In: Greco LA, Hayes SC, editors. Acceptance and mindfulness treatments for children and adolescents: a practitioner's guide. Oakland (CA): New Harbinger Publications; 2008. p. 187–214.
38. Murrell A, Coyne L, Wilson K. Treating children with acceptance and commitment therapy. In: Hayes SC, Strosahl K, editors. Acceptance and commitment therapy: a clinician's guide. New York: Guilford Press; 2004. p. 249–74.
39. Barlow D. Unraveling the mysteries of anxiety and its disorders from the perspective of emotion theory. Am Psychol 2000;55:1247–63.
40. Barlow D, Allen L, Choate M. Toward a unified treatment for emotional disorders. Behav Ther 2004;35:205–30.
41. Tiwari S, Podell J, Martin E, et al. Experiential avoidance in the parenting of anxious youth: theory, research, and future directions. Cognit Emot 2008;22:480–96.
42. Trosper S, Buzzella B, Bennett S, et al. Emotion regulation in youth with emotional disorders: implications for a unified treatment approach. Clin Child Fam Psychol Rev 2009;12:234–54.
43. McHugh L, Barnes-Holmes Y, Barnes-Holmes D. Perspective-taking as relational responding: a developmental profile. Psychol Rec 2004;54:115–44.
44. Wilson K, Murrell A. Values work in acceptance and commitment therapy: setting a course for behavioral treatment. In: Hayes SC, Follette VM, Linehan MM, editors. Mindfulness and acceptance: expanding the cognitive-behavioural tradition. New York: Guilford Press; 2004. p. 120–51.
45. Martell C, Addis M, Jacobson NS. Depression in context: strategies for guided action. New York: WW Norton & Co; 2001. p. 223.
46. Russ H, Hayes M. ACT made simple: an easy-to-read primer on acceptance and commitment therapy. Oakland (CA): New Harbinger; 2007. p. 265.
47. Ciarrochi J, Kashdan T, Leeson P, et al. On being aware and accepting: a one-year longitudinal study into adolescent well-being. J Adolesc, October 14, 2010 [online].
48. Armelie AP, Delahanty PL, Boarts JM. The impact of verbal abuse on depression symptoms in lesbian, gay, and bisexual youth: the roles of self-criticism and psychological inflexibility. Poster presented at the June 2010 Association for Contextual and Behavioral Science. Reno (NV), June 21, 2010.
49. McCracken LM, Gauntlett-Gilbert J, Eccleston C. Acceptance of pain in adolescents with chronic pain: validation of an adapted assessment instrument and preliminary correlation analyses. Eur J Pain 2010;2010(14):316–20.

50. Fields L, Prinz R. Coping and adjustment during childhood and adolescence. Clin Psychol Rev 1997;17:937–76.
51. Marsac M, Funk J, Nelson L. Coping styles, psychological functioning and quality of life in children with asthma. Child Care Health Dev 2007;33:360–7.
52. Ollendick T, Langley A, Jones R, et al. Fear in children and adolescents: relations with negative life events, attributional style, and avoidant coping. J Child Psychol Psychiatry 2001;42:1029–34.
53. Orsmond G, Kuo H, Seltzer M. Siblings of individuals with an autism spectrum disorder: sibling relationships and wellbeing in adolescence and adulthood. Autism 2009;13:59–80.
54. Reijntjes A, Steege H, Terwogt M, et al. Children's coping with in vivo peer rejection: an experimental investigation. An official publication of the International Society for Research in Child and Adolescent Psychopathology. J Abnorm Child Psychol 2006;34:877–89.
55. Steiner H, Erickson S, Hernandez N, et al. Coping styles as correlates of health in high school students. J Adolesc Health 2002;30:326–35.
56. Dempsey M, Overstreet S, Moely B. 'Approach' and 'avoidance' coping and PTSD symptoms in inner-city youth. Curr Psychol 2000;19:28–45.
57. Marx B, Sloan D. The role of emotion in the psychological functioning of adult survivors of childhood sexual abuse. Behav Ther 2002;33:563–77.
58. Simons L, Ducotte J, Kirkby K, et al. Childhood trauma, avoidance coping, and alcohol and other drug use among women in residential and outpatient treatment programs. Alcohol Treat Q 2003;21:37–54.
59. Laugesen N, Dugas M, Bukowski W. Understanding adolescent worry: the application of a cognitive model. An official publication of the International Society for Research in Child and Adolescent Psychopathology. J Abnorm Child Psychol 2003;31:55–64.
60. Moos R. Life stressors, social resources, and coping skills in youth: applications to adolescents with chronic disorders. J Adolesc Health 2002;30:22–9.
61. Barrett P, Rapee R, Dadds M, et al. Family enhancement of cognitive style in anxious and aggressive children. An official publication of the International Society for Research in Child and Adolescent Psychopathology. J Abnorm Child Psychol 1996;24:187–203.
62. Greco L, Heffner M, Poe S, et al. Maternal adjustment following preterm birth: contributions of experiential avoidance. Behav Ther 2005;36:177–84.
63. Coyne L, Miller A, Low C, et al. Mothers' empathic understanding of their toddlers: associations with maternal sensitivity and depression. J Child Fam Stud 2007;16:483–97.
64. Shea S, Coyne L. Maternal dysphoric mood, stress and parenting practices in mothers of preschoolers: the role of experiential avoidance. J Child Family Behav Therapy, in press.
65. Coyne L, Thompson A. Maternal depression, locus of control, and emotion regulatory strategy as predictors of child internalizing problems. J Child Fam Stud, February 1, 2011 [online].
66. Berlin K, Sato A, Jastrowski K, et al. Effects of experiential avoidance on parenting practices and adolescent outcomes. In: KS Berlin, AR Murrell (Chairs). Extending acceptance and mindfulness research to parents, families, and adolescents: process, empirical findings, clinical Implications, and future directions. Symposium presented to the 2006 Association for Behavioral and Cognitive Therapies. Chicago, November 17, 2006.

67. Blackledge J, Hayes S. Using acceptance and commitment training in the support of parents of children diagnosed with autism. Child Fam Behav Ther 2006;28:1–18.
68. Cheron D, Ehrenreich J, Pincus D. Assessment of parental experiential avoidance in a clinical sample of children with anxiety disorders. Child Psychiatry Hum Dev 2009;40:383–403.
69. Murrell A, Wilson K, LaBorde C, et al. Relational responding in parents. Behav Analyst Today 2009;9:196–214.
70. Coyne L, Cheron D, Ehrenreich J. Assessment of acceptance and mindfulness processes in youth. In: L Greco, editor. Acceptance and mindfulness interventions for children, adolescents, and families. Reno (NV): Context Press; 2008. p. 37–62.
71. Greco L, Baer R. Child acceptance and mindfulness measure (CAMM) available from the first author at Department of Psychology. St Louis (MO): University of Missouri.
72. McCracken LM, Vowles KE, Eccleston C. Acceptance of chronic pain: component analysis and a revised assessment method. Pain 2004;107:159–66.
73. Blackledge J, Ciarrochi J. Personal values questionnaire. Available from the first author at University of Wollongong. New South Wales (Australia); 2006.
74. Blackledge J, Ciarrochi J. Social values survey. Available from the first author at University of Wollongong. New South Wales (Australia); 2006.
75. Ciarrochi J, Bilich L. Acceptance and commitment measures packet: process measures of potential relevance to ACT. 2006. Available at: www.uow.edu.au/health/iimh/act_researchgroup/resources.html. Accessed July 11, 2010, from University of Wollongong website.
76. Greco L, Murrell A, Coyne L. Avoidance and fusion questionnaire for youth. Available at: www.contextualpsychology.org. The first author at Department of Psychology. Accessed September 5, 2010.
77. Greco L, Lambert W, Baer R. Psychological inflexibility in childhood and adolescence: development and evaluation of the avoidance and fusion questionnaire for youth. Psychol Assess 2008;20:93–102.
78. Ehrenreich J, Cheron D. Parental acceptance and action questionnaire. Boston (MA): Boston University.
79. Bond F, Bunce D. The role of acceptance and job control in mental health, job satisfaction, and work performance. J Appl Psychol 2003;88:1057–106.
80. Murrell A, Scherbath A. State of the Research & Literature address: ACT with children, adolescents and parents. International Journal of Behavioral Consultation and Therapy 2006;2:431–43.
81. Heffner M, Sperry J, Eiftert GH, et al. Acceptance and commitment therapy in the treatment of an adolescent female with anorexia nervosa: a case example. Cognit Behav Pract 2002;9:232–6.
82. Morris T, Greco L. Incorporating parents and peers in the assessment and treatment of childhood anxiety. In: VandeCreek L, Jackson TL, editors. Innovations in clinical practice: a source book, vol. 20. Sarasota (FL): Professional Resource Press/Professional Resource Exchange; 2002. p. 75–85.
83. Brown FJ, Hooper S. Acceptance and commitment therapy (ACT) with a learning-disabled young person experiencing anxious and obsessive thoughts. J Intellect Disabil 2009;13:195–201.
84. Ruiz-Jimenez, Luciano-Soriano. Improving chess performance with ACT. In: JT Blackledge (Chair). Applications of Acceptance and Commitment Therapy with children and adolescents. Symposium presented at the 32nd annual meeting of the Association for Behavior Analysis. Atlanta (GA): 2006.

85. Wicksell R, Dahl J, Magnusson B, et al. Using acceptance and commitment therapy in the rehabilitation of an adolescent female with chronic pain: a case example. Cognit Behav Pract 2005;12:415–23.

86. Wicksell R, Melin L, Olsson G. Exposure and acceptance in the rehabilitation of adolescents with idiopathic chronic pain-a pilot study. Eur J Pain 2007;11: 267–74.

87. Greco L. Acceptance and change among youth with chronic pain conditions. In: JT Blackledge (Chair). Applications of acceptance and commitment therapy with children and adolescents. Symposium presented at the 32nd annual meeting of the Association for Behavior Analysis. Atlanta (GA), May 24, 2006.

88. Wicksell RK, Melin L, Lekander M, et al. Evaluating the effectiveness of exposure and acceptance strategies to improve functioning and quality of life in longstanding pediatric pain—a randomized controlled trial. Pain 2009;141:248–57.

89. Merwin RM, Timko AC, Zucker NL, et al. ACT-based family intervention for adolescents with anorexia nervosa. Paper presented at the Association for Behavioral and Contextual Science. Reno (NV), July 23, 2010.

90. Garcia-Montes J, Pérez-Álvarez M. ACT as a treatment for psychotic symptoms: the case of auditory hallucinations. Análisis y Modificación 2001;27:455–72.

91. Veiga-Martinez C, Perez-Alvarez M, Garcia-Montes J. Acceptance and commitment therapy applied to treatment of auditory hallucinations. Clin Case Stud 2008;7:118.

92. Coyne L, Wilson K. Cognitive fusion in impaired parenting: an RFT analysis. Int J Psychol Psychol Ther 2004;4:469–86.

93. Eyberg S. Parent-child interaction therapy: integration of traditional and behavioral concerns. Child Fam Behav Ther 1988;10:33–46.

94. McNeil CB, Hembree-Kigin TL. Parent child interaction therapy. 2nd edition. New York: Springer; 2010. p. 445.

95. Metzler C, Biglan A, Noell J, et al. A randomized controlled trial of a behavioral intervention to reduce high-risk sexual behavior among adolescents in STD clinics. Behav Ther 2000;31:27–54.

Index

Note: Page numbers of article titles are in **boldface** type.

Child Adolesc Psychiatric Clin N Am 20 (2011) 401–411
doi:10.1016/S1056-4993(11)00025-3
1056-4993/11/$ – see front matter © 2011 Elsevier Inc. All rights reserved.

childpsych.theclinics.com

Moving?

Make sure your subscription moves with you!

To notify us of your new address, find your **Clinics Account Number** (located on your mailing label above your name), and contact customer service at:

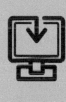

Email: journalscustomerservice-usa@elsevier.com

800-654-2452 (subscribers in the U.S. & Canada)
314-447-8871 (subscribers outside of the U.S. & Canada)

Fax number: 314-447-8029

Elsevier Health Sciences Division
Subscription Customer Service
3251 Riverport Lane
Maryland Heights, MO 63043

*To ensure uninterrupted delivery of your subscription, please notify us at least 4 weeks in advance of move.

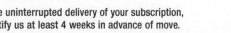

ELSEVIER

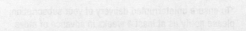

Printed and bound by CPI Group (UK) Ltd, Croydon, CR0 4YY

03/10/2024

01040447-0006